New Insights on Biofilm Antimicrobial Strategies

New Insights on Biofilm Antimicrobial Strategies

Editors

Luís Melo
Nuno F. Azevedo

MDPI • Basel • Beijing • Wuhan • Barcelona • Belgrade • Manchester • Tokyo • Cluj • Tianjin

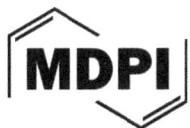

Editors
Luís Melo
Centre of Biological Engineering
University of Minho
Braga
Portugal

Nuno F. Azevedo
LEPABE – Dep. of Chemical
Engineering
Faculty of Engineering,
University of Porto
Porto
Portugal

Editorial Office
MDPI
St. Alban-Anlage 66
4052 Basel, Switzerland

This is a reprint of articles from the Special Issue published online in the open access journal *Antibiotics* (ISSN 2079-6382) (available at: www.mdpi.com/journal/antibiotics/special_issues/ biofilm_antimicro).

For citation purposes, cite each article independently as indicated on the article page online and as indicated below:

LastName, A.A.; LastName, B.B.; LastName, C.C. Article Title. *Journal Name* **Year**, *Volume Number*, Page Range.

ISBN 978-3-0365-1221-1 (Hbk)
ISBN 978-3-0365-1220-4 (PDF)

© 2021 by the authors. Articles in this book are Open Access and distributed under the Creative Commons Attribution (CC BY) license, which allows users to download, copy and build upon published articles, as long as the author and publisher are properly credited, which ensures maximum dissemination and a wider impact of our publications.

The book as a whole is distributed by MDPI under the terms and conditions of the Creative Commons license CC BY-NC-ND.

Contents

About the Editors vii

Luís D. R. Melo and Nuno F. Azevedo
New Insights on Biofilm Antimicrobial Strategies
Reprinted from: *Antibiotics* 2021, *10*, 407, doi:10.3390/antibiotics10040407 1

Cristina Uruén, Gema Chopo-Escuin, Jan Tommassen, Raúl C. Mainar-Jaime and Jesús Arenas
Biofilms as Promoters of Bacterial Antibiotic Resistance and Tolerance
Reprinted from: *Antibiotics* 2020, *10*, 3, doi:10.3390/antibiotics10010003 5

Abebe Mekuria Shenkutie, Mian Zhi Yao, Gilman Kit-hang Siu, Barry Kin Chung Wong and Polly Hang-mei Leung
Biofilm-Induced Antibiotic Resistance in Clinical *Acinetobacter baumannii* Isolates
Reprinted from: *Antibiotics* 2020, *9*, 817, doi:10.3390/antibiotics9110817 41

Andreia S. Azevedo, Gislaine P. Gerola, João Baptista, Carina Almeida, Joana Peres, Filipe J. Mergulhão and Nuno F. Azevedo
Increased Intraspecies Diversity in *Escherichia coli* Biofilms Promotes Cellular Growth at the Expense of Matrix Production
Reprinted from: *Antibiotics* 2020, *9*, 818, doi:10.3390/antibiotics9110818 57

Tânia Grainha, Andreia P. Magalhães, Luís D. R. Melo and Maria O. Pereira
Pitfalls Associated with Discriminating Mixed-Species Biofilms by Flow Cytometry
Reprinted from: *Antibiotics* 2020, *9*, 741, doi:10.3390/antibiotics9110741 71

Patrícia Alves, Joana Maria Moreira, João Mário Miranda and Filipe José Mergulhão
Analysing the Initial Bacterial Adhesion to Evaluate the Performance of Antifouling Surfaces
Reprinted from: *Antibiotics* 2020, *9*, 421, doi:10.3390/antibiotics9070421 89

Márcia R. Vagos, Marisa Gomes, Joana M. R. Moreira, Olívia S. G. P. Soares, Manuel F. R. Pereira and Filipe J. Mergulhão
Carbon Nanotube/Poly(dimethylsiloxane) Composite Materials to Reduce Bacterial Adhesion
Reprinted from: *Antibiotics* 2020, *9*, 434, doi:10.3390/antibiotics9080434 101

Renata Scheeren Brum, Luiza Gomes Labes, Cláudia Ângela Maziero Volpato, César Augusto Magalhães Benfatti and Andrea de Lima Pimenta
Strategies to Reduce Biofilm Formation in PEEK Materials Applied to Implant Dentistry—A Comprehensive Review
Reprinted from: *Antibiotics* 2020, *9*, 609, doi:10.3390/antibiotics9090609 117

Hannah Trøstrup, Anne Sofie Boe Laulund and Claus Moser
Insights into Host–Pathogen Interactions in Biofilm-Infected Wounds Reveal Possibilities for New Treatment Strategies
Reprinted from: *Antibiotics* 2020, *9*, 396, doi:10.3390/antibiotics9070396 139

James B. Doub
Bacteriophage Therapy for Clinical Biofilm Infections: Parameters That Influence Treatment Protocols and Current Treatment Approaches
Reprinted from: *Antibiotics* 2020, *9*, 799, doi:10.3390/antibiotics9110799 153

Viviane C. Oliveira, Ana P. Macedo, Luís D. R. Melo, Sílvio B. Santos, Paula R. S. Hermann, Cláudia H. Silva-Lovato, Helena F. O. Paranhos, Denise Andrade and Evandro Watanabe
Bacteriophage Cocktail-Mediated Inhibition of *Pseudomonas aeruginosa* Biofilm on Endotracheal Tube Surface
Reprinted from: *Antibiotics* **2021**, *10*, 78, doi:10.3390/antibiotics10010078 165

Lan Hoang, František Beneš, Marie Fenclová, Olga Kronusová, Viviana Švarcová, Kateřina Řehořová, Eva Baldassarre Švecová, Miroslav Vosátka, Jana Hajšlová, Petr Kaštánek, Jitka Viktorová and Tomáš Ruml
Phytochemical Composition and In Vitro Biological Activity of *Iris* spp. (Iridaceae): A New Source of Bioactive Constituents for the Inhibition of Oral Bacterial Biofilms
Reprinted from: *Antibiotics* **2020**, *9*, 403, doi:10.3390/antibiotics9070403 179

Virginie Lemoine, Clément Bernard, Charlotte Leman-Loubière, Barbara Clément-Larosière, Marion Girardot, Leslie Boudesocque-Delaye, Emilie Munnier and Christine Imbert
Nanovectorized Microalgal Extracts to Fight *Candida albicans* and *Cutibacterium acnes* Biofilms: Impact of Dual-Species Conditions
Reprinted from: *Antibiotics* **2020**, *9*, 279, doi:10.3390/antibiotics9060279 199

Dalila Mil-Homens, Maria Martins, José Barbosa, Gabriel Serafim, Maria J. Sarmento, Rita F. Pires, Vitória Rodrigues, Vasco D.B. Bonifácio and Sandra N. Pinto
Carbapenem-Resistant *Klebsiella pneumoniae* Clinical Isolates: In Vivo Virulence Assessment in *Galleria mellonella* and Potential Therapeutics by Polycationic Oligoethyleneimine
Reprinted from: *Antibiotics* **2021**, *10*, 56, doi:10.3390/antibiotics10010056 213

Mohammad Azam Ansari, Hani Manssor Albetran, Muidh Hamed Alheshibri, Abdelmajid Timoumi, Norah Abdullah Algarou, Sultan Akhtar, Yassine Slimani, Munirah Abdullah Almessiere, Fatimah Saad Alahmari, Abdulhadi Baykal and It-Meng Low
Synthesis of Electrospun TiO_2 Nanofibers and Characterization of Their Antibacterial and Antibiofilm Potential against Gram-Positive and Gram-Negative Bacteria
Reprinted from: *Antibiotics* **2020**, *9*, 572, doi:10.3390/antibiotics9090572 227

Joanna Verran, Sarah Jackson, Antony Scimone, Peter Kelly and James Redfern
Biofilm Control Strategies: Engaging with the Public
Reprinted from: *Antibiotics* **2020**, *9*, 465, doi:10.3390/antibiotics9080465 243

About the Editors

Luís Melo

With a degree and MSc in biology and a post-graduation qualification in nethods of DNA analysis, he obtained his PhD in biomedical engineering at the University of Minho, where he is currently a junior researcher. Luis D.R. Melo established his research on exploring phages' interactions with bacterial biofilms and has demonstrated the value of phage proteins on the control and detection of pathogenic bacteria. His experience in flow cytometry, genomics, transcriptomics, and proteomics has led to an increased knowledge on phage/host interactions. He has been involved in different scientifically funded projects, being the PI of two. He is also involved in the organization of international practical courses and conferences within this field of knowledge. The quality and innovative character of the research developed led to the publication of several internationally referenced papers and book chapters and enabled the creation of a patent.

Nuno F. Azevedo

Nuno F. Azevedo (PhD) is an assistant professor at the Faculty of Engineering of the University of Porto (FEUP) and a researcher at the Laboratory for Process Engineering, Environment, Biotechnology, and Energy (LEPABE). His main research interests include exploring the potential of nucleic acid mimics (NAMs) for rapid diagnosis and treatment of infectious agents in multispecies biofilms. He is currently leading the EU-funded project DelNAM, a project that aims to develop a novel therapeutic approach to solve bacterial resistance to antibiotics through the delivery of antibacterial NAMs into bacterial biofilms and cells within the human body. During his research career, he has authored or co-authored more than 100 papers in peer-reviewed international journals, submitted seven patents, and co-edited two books. He was also a co-founder of the biotech company Biomode SA, which was granted >1.5M€ in investment funds.

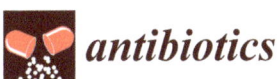

Editorial

New Insights on Biofilm Antimicrobial Strategies

Luís D. R. Melo [1],* and Nuno F. Azevedo [2],*

1. Centre of Biological Engineering, University of Minho, 4710-057 Braga, Portugal
2. LEPABE—Laboratory for Process Engineering, Environment, Biotechnology and Energy, Department of Chemical Engineering, Faculty of Engineering of the University of Porto, Rua Dr Roberto Frias, 4200-465 Porto, Portugal
* Correspondence: lmelo@deb.uminho.pt (L.D.R.M.); nazevedo@fe.up.pt (N.F.A.)

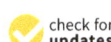

Citation: Melo, L.D.R.; Azevedo, N.F. New Insights on Biofilm Antimicrobial Strategies. *Antibiotics* **2021**, *10*, 407. https://doi.org/10.3390/antibiotics10040407

Received: 26 March 2021
Accepted: 6 April 2021
Published: 9 April 2021

Publisher's Note: MDPI stays neutral with regard to jurisdictional claims in published maps and institutional affiliations.

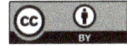

Copyright: © 2021 by the authors. Licensee MDPI, Basel, Switzerland. This article is an open access article distributed under the terms and conditions of the Creative Commons Attribution (CC BY) license (https://creativecommons.org/licenses/by/4.0/).

Over the last few decades, the study of microbial biofilms has been gaining interest among the scientific community. These microbial communities comprise cells adhered to surfaces that are surrounded by a self-produced exopolymeric matrix that protects biofilm cells against different external stresses. Biofilms can have a negative impact on different sectors within society, namely in agriculture, food industries, and veterinary and human health. As a consequence of their metabolic state and matrix protection, biofilm cells are very difficult to tackle with antibiotics or chemical disinfectants. Due to this problem, recent advances in the development of antibiotic alternatives or complementary strategies to prevent or control biofilms have been reported. This Special Issue includes different strategies to prevent biofilm formation or control biofilm development and includes full research articles, reviews, a communication, and a perspective.

Regarding the problem per se, Uruén and Chopo-Escuin et al. [1] reviewed the mechanisms by which biofilms are tolerant or resistant to antibiotics, emphasizing the role of the biofilm matrix, physiological heterogeneity of biofilm cells, quorum sensing, horizontal gene transfer, and other mutations on biofilms. In the second part of the review, several alternatives to combat biofilms were discussed. The problem of bacterial resistance was assessed in an original study by Shenkutie et al. [2], where the biofilm-forming ability of 104 *Acinetobacter baumannii* clinical strains was evaluated. Moreover, the authors observed that the minimum biofilm eradication concentrations were significantly higher than the minimum bactericidal concentrations for several antibiotics, a fact that led to an increase in persister cell detection on biofilms. In another study, the influence of *Escherichia coli* diversity in biofilms composed of up to six different strains isolated from urine was evaluated in urinary tract infection conditions. The authors detected that as the number of strains increased, the number of culturable cells also increased but overall the biofilms produced less matrix [3]. The impact of the biofilm matrix on flow cytometry in multi-species biofilms was one of the parameters evaluated by Grainha et al. [4]. Despite the potential of this technique to assess several aspects of biofilms, the authors reported that results are very dependent of the microbial strain used, the morphological state of the cells, and the biofilm matrix.

Another important topic covered in this Special Issue is the prevention of biofilm formation. Alves et al. studied the initial events of *E. coli* adhesion to polydimethylsiloxane and demonstrated that a proper tuning of operational parameters is required to avoid hydrodynamic blocking, which will allow the scientific community to obtain reliable data about cell–surface interactions [5]. In another study performed by the same group, the authors show the effect of pristine and functionalized carbon nanotube incorporation into poly(dimethylsiloxane) materials. Initial *E. coli* adhesion was assessed in conditions simulating urinary tract devices (catheters and stents). The results led the authors to conclude that the incorporation of carbon nanotubes, even at low loading values, might be beneficial for the application of biomedical devices for the urinary tract [6].

Trøstrup et al. and Brum et al. contributed to this Special Issue with two reviews [7,8]. The first is focused on the impact of Pseudomonas aeruginosa biofilms on the local and systemic host response observed in vitro and in vivo. The authors also discussed the implications for clinical wound healing and a possible therapeutic approach using an antimicrobial peptide as immunomodulatory topical treatment [8]. In the second review, a comparison between the use of polyether-ether-ketone (PEEK) and other commonly used materials in implant dentistry (titanium and zirconia) as biofilm-preventing or -controlling agents was comprehensively conducted. The authors concluded that despite pure PEEK being susceptible to biofilm formation, there are numerous strategies that can improve its antibiofilm properties, namely PEEK sulfonation, incorporation of therapeutic/bioactive agents in the PEEK matrix or surface, PEEK coatings, and, finally, the incorporation of reinforcement agents [7].

Different approaches to control biofilms using antibiotic alternative strategies were also submitted to this Special Issue. James D. Boub provided a perspective on the use of phage therapy to combat infectious biofilms [9]. The perspective referred to many aspects of bacteriophage therapy that should be taken into consideration before their broader use. The author suggested the development of standardized protocols that will allow for better and stricter testing of this therapeutic agent in the treatment of biofilm infections. Regarding this topic, Oliveira et al. used a bacteriophage cocktail to control *P. aeruginosa* biofilm formation on endotracheal tubes [10]. Despite some promising results on reducing bacterial colonization, the authors concluded that this strategy could have more potential with the development of new coating strategies. Several natural products are also commonly seen as promising antibiofilm agents. Hoang et al. analyzed the composition and antibiofilm activity of 15 methanolic extracts from *Iris* spp. [11]. *Iris pallida* s.l. leaf extract was the most effective at both preventing biofilm formation and controlling multi-species oral biofilms, with no toxicity observed, suggesting its potential application for oral biofilms. In another study, the antibiofilm activity of cyanobacteria *Arthrospira platensis* extracts (free and nanovectorized) was studied on *Candida albicans* and *Cutibacterium acnes* (single- and dual-species biofilms). Efficacy results varied depending on the microbial species and on the type of biofilm, emphasizing the importance of studying more complex communities such as polymicrobial biofilms [12].

Using a different approach, Mil-Homens et al. reported the application of a synthetic polycationic oligomer (L-OEI-h) as an alternative to treat *Klebsiella pneumoniae* infections [13]. The authors showed that L-OEI-h caused lysis of the cytoplasmic membrane in a panel of different species. This promising compound showed no visible cytotoxicity on the *Galleria mellonella* in vivo model; however, its antibiofilm capacity is yet to be tested.

The last approach published in this Special Issue was the use of electrospun titanium dioxide (TiO_2) nanofibers and their activity against *Staphylococcus aureus* and *P. aeruginosa* [14]. Although, on planktonic cultures, TiO_2 nanofibers were more active against *P. aeruginosa* than *S. aureus*, biofilms were prevented in both species in the same order of magnitude, suggesting their potential use for coating inanimate objects.

From a different perspective, Verran et al. provided a communication discussing the relevance of public engagement activities in complex phenomena such as biofilms and Antimicrobial resistance (AMR) [15]. The authors describe three different public engagement activities focused on biofilm control, namely hand hygiene, plaque control, and an externally applied antimicrobial coating using quantitative and/or qualitative methods.

This Special Issue collects high-quality original articles and reviews that demonstrate the relevance of biofilm infections as well as the potential of numerous antibiotic alternative strategies to prevent or control them. We hope that these articles will encourage researchers to investigate new antibiofilm strategies and implement them using standardized protocols that will help research to more effectively move towards clinical implementation.

References

1. Uruén, C.; Chopo-Escuin, G.; Tommassen, J.; Mainar-Jaime, R.C.; Arenas, J. Biofilms as Promoters of Bacterial Antibiotic Resistance and Tolerance. *Antibiotics* **2020**, *10*, 3. [CrossRef]
2. Shenkutie, A.M.; Yao, M.Z.; Siu, G.K.-H.; Wong, B.K.C.; Leung, P.H.-M. Biofilm-Induced Antibiotic Resistance in Clinical *Acinetobacter baumannii* Isolates. *Antibiotics* **2020**, *9*, 817. [CrossRef] [PubMed]
3. Azevedo, A.S.; Gerola, G.P.; Baptista, J.; Almeida, C.; Peres, J.; Mergulhão, F.J.; Azevedo, N.F. Increased Intraspecies Diversity in *Escherichia coli* Biofilms Promotes Cellular Growth at the Expense of Matrix Production. *Antibiotics* **2020**, *9*, 818. [CrossRef] [PubMed]
4. Grainha, T.; Magalhães, A.P.; Melo, L.D.R.; Pereira, M.O. Pitfalls Associated with Discriminating Mixed-Species Biofilms by Flow Cytometry. *Antibiotics* **2020**, *9*, 741. [CrossRef] [PubMed]
5. Alves, P.; Moreira, J.M.; Miranda, J.M.; Mergulhão, F.J. Analysing the Initial Bacterial Adhesion to Evaluate the Performance of Antifouling Surfaces. *Antibiotics* **2020**, *9*, 421. [CrossRef] [PubMed]
6. Vagos, M.R.; Gomes, M.; Moreira, J.M.R.; Soares, O.S.G.P.; Pereira, M.F.R.; Mergulhão, F.J. Carbon Nanotube/Poly(dimethylsiloxane) Composite Materials to Reduce Bacterial Adhesion. *Antibiotics* **2020**, *9*, 434. [CrossRef] [PubMed]
7. Brum, R.S.; Labes, L.G.; Volpato, C.Â.M.; Benfatti, C.A.M.; Pimenta, A.D.L. Strategies to Reduce Biofilm Formation in PEEK Materials Applied to Implant Dentistry—A Comprehensive Review. *Antibiotics* **2020**, *9*, 609. [CrossRef] [PubMed]
8. Trøstrup, H.; Laulund, A.S.B.; Moser, C. Insights into Host–Pathogen Interactions in Biofilm-Infected Wounds Reveal Possibilities for New Treatment Strategies. *Antibiotics* **2020**, *9*, 396. [CrossRef] [PubMed]
9. Doub, J.B. Bacteriophage Therapy for Clinical Biofilm Infections: Parameters That Influence Treatment Protocols and Current Treatment Approaches. *Antibiotics* **2020**, *9*, 799. [CrossRef] [PubMed]
10. Oliveira, V.; Macedo, A.; Melo, L.; Santos, S.; Hermann, P.; Silva-Lovato, C.; Paranhos, H.; Andrade, D.; Watanabe, E. Bacteriophage Cocktail-Mediated Inhibition of *Pseudomonas aeruginosa* Biofilm on Endotracheal Tube Surface. *Antibiotics* **2021**, *10*, 78. [CrossRef] [PubMed]
11. Hoang, L.; Beneš, F.; Fenclová, M.; Kronusová, O.; Švarcová, V.; Řehořová, K.; Švecová, E.B.; Vosátka, M.; Hajšlová, J.; Kaštánek, P.; et al. Phytochemical Composition and In Vitro Biological Activity of *Iris* spp. (Iridaceae): A New Source of Bioactive Constituents for the Inhibition of Oral Bacterial Biofilms. *Antibiotics* **2020**, *9*, 403. [CrossRef] [PubMed]
12. Lemoine, V.; Bernard, C.; Leman-Loubière, C.; Clément-Larosière, B.; Girardot, M.; Boudesocque-Delaye, L.; Munnier, E.; Imbert, C. Nanovectorized Microalgal Extracts to Fight Candida albicans and Cutibacterium acnes Biofilms: Impact of Dual-Species Conditions. *Antibiotics* **2020**, *9*, 279. [CrossRef] [PubMed]
13. Mil-Homens, D.; Martins, M.; Barbosa, J.; Serafim, G.; Sarmento, M.J.; Pires, R.F.; Rodrigues, V.; Bonifácio, V.D.; Pinto, S.N. Carbapenem-Resistant *Klebsiella pneumoniae* Clinical Isolates: In Vivo Virulence Assessment in *Galleria mellonella* and Potential Therapeutics by Polycationic Oligoethyleneimine. *Antibiotics* **2021**, *10*, 56. [CrossRef] [PubMed]
14. Ansari, M.A.; Albetran, H.M.; Alheshibri, M.H.; Timoumi, A.; Algarou, N.A.; Akhtar, S.; Slimani, Y.; Almessiere, M.A.; AlAhmari, F.S.; Baykal, A.; et al. Synthesis of Electrospun TiO_2 Nanofibers and Characterization of Their Antibacterial and Antibiofilm Potential against Gram-Positive and Gram-Negative Bacteria. *Antibiotics* **2020**, *9*, 572. [CrossRef] [PubMed]
15. Verran, J.; Jackson, S.; Scimone, A.; Kelly, P.; Redfern, J. Biofilm Control Strategies: Engaging with the Public. *Antibiotics* **2020**, *9*, 465. [CrossRef] [PubMed]

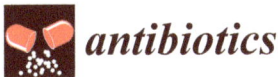

Review

Biofilms as Promoters of Bacterial Antibiotic Resistance and Tolerance

Cristina Uruén [1,†], Gema Chopo-Escuin [1,†], Jan Tommassen [2], Raúl C. Mainar-Jaime [1] and Jesús Arenas [1,*]

1. Unit of Microbiology and Immunology, Faculty of Veterinary, University of Zaragoza, Miguel Servet, 177, 50017 Zaragoza, Spain; 700469@unizar.es (C.U.); 721072@unizar.es (G.C.-E.); rcmainar@unizar.es (R.C.M.-J.)
2. Department of Molecular Microbiology, Institute of Biomembranes, Utrecht University, 3584 CH Utrecht, The Netherlands; J.P.M.Tommassen@uu.nl
* Correspondence: jaarenas@unizar.es
† These authors contributed equally to this work.

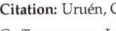

Citation: Uruén, C.; Chopo-Escuin, G.; Tommassen, J.; Mainar-Jaime, R.C.; Arenas, J. Biofilms as Promoters of Bacterial Antibiotic Resistance and Tolerance. *Antibiotics* **2021**, *10*, 3. https://dx.doi.org/10.3390/antibiotics10010003

Received: 28 September 2020
Accepted: 19 December 2020
Published: 23 December 2020

Publisher's Note: MDPI stays neutral with regard to jurisdictional claims in published maps and institutional affiliations.

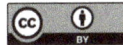

Copyright: © 2020 by the authors. Licensee MDPI, Basel, Switzerland. This article is an open access article distributed under the terms and conditions of the Creative Commons Attribution (CC BY) license (https://creativecommons.org/licenses/by/4.0/).

Abstract: Multidrug resistant bacteria are a global threat for human and animal health. However, they are only part of the problem of antibiotic failure. Another bacterial strategy that contributes to their capacity to withstand antimicrobials is the formation of biofilms. Biofilms are associations of microorganisms embedded a self-produced extracellular matrix. They create particular environments that confer bacterial tolerance and resistance to antibiotics by different mechanisms that depend upon factors such as biofilm composition, architecture, the stage of biofilm development, and growth conditions. The biofilm structure hinders the penetration of antibiotics and may prevent the accumulation of bactericidal concentrations throughout the entire biofilm. In addition, gradients of dispersion of nutrients and oxygen within the biofilm generate different metabolic states of individual cells and favor the development of antibiotic tolerance and bacterial persistence. Furthermore, antimicrobial resistance may develop within biofilms through a variety of mechanisms. The expression of efflux pumps may be induced in various parts of the biofilm and the mutation frequency is induced, while the presence of extracellular DNA and the close contact between cells favor horizontal gene transfer. A deep understanding of the mechanisms by which biofilms cause tolerance/resistance to antibiotics helps to develop novel strategies to fight these infections.

Keywords: biofilms; antibiotic resistance; antibiotic tolerance; multidrug-resistant bacteria; recalcitrance; biofilm control

1. Introduction

During the last few decades, a significant increase in the number of clinical and environmental multidrug-resistant (MDR) bacteria, also called superbugs, has been reported. Particularly problematic in this respect are the major human pathogens, e.g., *Enterococcus faecium*, *Staphylococcus aureus*, *Klebsiella pneumoniae*, *Acinetobacter baumannii*, *Pseudomonas aeruginosa*, and *Enterobacter* spp. Additionally, among veterinary pathogens, particularly those associated with livestock farming and poultry production, the rate of drug resistance has increased. Some of them, such as *Salmonella enterica* and *Campylobacter* spp., are also important zoonotic pathogens.

About 700,000 human deaths are attributed to MDR bacteria each year globally, and this number is expected to exceed 10 million deaths by 2050, at a cumulative global cost of USD 100 trillion [1]. Additionally, the Global Antimicrobial Surveillance System from the World Health Organization (WHO) reported a widespread occurrence of MDR in 2018 among 2,164,568 people with suspected bacterial infections across 66 countries (ranging from high to low income). The proportion of people infected with MDR bacteria varies among countries, with higher levels of resistance to those drugs more widely utilized for treating infections (e.g., ciprofloxacin) [2], and many pathogens have developed mechanisms to survive to practically all of the antibiotic families available on the market, for example *K. pneumoniae*. Despite the apparent exacerbation of this global issue, the high costs of the development of new antibiotics and the unavoidable emergence of antimicrobial resistances (AMR) have caused antibiotic development to lack economic appeal to the pharmaceutical industry.

MDR infections have been extensively associated with hospital and healthcare settings, for example those caused by *P. aeruginosa, A. baumannii,* or *K. pneumoniae*. However, MDR pathogens can also be transmitted within the community, for example *Neisseria gonorrhoeae*. In addition, people can be infected by MDR zoonotic bacteria that were selected through the use of antibiotics in food animals. In fact, antimicrobial resistance (AMR) in zoonotic bacteria recovered either from food animals or their carcasses is widespread. For instance, among *Salmonella enterica* recovered from pig carcasses in the EU in 2017, 53%, 59.5%, and 56.8% were resistant to ampicillin, sulfamethoxazole, and tetracycline, respectively. In the case of *Campylobacter* spp. recovered from poultry meat, high levels of resistance were noted for ciprofloxacin, nalidixic acid, and tetracycline in 54–83% of the isolates [3]. In fact, the relation between the use of some antibiotics in food animals and the subsequent detection of AMR in bacteria isolated from humans has been suggested in several studies [4,5]. Thus, the wide spreading of AMR, the high mortality rates, and the lack of initiatives to discover new antibiotics together make MDR bacteria a critical problem for modern medicine.

In addition to the well-known genetic mechanisms behind the AMR phenomenon and the transfer of antibiotic-resistance genes by horizontal gene transfer (HGT), bacteria are capable of displaying other strategies to withstand an exposure to antimicrobials, one of which is the ability to produce biofilms. Biofilms are highly structured associations of microorganisms embedded in a self-produced extracellular matrix (ECM) and adhered to a biotic or an abiotic surface. The biofilm confers many benefits to the members of the community, including collective recalcitrance. Recalcitrance is a term defined as *"the ability of pathogenic biofilms to survive in presence of high concentrations of antibiotics"* [6]. Indeed, biofilm cells are 10–1000 fold less susceptible to various antimicrobial agents than their planktonic forms [7–9]. Recalcitrance to antibiotics is achieved in biofilms through a variety of mechanisms, some of which can lead to an increase in the number of MDR bacteria, since processes such as HGT or hypermutability are favored within the biofilm environment. In fact, the biofilm is recognized as a reservoir of antibiotic-resistance genes [10].

Biofilms are involved in a broad range of infections. Indeed, about 80% of the chronic and recurrent microbial infections in humans are caused by biofilms, some of which result in high mortality and morbidity rates [11,12], particularly those caused by MDR bacteria. Patients with cystic fibrosis or with assisted ventilation are susceptible to chronic infections by biofilm-forming *P. aeruginosa* [13] and *A. baumannii* [14], respectively. These bacteria are also well-known for acquiring MDR, and the resulting biofilms are almost impossible to treat [15]. In addition, biofilms are highly resistant to the host immune defenses and clearance mechanisms. Other nocosomial infections include those caused by biofilms strongly adhered to implants and catheters or medical devices. They are generated by different pathogens, such as *Escherichia coli, Proteus mirabilis,* or *K. pneumoniae* [16,17], which can also become MDR. Additionally, *N. gonorrhoeae* forms biofilms on genital mucosa causing chronic infections [18]. The WHO classified this pathogen as high priority because of its extraordinary capacity to persist against all recommended antibiotics to treat the infection [19]. Together, these and many other studies have related the high capacity of several bacteria to survive to antibiotics through biofilms. Understanding the mechanisms that these pathogens utilize to survive antibiotics will help to design adequate surveillance methods and novel strategies to combat these infections. This review focuses on the role of biofilms in the poor susceptibility of bacteria to antibiotics. We will describe the mechanisms responsible for recalcitrance and the currently proposed solutions to treat or prevent biofilm infections.

2. Basis of Biofilm-Mediated Antibiotic Survival

The recalcitrant nature of biofilms to antibiotics depends mostly on (i) the developmental stage of the biofilm, (ii) the ECM composition, and (iii) the biofilm architecture.

2.1. Biogenesis of Biofilms

Biofilm formation is a dynamic process that takes place in a series of sequential steps. It is initiated by the interaction of the bacteria with a surface. Exposure of planktonic cells to stress, which may be provoked by antibiotics, starvation, or other adverse environmental conditions, can initiate biofilm formation by activating gene expression [20]. Additionally, molecules involved in cell-to-cell communication accumulate at high cell density. These molecules, generally referred to as autoinducers, can activate and regulate the process [21] and allow for a coordinated response of the population members, which is known as quorum sensing (QS). The first step of biofilm formation consists of the adhesion of the bacteria to the substratum. This process is often mediated by long, proteinaceous, filamentous fibers that protrude from the bacterial cell surface, such as flagella, fimbriae, or pili. After initial interaction is established, shorter cell surface-exposed structures interact with the substratum, thereby increasing the contact between bacteria and the substratum [12]. Strains of *E. coli* and *Salmonella* produce curli fimbrae that mediate both cell-to-substratum and cell-to-cell interactions [22]. Other proteins such as Bap-family proteins in *S. epidermidis* [23] or CdrA in *P. aeruginosa* [24] are large proteins that interact with ECM components and the bacterial cell surface thereby strengthening the matrix. Autotransporters are proteins secreted through the Type V secretion system in many Gram-negative bacteria and often have demonstrated roles in interbacterial interactions [25]. Then, the bacteria secrete ECM components and proliferate to form a microcolony. ECM serves as a glue element that helps to stabilize interbacterial interactions. Bacteria within the microcolony communicate and organize spatially. Type IV pili act at the junction between cells to form microcolonies and can also contribute to the reorganization of bacteria within the biofilm [26]. Cell-to-cell communication, including QS [21] and also cell-contact-dependent communication systems [27], seem to be relevant for this process. At this stage, the expression of genes for the formation of the ECM increases [12], and biofilms become less vulnerable to antibiotics than earlier biofilm stages [28].

2.2. Composition of the ECM

The ECM consists of a conglomerate of different substances that together provide structural integrity to the biofilm. In general, the ECM can be composed of water, polysaccharides, proteins, lipids, surfactants, glycolipids, extracellular DNA (eDNA), extracellular RNA, membrane vesicles, and ions such as Ca^{2+}. In many bacteria, extracellular polysaccharides and eDNA are prominent components of the ECM [29].

eDNA is constituted of chromosomal DNA that is released into the extracellular milieu through cell lysis, dedicated secretion systems, or membrane vesicles. eDNA is often involved in adhesion, particularly after the first interaction of the cell with the substratum. It mediates acid–base interactions and increases the hydrophobicity of bacterial cells which are favorable for the cell–substratum interaction [30,31]. Indeed, eDNA is used for initiation of biofilm formation in many pathogenic bacteria, including Gram-positive and Gram-negative bacteria and mycobacteria [32–34]. In addition, eDNA facilitates the interaction of the bacteria in the ECM. This is achieved by binding of positively charged segments of cell surface-exposed proteins with the negatively charged eDNA molecules [35]. Various proteins can be implicated in this interaction, such as autotransporters, lipoproteins or two-partner secretion protein A of Gram-negative bacteria, and cell wall-associated proteins in Gram-positive bacteria and fungi [35]. Thus, anchoring the eDNA to the cell surface by DNA-binding proteins is a widespread mechanism for biofilm formation that may also facilitate multispecies biofilms. eDNA can also mediate interactions with other ECM components such as polysaccharides [36]. Together, these interactions are relevant for the structural integrity of biofilms.

The composition of the polysaccharides present in the ECM varies between different bacterial species and even between different isolates of the same species. Most are long linear or branched molecules formed by one (homopolysaccharides) or several different (heteropolysaccharides) residues. They may contain substituents that greatly affect their biological properties. One of the most commonly studied polysaccharides is poly-β-1,6-N-acetyl-D-glucosamine, often named PGA or PNAG. It is synthetized by *E. coli* [37] and *S. aureus* [38], among others. In *E. coli*, PGA is required for initial cell-to-cell and cell-to-substratum attachment [37]. Another polysaccharide present in ECM is cellulose, a linear polymer of β-1,4 linked D-glucose. It is a major component of the ECM of some *E. coli* [39], *Salmonella* [40], and *Pseudomonas* strains [41]. Some *E. coli* strains produce a complex branched polysaccharide called colanic acid [42]. Additionally, *P. aeruginosa* can produce diverse exopolysaccharides. Mucoid *P. aeruginosa* strains produce alginate, a polymer of β-1-4-linked mannuronic acid and α-L-guluronate. Production of alginate confers a mucoid phenotype [43,44], typical of strains isolated from lungs of cystic fibrosis patients with *Pseudomonas* infections that underwent several rounds of antibiotic treatment. Therefore, secretion of alginate is related to pathogenic biofilms [45]. Alginate mediates the establishment of microcolonies at early stages of biofilm formation and provides stability to mature biofilms. Nonmucoid *P. aeruginosa* strains can produce other exopolysaccharides, e.g., Psl or Pel. Pel is a linear, cationic exopolysaccharide formed by 1→4 glycosidic linkages of *N*-acetylglucosamine and *N*-acetylgalactosamine. It has a critical role in maintaining cell-to-cell interactions and pellicle formation [46]. In contrast, Psl is composed of repeating pentasaccharide subunits of D-glucose, D-mannose, and L-rhamnose [47]. Psl mediates attachment to biotic surfaces such as mucin-coated epithelial surfaces and epithelial cells, indicating its relevance for the establishment of *P. aeruginosa* infection [48]. Additionally, *P. aeruginosa* strains can secrete cyclic and linear glucans [49,50] that are formed by β-1,3 linked glucose residues.

The proteinaceous content of the ECM includes proteins that are secreted through active secretion systems or released during cell lysis. The role of many of these proteins in the biofilm matrix is unknown, but some of them have been identified as important contributors to biofilm formation or restructuring in many pathogens. Various are extracellular enzymes. Their substrates can be polysaccharides, proteins, and nucleic acids, present in the ECM. They can function in remodeling of the ECM, detachment of cells from the biofilm, or degradation of polymers for nutrient acquisition.

ECM biogenesis and composition are dynamic and vary between strains of a given species and also depend on environmental conditions, such as nutrient availability and the presence of stressors, and on social crosstalk. Several functions have been attributed to the ECM based on its extraordinary capacity to establish intermolecular interactions between its components, and with surface-exposed structures of the cells, biotic and abiotic substrata, and many environmental molecules [29]. Thereby, the ECM immobilizes cells and keeps them in the biofilm community. By retaining the cells in close proximity, the ECM establishes the optimal conditions for interbacterial communication and exchange of genetic material, which is relevant, amongst others, for the dispersion of antibiotic-resistance genes. The ECM additionally retains water and thereby protects the cells against desiccation. Furthermore, the extracellular enzymes in that hydrated environment generate an external digestive system. In addition, ECM retains several other substances, for instance, nutrients, energy sources, antibiotics, antibiotic-degrading enzymes, and molecules released by cell lysis, thereby constituting a recycling unit [29]. In general, the ECM acts as a protective scaffold.

2.3. Biofilm Architecture

The architecture of biofilms is defined by the organization of the biomass and the spaces in between. The development of this structure depends on the composition of cell-surface structures mediating mutual interactions between cells and interactions of cells with ECM components and with the substratum [35]. The biofilm architecture is responsible for the generation of gradients of dispersion of substances within the biofilm. This will influence the accessibility of these substances to particular niches inside the biofilm, and determines, amongst others, the variation in antibiotic susceptibility of cells within biofilms. Figure 1 illustrates the biofilm architecture of different bacterial species. *P. aeruginosa* strain ATCC 15,692 forms complex biofilms with mushroom-like architectural features consisting of well-defined stalks and caps. *Enterococcus faecalis* ATCC 51,299 biofilms, however, are flat and compact [51], while *Salmonella enterica* strain S12 and *E. coli* strain ESC.1.16 form biofilms constituted of small cell clusters (Figure 1A) [51]. In contrast, biofilms of *Neisseria meningitidis* strain HB-1 are constituted of cell aggregates of different sizes forming defined channel-like structures [33] (Figure 1B).

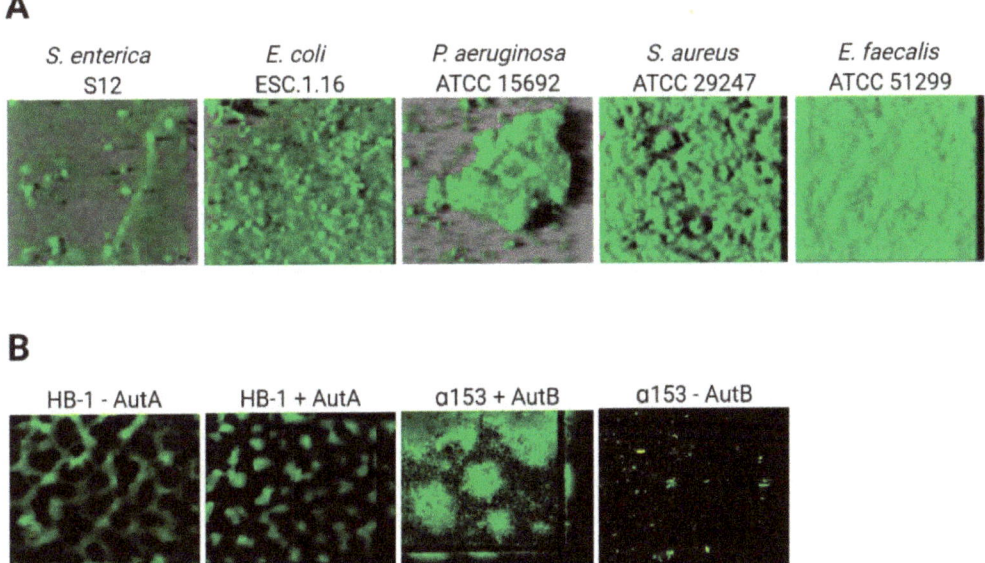

Figure 1. Variable architecture of biofilms. (**A**) Biofilms of five species (*Salmonella enterica, Escherichia coli, Pseudomonas aeruginosa Staphylococcus aureus, Enterococcus faecalis*) were formed under static conditions on abiotic surfaces during 24 h and were stained with Syto9, a green fluorescent nucleic acid marker. Reprinted from [51] with permission from Elsevier. (**B**) Strains of *Neisseria meningitidis* HB-1 and α153 and derivatives, which do or do not produce the autotransporters AutA and AutB (as indicated), formed biofilms under flow conditions during 14 h and were stained with the LIVE/DEAD Backlight bacterial viability stain (where red cells are dead and green cells are live). Reproduced from [52,53].

Thus, in general, based on their architecture, biofilms can be classified into (i) monolayer biofilms, formed by a compact layer with high surface coverage, or (ii) multilayer biofilms, formed by bacterial clusters of different morphology with a low surface interaction. The biofilm architecture can vary depending on different factors, for instance the expression of surface-exposed proteins. Examples are the meningococcal autotransporters AutA and AutB, whose expression is phase variable and significantly alters the biofilm (Figure 1B) [52,53]. Additionally, the medium composition influences the biofilm architecture. *P. aeruginosa* PAO1 makes monolayer biofilms in the presence of citrate benzoate and casamino acids and multilayer biofilms in presence of glucose [54].

3. Mechanisms of Biofilm Recalcitrance
3.1. Types of Antibiotic Recalcitrance

Biofilm recalcitrance comprises two independent phenomena: antibiotic resistance and antibiotic tolerance. Resistance refers to the capacity of a microorganism to survive and grow at increased antibiotic concentrations for long periods of time and is quantifiable by assessing the minimum inhibitory concentration (MIC) [55]. It involves mechanisms that prevent the binding of an antibiotic to its target, including enzymatic deactivation, active efflux of a drug once it is in the cytoplasm or the cytoplasmic membrane, or reduced influx, among others, and can be generated by HGT or mutations. Together, they preclude antibiotics from altering their target's function and they prevent the production of toxic products that would end up damaging the cell. Resistance can be further classified into intrinsic, acquired, and/or adaptive resistance (expanded in Box 1).

Box 1. Types of antibiotic resistance.

Intrinsic resistance. This is the inherent/natural property of the bacteria to withstand antibiotics. For example, Gram-negative bacteria are, in general, more resistant to antibiotics than Gram-positive ones due to the presence of the outer membrane, which reduces the permeability to many antibiotics [56]. Another example is the wall-less bacterial genus Mycoplasma, which is not affected by antibiotics whose target is the cell wall.

Acquired resistance. This arises through genetic modifications of originally sensitive bacteria, either through mutations or by the incorporation of new genes via HGT. Thus, microorganisms that are initially sensitive to an antibiotic become resistant due to spontaneous or induced mutations that alter, for example, the target of the antibiotic or its uptake by the cell or after the acquisition of one or more molecular mechanisms for AMR, such as antibiotic inactivation or, increased antibiotic efflux [57]. These genetic modifications are heritable and will result in a permanent effect if the fitness-cost associated with them is low or null or compensation mechanisms exists [58].

Adaptive resistance. This is the capacity of bacteria to vary rapidly gene expression or protein production in response to antibiotics or adverse environmental conditions. The molecular mechanism behind involves epigenetic inheritance, population heterogeneity, gene amplification, and efflux pumps that are regulated by intricate regulatory pathways [59].

Heteroresistance. This is the presence, within a given population of bacteria, of one or several subpopulations displaying increased levels of antibiotic resistance compared with the main population [60]. This phenomenon is often related with the presence of unstable genes which would give the bacteria a high likelihood for reversion to susceptibility in the absence of antibiotic selective pressure [61]. This instability makes its detection difficult, increasing thus the risk for treatment failure [62].

By contrast, antibiotic tolerance is the capacity of bacteria to survive a transient exposure to increased antibiotic concentrations, even those above the MIC. Tolerance is assessed by the minimum bactericidal concentration, that is, the minimum concentration of antibiotic required to kill 99.9% of the cells [63]. Unlike resistance, tolerance is only temporary and after longer exposure periods, the antibiotic will kill the bacteria. It is an adaptive phenomenon that implies a change in cellular behavior, from an active (growing) state to a quiescent (dormant) state [57], and requires large metabolic rearrangements affecting, for example, energy production and nonessential functions. These changes are triggered during poor growth conditions or exposure to stress factors or antibiotics [55,64]. In this case, antibiotics can usually attach to the target molecules, but because their function is no longer essential, the microorganism survives [65]. Tolerance in biofilms is also caused by entrapment of the antibiotics in the ECM, in this case, the antibiotic does not reach its target. In contrast to resistant cells, tolerant cells within the biofilm cannot grow in presence of a bactericidal antibiotic. Persistence is an especial phenomenon of tolerance [64]. Indeed, persistence is a phenomenom that increase the survival of a given population in the presence of bactericidal antibiotics without enhancing the MIC, but in contrast to tolerance, persistence only affects a subset of cells of the population called persisters [64]. Persisters cells are tolerant cells that eventually can be killed at longer exposure times. There are two types of persisters, e.g., type I or triggered persistence, which is induced upon environmental signals, such as starvation, and type II or spontaneous persistence, where a subpopulation of growing bacteria converts into the persister state by a stochastic process [66]. Any how, persistence can be also refereed to as heterotolerance, which is different than heteroresistance (Box 1), as persisters can eventually be killed at longer exposure times. Figure 2 illustrates the mechanisms that govern antibiotic tolerance and antibiotic resistance of biofilms, and they will be further discussed in the next section.

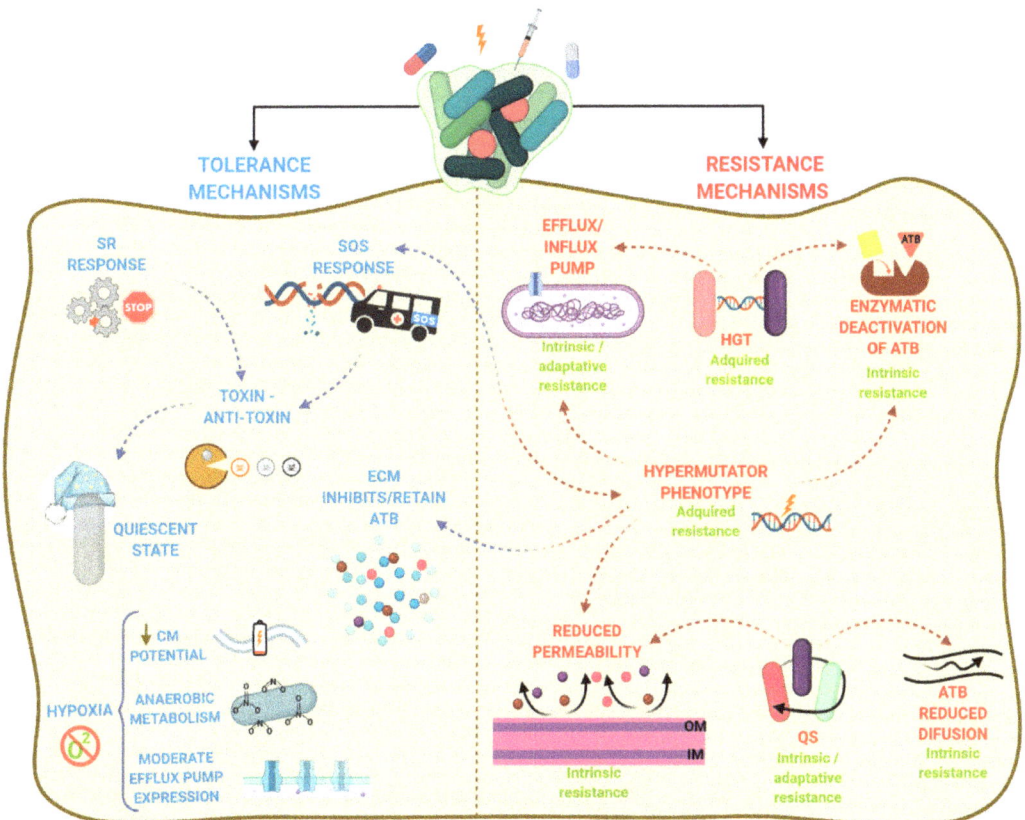

Figure 2. Mechanisms of biofilms recalcitrance. Biofilm recalcitrance comprises a combination of antibiotic (ATB) resistance mechanisms (right panel) and ATB tolerance mechanisms (left panel). Resistance mechanisms confer the ability to survive and grow at increased ATB concentrations for long periods and involve horizontal genetic transfer (HGT), hypermutation, and quorum sensing (QS), leading to transport of antibiotics via efflux pumps, reduced permeability of the outer membrane, or production of enzymes that inactivate ATB. The type of AMR (Box 1) is indicated in green. In contrast, tolerance mechanisms lead microorganisms to survive at increased ATB concentrations temporally, and involve activation of stress responses (SOS response, stringent response SR)) and hypoxia, leading to activation of a quiescent state, anaerobic metabolism, decrease of membrane potential, and moderate increase in efflux pump expression. Arrowhead lines indicate the interrelation between mechanisms. CM: cytoplasmic membrane.

Overall, biofilm recalcitrance does not depend on one unique mechanism but is a combination of both antibiotic tolerance and antibiotic resistance mechanisms. Such combination varies depending upon aspects such as the bacterial species or strain, the antimicrobial agent, the developmental stage of the biofilm, and the biofilm growth conditions [63].

3.2. The Protective ECM Barrier

The components of the ECM can impact the efficacy of antibiotics on biofilm-forming cells. ECM influences the biofilm architecture, which in turn generates gradients of dispersion that affect the access of antibiotics to the biofilm members. The flow of substances through biofilm varies. In the channels, the flow is convective while it occurs by diffusion within cell clusters [67]. Thus, antibiotics can penetrate rapidly through the channels of the biofilm but may be retained locally in cell aggregates. Due to the differences in biofilm architecture (Figure 1), the time for an antibiotic to reach the interior of the biofilm varies between strains [68].

The diffusion of antibiotics through the biofilm can also be limited by their interaction with particular ECM components, which affects antibiotic effectivity. This is illustrated in the literature by several examples including *P. aeruginosa*. Alginate is a polyanionic exopolysaccharide that protects *Pseudomonas* biofilms from aminoglycosides [44]. Additionally, the highly anionic cyclic glucans present in these biofilms interact with the aminoglycoside kanamycin [69]. Presumably, the high negative charge of alginate and the cyclic glucans helps to establish ionic interactions with these positively charged antibiotics. However, in strains that do not secrete alginate, the polysaccharides Pel and Psl are involved in the establishment of biofilms. Pel provides protection against the aminoglycosides tobramycin and gentamicin, but not against ciprofloxacin [70]. Unlike alginate, Pel is a cationic exopolysaccharide, and, therefore, resistance to aminoglycosides cannot be explained by direct charge interaction. However, Pel binds eDNA [46], which is negatively charged and can interact with aminoglycosides. Additionally, Pel could bind negatively charged portions of other antibiotics such as ampicillin, though this hypothesis has not been explored yet. The exopolysaccharide Psl also binds eDNA [71] and plays a role in resistance to colistin, polymyxin B, tobramycin, and ciprofloxacin at early stages of biofilm formation [72]. This protective effect was also observed in the non-Psl producing species *E. coli* and *S. aureus* if they were present in a mixed biofilm together with *P. aeruginosa* [72].

Studies in *Pseudomonas* evidence that eDNA enhances resistance of biofilms to aminoglycosides but not to fluoroquinolones or β-lactams [73,74]. eDNA also enhances resistance of biofilms of *Staphylococcus epidermidis* to the glycopeptide antibiotic vancomycin [75]. Likely, the negatively charged eDNA binds positively charged aminoglycosides and glycopeptides. The latter study [75] also demonstrated that the binding constant of vancomycin and eDNA is up to 100-fold higher than that of vancomycin and its target, the D-Ala-D-Ala peptide in peptidoglycan precursors. Thus, within the biofilm environment, eDNA may compete with D-Ala-D-Ala peptide, and, because of the higher affinity of vancomycin for eDNA, it may be retained in the ECM. Besides direct interaction of eDNA with antibiotics, accumulation of eDNA creates a cation-limited environment by chelating cations such as Mg^{2+}. In *P. aeruginosa* and *S. enterica* serovar Typhimurium (*S.* Typhimurium), reduction of the Mg^{2+} concentration triggers the two-component regulatory systems PhoPQ and PmrAB, which are linked to AMR [74,76]. Activation of these systems generates modifications in the lipid A moiety of lipopolysaccharides (LPS) through (i) the expression of the outer membrane (OM) protein PagP, which adds a palmitoyl residue to the lipid A, (ii) the substitution of the phosphate groups with 4-amino-4-deoxy-L-arabinose and/or phophoethanolamine, and (iii) the production of LpxO, which adds a hydroxyl group onto the second carbon atom of one of the fatty acyl chains. The first stage of aminoglycoside uptake involves the binding of the polycationic antibiotics to the negatively charged components of the bacterial membrane, such as LPS of Gram-negative organisms. This is followed by displacement of Mg^{2+} ions [77,78], which leads to disruption of the OM and initiation of aminoglycoside uptake [79,80]. The modifications in the lipid A generated by the activation of PhoPQ and PmrAB alter considerably the lipid A charge and the OM permeability, which could explain the involvement of eDNA in aminoglycoside resistance. On the other hand, the activity of antimicrobials can also promote the release of eDNA to the ECM. For instance, the amount of eDNA in biofilms of *S. epidermidis* doubled by treatment with vancomycin [75]. The released eDNA can then bind the positively charged antibiotics and prevent them from reaching the cells and exerting their activity. Considering that eDNA is a constituent of the ECM of many bacteria, it is tempting to speculate that this phenomenon could also occur in other bacteria. Additionally, antibiotic-modifying enzymes can be released and located into the biofilm matrix. In mixed-species biofilms, the presence of a single species that secretes such enzymes would be beneficial for antibiotic-sensitive species in the same biofilm. Examples include *Moraxella catarrhalis* which secretes β-lactamases and, thereby, protects *S. pneumoniae* [81] and *H. influenzae* [82] from amoxicillin and ampicillin treatments, respectively, in mixed biofilms.

To summarize, components of the ECM alter the biomass organization affecting diffusion of certain antibiotics within the biofilm and, thus, altering the level of exposition of cells located in specific biofilm niches particularly those within dense biomass. Additionally, certain ECM components can interact with antibiotics, preventing them from reaching their targets within cells. Furthermore, the ECM can retain antibiotic-modifying enzymes, which is particularly relevant in mixed biofilms, where susceptible bacteria can be protected by such enzymes released from resistant cohabitants.

3.3. Physiological Heterogeneity

The architecture and organization of the biofilm also generates gradients of dispersion of nutrients, oxygen, pH, signaling molecules, and waste products. Oxygen and nutrient depletion occur in particular niches, such as inside the microcolonies and in the lower cell layers, and these conditions can induce a variety of physiological states involving different metabolism (aerobic, microaerobic, and fermentative) and growth rates (fast and slow growth, dormant cells, and persister cells) [83,84]. Nongrowing and slowly growing bacteria are less vulnerable to antibiotics as a consequence of the inactivity of antibiotic targets, a phenomenon called "drug indifference". In contrast, persister cells are phenotypic variants that constitute a part of the population with tolerance to antibiotics (see Section 3.1) that can resume growth after antibiotic removal. Persisters are present in both biofilm and planktonic cultures; however, biofilms typically harbor more persisters than planktonic cultures [66]. Ultimately, the biofilm is constituted of cells with different physiological states and chances to survive an external drug insult. Indeed, this repertoire of physiological cell states is relevant for tolerance to multiple antibiotics. For example, slowly growing cells are tolerant to antibiotics such as tobramycin and ciprofloxacin [85], which target protein synthesis machinery and DNA gyrase, respectively, and thus, exert their activity on fast-growing cells. In contrast, slowly growing cells are susceptible to antibiotics such as colistin [86] that act on the membrane.

Bacteria respond to starvation and stress conditions through specific adaptative mechanisms, such as activation of the stringent response (SR) and the SOS response. The SR is induced by amino-acid, carbon, and iron starvation [87]. Under amino-acid deprivation, the ribosomes are stalled by the presence of uncharged tRNA in the A site (Figure 3A). (p)ppGpp synthetases, e.g., RelA and SpoT in β- and γ-proteobacteria, sense stalled ribosomes and synthetize (p)ppGpp, also known as *alarmone*, which initiates transcriptional reprogramming and regulates various metabolic pathways, such as phosphate, amino-acid and lipid metabolism, among others [87] (Figure 3A). (p)ppGpp also modulates the repressor CodY, a master regulator of many genes triggered during environmental stress. Ultimately, the SR shuts down almost all metabolic processes, and, thus, cells become tolerant to antibiotics that target such processes. For example, the SR in *E. coli* has been linked to tolerance to inhibitors of cell-wall biosynthesis, such as penicillins [88], cephalosporins and carbapenems [89], and of cell division, such as norfloxacin [90] and ofloxacin [91]. The SR has been related to reduced susceptibility to ofloxacin [92,93], meropenem, colistin [92], and gentamicin [92,94,95] in *P. aeruginosa* biofilms, and to tolerance to ampicillin and vancomycin in *S. aureus* [96].

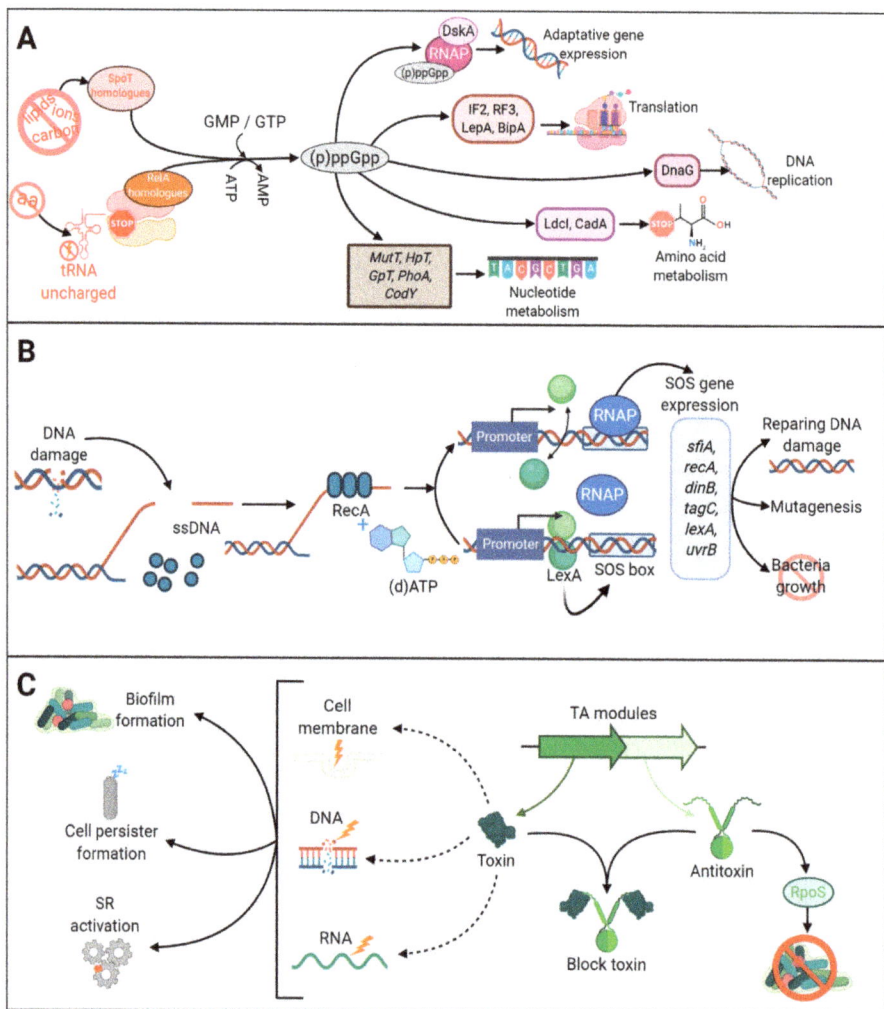

Figure 3. The stringent response, toxin-antitoxin, and SOS response pathways. (**A**) The stringent response (SR) is triggered by several stress conditions (amino-acid, carbon and iron deprivation or membrane damage) that activate the production (p)ppGpp by the synthetases RelA and SpoT and homologues. (p)ppGpp reprograms cell metabolism through the interaction with proteins involved in translation, transcription, replication, amino-acid metabolism, and nucleotide metabolism. (**B**) The SOS response is triggered by damaged DNA. Single-stranded (ssDNA) is detected by RecA. In the presence of (d)ATP, RecA is activated causing self-cleavage of LexA. LexA is a dimer that represses the transcription of SOS genes, which harbor an SOS box in their promoter. Cleavage of LexA leads to activation of the SOS genes inducing a repertoire of activities as indicated. The *lexA* gene also contains an SOS box; therefore, LexA production is self-regulated. Once the DNA is repaired, LexA represses the SOS response. (**C**) Several toxin-antitoxin (TA) modules are dispersed on the chromosome and are further classified according to the nature of the antitoxin and its mechanism of action. They are constituted by two genes, one encoding a toxin, with specific activities against target molecules (DNA, RNA, membrane, cell wall synthesis, ATP), and the other an antitoxin that binds to the toxin and inhibits its toxic activity. Under normal conditions, toxin and antitoxin are equally produced and thus the toxin does not exert its function. However, under stress conditions, the antitoxin can be degraded, and the toxin is free for toxic reactions. SR and SOS responses increase the production of ClpXP and Lon proteases, which activates the toxin by degradation of the antitoxin TA modules production. The toxic activity has several repercussions on cell biology.

The SOS response also contributes to antibiotic tolerance. It is generated by stress conditions such as DNA damage. Single-stranded DNA, generated by disruption of the DNA, activates RecA, which, in the presence of (d)ATP, stimulates self-cleavage of the repressor LexA leading to de-repression of SOS genes [97] (Figure 3B). Under regular physiological conditions, LexA is bound to a specific DNA sequence (SOS box) located upstream of several genes participating in DNA repair, mutagenesis and cell growth, and represses SOS gene expression (Figure 3B). The SOS response plays an important role in tolerance to antibiotics that cause DNA damage such as fluoroquinolones [98]. Studies in *E. coli* have demonstrated the function of the SOS response in enhancing biofilm tolerance to fluoroquinolones [91]. Together with the SR, the SOS response can also activate the expression of toxin-antitoxin (TA) modules [91,99], although TA modules can also be activated by stress-induced proteases like ClpXP and Lon in response to antibiotics. TA modules are genetic elements composed of two genes. One gene encodes a stable toxin protein that inhibits bacterial growth by interfering with essential cellular processes such as DNA replication, translation, cell wall synthesis, and membrane homeostasis, among others [100] (Figure 3C). The other gene encodes a cognate antitoxin that typically prevents or impairs toxin function. Antitoxins can be labile molecules that are degraded under stress conditions, a circumstance that allows the toxins to exert their harmful effects in cellular functions. Thus, by inactivating antibiotic targets, TA confers antibiotic tolerance [101] and increases persister formation [102] (Figure 3C). Several studies have shown upregulation of TA modules in persister cells. A well-studied example is MqsA and MqsR, a classical TA module where the MqsR functions as the toxin and MqsA as the antitoxin [103,104]. MqsR production is stimulated during biofilm formation and enhances cell motility in *E. coli* [103], and MqsA has been linked to the regulation of the general stress responses, such as oxidative stress [104]. MqsA represses the stress regulator RpoS, which decreases the concentration of the messenger 3,5-cyclic diguanylic acid and, consequently, biofilm formation is inhibited. However, upon stress conditions, such as oxidative stress, MqsA is unstable and rapidly degraded by Lon and ClpXP proteases, causing the accumulation of RpoS [104]. Then, SR is activated, and bacteria initiate biofilm formation. However, this has recently been disputed. Frainkin et al. (2019) reported that MqsA is not a global regulator and does not regulate *rpoS* expression. Moreover, authors showed that *mpsRA* production is not regulated by stress and that mutation of mpsRA has no clear effect on biofilm formation [105].

TAs are often involved in the stabilization of plasmids [106] and genomic islands that carry integrative and conjugative elements, which can mediate resistance to multiple antibiotics [107]. Considering that these genomic elements are commonly involved in promoting HGT [108], the role of TAs in antibiotic resistance can be notable. The SOS response and the SR participate in the dissemination of antibiotic resistance through integrons. Integrons are genetic elements involved in the capture antibiotic resistance genes. As they are located on mobile genetic elements, such as transposons, they contribute to the dissemination of these genes among Gram-negative bacteria [109]. An integron is composed of a gene encoding an integrase, a specific recombination site, and a promoter that controls the expression of promoter-less genes embedded within gene cassettes [110], some of which can be located in genetic mobile elements and contain antibiotic resistance-gene cassettes. Within the biofilm environment, transposases are activated under SOS response and SR regulates integrase expression [111], thereby promoting the dissemination of the antibiotic resistance genes located in mobile elements within members of the biofilm.

Depletion of oxygen in the interior of biofilms [112,113] and the presence of oxygen gradients have been demonstrated in different biofilm models [114,115]. Hypoxia affects metabolism substantially, because it shifts aerobic respiration to alternative metabolic routes such as denitrification and fermentation. Consistent with the hypoxic conditions in biofilms is the detected production of nitrous oxide, an intermediate of denitrification, in sputum of cystic fibrosis patients with chronic *P. aeruginosa* infection [116]. Earlier work using 70 different Gram-negative and 23 Gram-positive bacteria growing in aerobic and anaerobic conditions showed that microorganisms were more tolerant to aminoglycosides and highly tolerant to tobramycin under anaerobic conditions [117]. Accordingly, *Pseudomonas* biofilms formed under anaerobic conditions were more tolerant to antibiotics such as tobramycin, ciprofloxacin, carbenicillin, ceftazidime, chloramphenicol, and tetracycline than those formed in aerobiosis [112]. Indeed, hypoxia reduces membrane potential conferring tolerance to antibiotics such as aminoglycosides that require an intact membrane potential to be transported into the cytoplasm [118].

Antibiotics can induce oxidative stress by increasing cellular hydroxyl radical levels and enhancing production of lethal reactive oxygen species (ROS) [119,120]. This could be caused by an increased oxidation rate of tricarboxylic-acid cycle-derived NADH that perturbs iron homeostasis. Ferrous iron from iron-sulfur clusters is oxidized to ferric iron in the Fenton reaction which yields extremely reactive and harmful hydroxyl radicals that oxidize vital macromolecules such as DNA, proteins, and lipids [120,121]. To counteract, bacteria stimulate production of catalases and superoxide dismutases. Indeed, *Pseudomonas* mutants lacking catalase generate biofilms more susceptible to ciprofloxacin than wild-type biofilms [122]. The SR increases catalase and superoxide dismutase levels and represses the production of 4-hydroxy-2-alkylquinolines, which are intercellular signaling molecules with prooxidant properties [92]. Additionally, persisters downregulate genes encoding proteins involved in the generation of ROS, including a ferredoxin reductase, which is involved in recycling Fe^{3+} to Fe^{2+} and thus drives the Fenton reaction, and upregulates genes involved in ROS detoxification. Thus, persister cells are, to some extent, protected against the detrimental effects of ROS produced upon antibiotic treatment. Considering that the SR and persister formation are more highly activated in biofilm cells than in planktonic cultures, biofilm cells can better deal with ROS induced by antibiotics.

3.4. Traffic of Substances across the Cell Envelope

Several proteins in the bacterial membranes function in the recognition and transport of substances, including antibiotics, into or out of the cell. This activity is facilitated by efflux pumps and porins (in Gram-negative bacteria) that mediate an active and passive transport, respectively. Efflux pumps can be divided into six families, e.g., the multidrug- and toxin-extrusion (MATE), small multidrug-resistance (SMDR), major facilitator (MF), ATP-binding cassette (ABC), resistance-nodulation-division (RND) and proteobacterial antimicrobial compound-efflux (PACE) families. These families display large differences concerning transporter structure, function, and substrate specificity and energy source [123]. All families use protein motif force for as driving force except for the ABC transporters, which use ATP hydrolysis, and some members of MATE family that use sodium gradient instead.

The MATE family comprises proteins of 400–700 amino-acid residues organized in 12 α-helices [124]. These pumps participate in the extrusion of diverse antibiotics, such as ciprofloxacin, chloramphenicol, streptomycin, kanamycin, norfloxacin, and ampicillin [125]. Representative examples of this family in MDR bacteria are YdhE in *E. coli*, which transports kanamycin and acriflavin, amongst others [126], PmpM in *P. aeruginosa* [127], and AbeM in *A. baumannii* [128]. The SMR family is constituted of small proteins composed 100–120 amino-acid residues organized as homodimers with four transmembrane helices in each subunit. EmrE [129] of *E. coli* and Smr/QacC in *S. aureus* [130], both transporters of acriflavine, belong to this family. The MF family is constituted of membrane proteins with 400–600 amino-acid residues organized in 12–14 transmembrane α-helices. This family of transporters facilitates the passage of ions and carbohydrates across membranes, as well as antimicrobial agents such as tetracyclines and fluoroquinolones [131,132]. NorA, LmrS, and MdeA of *S. aureus* are well-known members of this family [133]. The ABC transporters are active transporters, often constituted of a transmembrane channel, formed by one or two proteins, and a dimeric cytoplasmic ATPase. The MacB transporter of *E. coli*, which operates in concert with the outer-membrane protein TolC and transports azithromycin, clarithromycin, and erythromycin, belongs to the ABC family [134]. Members of the PACE family transport acriflavine, proflavine, benzalkonium, acriflavine, and chlorhexidine [135]. Transporters of the RND family form a protein complex constituted of about 1000 amino-acid residues organized in a 12-helical structure in the membrane, but, in contrast to MF transporters, RND proteins possess large periplasmic domains. In Gram-negative bacteria, members of MF (e.g., EmrB), RND (e.g., MdtK), and ABC (e.g., MacB) families can be organized in a tripartite protein complex formed of an inner membrane protein, a membrane fusion protein, and an OM protein [123]. Collectively, this complex spans the entire cell envelope and allows for efficient excretion of antibiotics into the external medium. The AcrAB-TolC complex of *E. coli* [136], MexAB-OprM of *P. aeruginosa* [137], and AdeABC of *A. baumannii* [138], all RND family members that participate in tripartite transporters, have been implicated in bacterial biofilm resistance and biofilm formation.

Several lines of evidence relate efflux-pump production to biofilm formation and, directly or indirectly, to AMR/tolerance. First, some efflux-pump-encoding genes are upregulated in biofilms as compared to planktonic cells. This was detected in different transporter families. Examples are the *mdpF* gene of *E. coli*, which encodes a component of the MdtEF efflux pump (RND family) that participates in the tolerance to nitrosyl-mediated toxicity and that was upregulated in anaerobic conditions [139], a condition found in biofilms. Another example is the multidrug efflux genes *acrA* and *acrB* of *S.* Typhimurium [140]. Second, the exposition of cells to efflux-pump inhibitors reduces biofilm formation in several pathogens such as *E. coli* and *K. pneumoniae* [141], *P. aeruginosa* [142], and *S.* Typhimurium [143]. Third, mutants lacking known efflux systems exhibit a marked reduction in biofilm formation, for instance pump mutants in *Salmonella* showed reduced production of curli [143], which are implicated in biofilm formation. Fourth, several studies link efflux-pump production and acquired resistance of biofilms to antibiotics. Within *Pseudomonas* biofilms, MexAB-OprM and MexCD-OprJ are essential for resistance to azithromycin [144], and MexAB-OprM also mediates resistance to colistin [145]. Additionally, the ABC transporter encoded by the PA1874–1877 operon conferred protection to tobramycin in biofilms [146]. Biofilms of *E. coli* formed by mutants in genes that participate in the AcrAB-TolC system exhibited sensitivity to tobramycin, tetracycline, and the antiseptic benzalkonium, while mutants in the EmrAB system exhibited sensitivity to tobramycin [147]. Overall, these studies evidence that efflux pumps can directly contribute to expel antibiotics during biofilms that contribute to AMR but also ECM components that ultimately contribute to biofilm tolerance.

The OM of Gram-negative bacteria forms a barrier for both hydrophobic and hydrophilic solutes. Porins control the access of antibiotics from the environment to the periplasm. Porins are trimers of 16-stranded β-barrels located in the OM that provide selective access of small hydrophilic molecules to periplasm by diffusion through a water-filled channel present in each of the subunits [148]. Not surprisingly, MDR clinical isolates of *Enterobacteriaceae* often exhibit loss of porin production [149,150]. Several genetic mechanisms reduce or prevent porin synthesis, including downregulation of expression, premature stop codons or insertion elements. Besides, missense mutations can alter the permeability properties. Efflux pumps and porin production act in synergy and have been associated to biofilm production, particularly in *Enterobacteriaceae* [141,151]. In *K. pneumoniae*, the gene coding for the porin OmpK36 was downregulated and the *acrB* gene, coding for a component of a major multidrug-efflux pump, was upregulated in biofilms as compared to planktonic cells [152].

The production of efflux pumps and porins can be up- and downregulated, respectively, to reduce the intracellular accumulation of antibiotics, an adaptive phenomenon based on the transport regulation. Curiously, upregulation of the MDR transporter MdfA of *E. coli* not only makes cells resistant to the aminoglycosides neomycin and kanamycin but also increases their susceptibility to spectinomycin by an, as yet, unexplained mechanism [153,154]. In general, efflux pump production could be regulated by local and global transcriptional regulators, modulators, various substances, including antibiotics, small RNAs and two-component regulatory systems whose activation depends on environmental stimuli [155]. MarA, BrlR, SoxS, Rob, and AcrR are very well-known regulators of pump production in pathogenic bacteria [155]. Pump production can be regulated at multiple levels. AcrAB-TolC of *E. coli* is the best-studied example of regulation under a complex regulatory network. AcrAB synthesis is negatively regulated by the local repressor AcrR that represses *acrAB* expression [156]. In addition, the repressor AcrS regulates *acrAB* negatively [157], while the histone-like nucleoid structuring protein H-NS has a role in the network repressing the expression *acrS* [158]. Therefore, by negatively regulating *acrS*, H-NS is a positive regulator of *acrAB*. Furthermore, the two-component regulatory systems EvgAS and/or PhoQP activate *tolC* expression, while EvgAS also activates *acrAB* expression [159]. Finally, the global regulators SdiA [160], MarA, SoxS, and Rob activate expression of *acrAB*, and the latter three regulators also activate *tolC* and *micF* expression [155]. *micF* transcripts inhibit the translation of the mRNA of porin OmpF. As OmpF plays an important role in the influx of antibiotics, the bacterium thus controls the efflux and influx of antibiotics by activating AcrAB-TolC and abolishing OmpF production, respectively. Interestingly, while MarA upregulates pump production, it downregulates biofilm formation through activation of the *ycgZ-ymgABC* operon which eventually reduces curli formation [161]. Possibly, MarA helps to activate a mechanism for cells to escape from biofilms as defence to the antibiotic insult. However, since pump expression is regulated by multiple mechanisms, it is difficult to speculate about the precise biological role of MarA within the complex regulatory network. In *P. aeruginosa*, the production of the efflux pumps MexAB-OprM and EmrAB is differentially regulated by the regulators MdrR1 and MdrR2 [162]. These regulators activate EmrAB but repress MexAB-OprM. Their expression varies between cells located in different layers of a biofilm, which leads to different susceptibility to antibiotics dependent on the position within the biofilm biomass. As these efflux pumps have different substrate specificities, it has been proposed that MdrR1 and MdrR2 could act as master modulators controlling the activities of various pumps in different microenvironments within the stratified biofilm structure [162]. All together, these studies illustrate that the regulation of pump production can be controlled by a complex repertoire of regulators, some of which act on a variety of genes that participate in biofilm production, and/or by varying conditions, which are generated within the biofilm environment.

3.5. Interbacterial Communication

QS is a population-density-dependent regulatory mechanism by which bacteria communicate via signaling molecules, called autoinducers. Bacteria produce autoinducers, which accumulate in the environment with the increase in the cell density. These autoinducers are recognized by cell-surface receptors or in the cytoplasm. After receptor recognition, gene transcription is activated, involving genes coding for surface proteins, transcription factors, virulence factors, and proteins involved in biofilm development [163,164]. Peptides are used as autoinducers in Gram-positive bacteria in contrast to the acylated homoserine lactones used in Gram-negative bacteria. Autoinducer 2 is used in Gram-negative and Gram-positive bacteria for intra- and interspecies communication.

QS seems to contribute to biofilm recalcitrance. Biofilms formed by QS mutants or wild-type bacteria treated with QS inhibitors are more susceptible to antibiotics. For example, *P. aeruginosa* biofilms formed by a mutant strain lacking *lasR* and *rhlR*, which is deficient in QS, were significantly more susceptible to tobramycin than wild-type biofilms [165]. Additionally, mixed *Pseudomonas* biofilms formed by QS mutants and wild-type bacteria exhibited a decreased resistance to tobramycin as compared to those formed only with wild-type bacteria [166]. In *S. aureus*, a QS-deficient *agrD* mutant exhibited a biofilm-specific decrease in resistance to rifampin compared to wild type [167]. Additionally, *fsrA* and *gelE* mutants of *E. faecalis*, which are deficient in QS and a QS-controlled protease, respectively, were impaired in biofilm formation in the presence of gentamicin, daptomycin, or linezolid, but not in the absence of these antibiotics [168]. The involvement of QS in biofilm recalcitrance may have multiple origins. QS is involved in biofilm formation and structuration; therefore, QS-defective mutants produce less structured biofilms.

Considering that the architecture of the biofilm is relevant for its recalcitrant properties, the resulting biofilms would be more susceptible to antibiotics. Alternatively, QS may have other contributions. For instance, QS in *P. aeruginosa* regulates the production of 2-n-heptyl-4-hydroxyquinoline-N-oxide (HQNO), which inhibits the respiratory chain by binding to the cytochrome bc_1 complex [169]. This results in the accumulation of ROS and the reduction in membrane potential and eventually in autolysis. Autolysis releases DNA, which, as previously discussed, promotes biofilm formation and confers resistance against positively charged antibiotics. Additionally, by reducing the electrochemical gradient, the sensitivity to aminoglycosides [170], tetracycline, and macrolides [171] is reduced. QS can also contribute to drug resistance within mixed species biofilms. *Stenotrophomonas maltophilia* and *P. aeruginosa* can form mixed biofilms when they coinfect cystic fibrosis patients. *P. aeruginosa* recognizes signal factors produced by *S. maltophilia* and induces the PmrAB two-component system that regulates resistance to cationic antimicrobial peptides [172]. Thus, QS signals and the resulting downstream consequences can elicit an ample range of physiological changes that alter the antimicrobial susceptibility of cells within a biofilm.

Some intercellular communication requires direct cell-to-cell contact. Well-described examples are the two-partner secretion system (TPS). In the TPS system, a large surface-exposed protein, generically called TpsA, is secreted by an OM protein, called TpsB [173]. Some bacteria produce several TPS systems. TpsAs can have several functions in biofilm formation. They can function in adhesion to biotic surfaces and in interbacterial interactions [173,174]. In *N. meningitidis*, TpsA contributes to the maturation of biofilms, and its synthesis is upregulated during biofilm formation [175]. In many microorganisms, TpsA functions in inhibiting the growth of related bacteria [176,177]. In the proposed model, TpsA interacts with a conserved receptor on a target cell, after which a small C-terminal part is proteolytically released and transported into the target cell where it displays toxic activities [174]. Kin target cells produce an immunity protein that inhibits the toxic activity by specifically binding to the toxin. In this case, the imported toxin moiety functions as a signaling molecule and stimulates community associated behaviors, such as biofilm formation, as was demonstrated in *Burkholderia* [178]. Killed target bacteria release intracellular components, including DNA, which contributes to the biofilm formation. Additionally, this activity mediates resistance to cefotaxime in *E. coli* [179]. TpsA induces persister formation upon direct contact with cells lacking sufficient levels of immunity protein [179]. Very likely, more recently discovered secretion systems that deliver toxins to the target cells [180,181] also contribute to biofilm formation and recalcitrance, a research area that needs to be addressed.

3.6. HGT in Biofilms

HGT can involve the exchange of AMR genes between bacteria and is carried out through five different mechanisms. Three of them are generally known, namely conjugation (a direct transfer of genes between cells), transformation (acquisition of DNA from the environment), and transduction (gene transfer between cells via bacteriophages). The other mechanisms involve the release of membrane vesicles (MVs), which act as DNA reservoirs, or elongated membranous structures called nanotubes, which are employed for direct cell-to-cell contact. HGT can occur at a higher rate in biofilms than in planktonic cells [182]. Indeed, biofilms play an important role in the dissemination of AMR genes, and they are considered as reservoirs of resistance genes [10]. HGT would be favored within a biofilm for three main reasons: (i) the polymicrobial nature of biofilms that make them reservoirs of genetic diversity, (ii) the structure of biofilm, which restricts bacterial motility, increases cell density and promotes interbacterial interactions, and (iii) the presence of eDNA, which is released by cell lysis or by active secretion systems and that is retained in the ECM and establishes contacts among biofilm members. Probably even more important than its role as a glue for bacterial interactions, the eDNA can be taken up by transformation, one of the main HGT mechanisms. In addition, other factors involved in HGT would be the biomass surface, as it has been shown that high surface/volume ratios (in well-structured biofilms) increase the efficiency of plasmid transfer [183,184].

Conjugative plasmids and integrative and conjugative elements (ICEs) are transferred mostly via conjugation. Conjugation is carried out by a conjugation system based on sex pili that mediate direct contact between two cells, the donor and the recipient. After pilus retraction, intimate contact between donor and recipient allows for DNA transfer. This is probably the most common mechanism for the transfer of AMR genes within the biofilm environment. A study in *S. aureus* that showed a 16,000-fold higher transfer rate of the conjugative plasmid pGO1, which includes trimethoprim- and gentamicin-resistance genes, in biofilms than in planktonic cells, serves as a good example [185]. Likewise, in vitro biofilm experiments have demonstrated inter-family transfer by conjugation of a bla_{NDM-1} gene encoding a carbapenemase from *Enterobacteriaceae* into *P. aeruginosa* and *A. baumannii* [186]. This mechanism occurs more intensely in biofilms than in free-living bacteria because of the proximity between cells in this structure. Apart from conjugation, where cell–cell contact is established by pili, nanotubes can transport nonconjugative plasmids between closely related strains of *Bacillus subtilis* and of *E. coli* [187]. These structures have also been detected in MDR-related bacteria, such as *Acinetobacter baylyi* [188]. Future research will elucidate their involvement in HGT among biofilm members.

Chromosomal DNA and nonconjugative plasmids are exchanged through transformation. Additionally, this mechanism is favored within biofilms because of the presence of large amounts of eDNA in the ECM. An experiment that compared the transformation rate in planktonic and biofilm cells of *N. gonorrhoeae* demonstrated that the transfer efficiency of two resistance genes, *ermC* and *aadA*, was higher at early stages of biofilm formation but decreased with biofilm age [189]. However, the transformation efficiency was shown not to depend on biofilm architecture. Spreading of transformants was observed in loose biofilms under selection pressure but was hardly observed from dense biofilms. Interestingly, even conjugative transposons of the Tn916 family, coding for tetracycline resistance, were shown to be transferred through this mechanism in in vitro grown biofilms of a multispecies consortium of oral bacteria [190].

Alternatively, genomic DNA, which may include AMR genes, can be transferred by transduction, although the diffusion of some phages through biofilms could be hampered by the biofilm matrix (discussed in Section 4). It can serve as an example, as a study showed that a temperate, Shiga-toxin (Stx)-encoding bacteriophage with a chloramphenicol-resistance gene (*cat*) inserted as a marker into the *stx* gene, could transfer this gene to *E. coli* within a biofilm [191]. Finally, although MV are released within biofilms and were demonstrated to transfer AMR genes, such as the β-lactamase-encoding bla_{OXA-24} gene in *A. baumannii* [192], their relevance in HGT in a biofilm environment remains to be studied.

3.7. Mutation and Biofilms

Mutations in the bacterial genome can also give rise to AMR [193]. They may occur spontaneously, that is, in the absence of strong selective pressure. Spontaneous mutations are found to occur at a common rate of 10^{-10}–10^{-9} per nucleotide per generation for many bacteria; therefore, mutants are usually already present as a minority within a population [194]. The mutation rate can increase significantly by exposure to agents that elicit oxidative stress. Oxidative stress is associated with the build-up of ROS, which may cause direct DNA damage and mutations. In certain circumstances, such as the exposure to sub lethal doses of bactericidal antibiotics, the accumulation of ROS is low, and it may promote resistance by the induction of the synthesis of multidrug efflux pumps and by mutagenesis [195]. This is a common situation when, for instance, subtherapeutic doses of antibiotics are used as growth promoters in animal production. However, more importantly, this may also occur within biofilms where antibiotic diffusion depends on the biofilm architecture. Additional mutations can also appear as a consequence of the SOS response, which induces the synthesis of error-prone DNA polymerases. Thus, stress responses can induce high mutation frequencies through different pathways. The mutation frequency may further increase after mutations are generated in the DNA failure-prevention or repair systems. The most frequent cause is related to defects in the methyl-directed mismatch repair system, e.g., in genes such as *mutS*, *mutL*, and *uvrD*. This can lead to a 100- to 1000-fold increase in the mutation rate [196,197]. The occurrence of microorganisms with this phenotype, called hypermutators, can represent an evolutionary advantage under selective pressure by increasing the possibility of acquiring favorable mutations, including mutations leading to AMR [198].

The hypermutator phenotype in biofilms has been detected in chronic infections in patients with cystic fibrosis, where 53% of the *Pseudomonas* isolates were hypermutable [199]. The frequency of mutants resistant to rifampicin and ciprofloxacin was higher in *Pseudomonas* biofilms than in free-living bacteria [200]. This state of hypermutability has also been reported in other bacteria isolated from cystic fibrosis patients, such as *S. aureus* and *H. influenzae* [201,202] but not in clinical isolates of the *Enterobacteriaceae* family from acute urinary tract infections governed by biofilms [203]. Thus, the hypermutation may be favored in some biofilm environments but is not a general mechanism. Altogether, bacteria in biofilms could be in a highly mutable state due to growth restrictions and nonlethal selective pressure, possibly further increased by antibiotic treatment, high- and hypermutability is also disadvantageous due to the accumulation of deleterious mutations. A solution could be transient hypermutability [204], where always a part of a population is transiently in a hypermutable state and prone to selection for favorable mutations, whereas the rest is rather stable. To the best of our knowledge, a transient hypermutator stage has not been experimentally demonstrated in biofilms. However, main conditions are accomplished: slow growth and nonlethal selective pressure. This raises the question whether transient hypermutability is a natural biological phenomenon that contributes to biofilm resistance.

In general, mutations that affect the bacterial susceptibility to antibiotics were described (i) to alter an antibiotic target, (ii) to increase the production of efflux pump, (iii) to lead to changes in the cell membranes, or (iv) to increase the production or alter the substrate specificity of enzymes that inactivate antibiotics. For example, mutations affecting the antibiotic target of aminoglycosides were in the *rspL* gene [205], which code for 16S rRNA and the S12 ribosomal protein, respectively. Mutations in the *mexZ* gene in clinical isolates of *Pseudomonas* resulted in overproduction of the efflux system MexXY-OprM [206]. Colistin resistance has been associated with mutations in the genes coding for the PmrAB two-component regulatory system that regulates the addition of aminoarabinose to lipid A [207]. Additionally, mutations resulting in increased production of β-lactamases, e.g., by mutations in the promoter of the chromosomal *ampC* gene [208] or by increase of plasmid copy number [150] have been described, among others. In addition, the genes have evolved over the years, showing a large number of β-lactamase variants with point mutations in the gene resulting in changes in the amino-acid sequence [209]. This has led to the development of extended-spectrum β-lactamases (ESBLs) that degrade also first, second, and third generation cephalosporins and/or became resistant to β-lactamase inhibitors [210].

4. Control of Biofilm Infections

4.1. Lessons from Recalcitrant Mechanisms

As biofilms contribute to bacterial pathogenicity and recalcitrance, novel strategies and agents are required to deal with this issue. We have now clear evidence that the antibiotics used for the treatment of biofilm infections should be carefully selected, and such selection should consider the mechanisms of resistance and tolerance of biofilms. The use of cocktails of antibiotics would probably be more successful than a single antibiotic, but the antibiotic combination should also be thoroughly considered. Antibiotics should cover the heterogenic nature of biofilms. While one of the antibiotics in the combination should be active against persisters (e.g., colistin), others should target growing cells (e.g., ciprofloxacin, tobramycin, or β-lactams). In addition, the selection of antibiotics will benefit from the characterization of ECM composition, particularly the sorption and charge of the matrix, as these properties are relevant contributors to AMR.

Many alternatives to antibiotics have been proposed to inhibit and/or eradicate biofilms. Their nature and their mechanisms of action are ample. In general, they possess one or several activities as (i) biofilm inhibitors, (ii) biofilm dispersers, and (iii) antimicrobials. An overview of these substances is listed in Table 1 and briefly discussed here. QS inhibitors can act as biofilm inhibitors or biofilm dispersers. Several plant-derived compounds exhibit this property, including halogenated furanones, which are molecules similar to N-acyl-homoserine lactones that prevent these QS signaling molecules to interact with their receptor, e.g., a LuxR family member. Thus, they function as antagonist of LuxR and repress expression of QS-induced genes [211,212]. Flavonoids, such as quercetin, can also interfere with QS. Quercetin represses the production of exopolysaccharides in *S. aureus*, required for initiation of biofilm formation [213,214]. However, QS involves a large variety of molecules in different organisms and their role in biofilm formation is species specific, thus, the activity of QS inhibitors is limited. Alternatively, enzymes that degrade QS signaling molecules such as lactonases that degrade lactone rings or phosphorylases have shown great promise [215,216], but again substrate specificity may limit their use. Other substances could contribute to inhibiting biofilm formation by interfering with the SR. For example, the 12-residue peptide 1018 interacts with (p)ppGpp and inhibits the accumulation of the alarmone and, thereby, persister formation, although this mechanism was later disputed [217]. The peptide prevents biofilm formation of different Gram-negative and Gram-positive bacteria [218] and revealed significant synergistic activity to eradicate biofilms in combination with antibiotics [219]. Eugenol is a secondary metabolite from clove (*Syzygium aromaticum*) with antibacterial activity. It inhibits biofilm formation and downregulates *relA* [220] leading to inhibition of the alarmone activation.

Table 1. Proposed alternatives to antibiotics with antimicrobial or antibiofilm activities. The substance, the mechanism of action (including anti-biofilm activity), and the target bacterial species are indicated for each agent.

Substance(s)	Mechanism of Action	Targets	References
Antimicrobial Peptides			
Natural Antimicrobial Peptides			
Melittin	Formation of short-lived pores in the membrane and increase of permeability of OM	*P. aeruginosa, S. aureus, E. coli, K. pneumoniae, A. baumannii*	[220–224]
Japonicin-2LF	Detergent-like activity against components of biofilm matrix; higher activity in inhibiting than in eradicating biofilms	*S. aureus*, MRSA, *E. coli*	[225]
Magainin 2	Destabilizes the bacterial membrane and intracellular processes	*A. baumannii, P. aeruginosa, E. coli*	[226–228]
LL-37	Membrane disruption; inhibits twitching and QS; interferes in bacterial attachment; downregulates *rhlA* and *rhlB* genes	*P. aeruginosa, A. baumanni, S. aureus*	[229–231]
Temporin 1Tb	Disruption of cell membrane integrity; capable of penetrating biofilm and killing bacteria; hemolytic activity	*S. epidermidis, S. aureus, K. pneumoniae, P. aeruginosa, E. faecium*	[232,233]

Table 1. Cont.

Substance(s)	Mechanism of Action	Targets	References
Synthetic Antimicrobial Peptides			
1037	Downregulates genes of biofilm development; reduces swimming and swarming motilities	*P. aeruginosa, L. monocytogenes, Burkolderia cenocepacia*	[218]
Esculentin (1–21)	Biofilm eradication	*P. aeruginosa*	[234]
1018	Binds (p)ppGpp and inhibits SR; inhibits attachment, QS, and twitching motility	*E. coli, S. aureus*, MRSA, *P. aeruginosa, A. baumannii, K. pneumoniae, A. baumannii, S.* Typhimurium, *E. faecium*	[218,219,235]
STAMP G10KHc	Disrupts and permeabilizes OM and IM	*P. aeruginosa*	[236]
$F_{2,5,12}W$	Reduces initial adhesion of bacteria; eliminates mature biofilms; suppresses biofilm formation	*S. epidermidis*	[237]
Combined Therapies			
1018 + antibiotics (e.g., ciprofloxacin)	Inhibition of (p)ppGpp activation; downregulation of genes that interfere with antibiotic resistance and biofilm formation	*E. coli*, MRSA, *P. aeruginosa, K. pneumoniae, A. baumannii, S. enterica*	[219]
Esculentin (1–21) + AuNPs (AuNPs@Esc(1–21))	Disruption of membrane forming clusters	*P. aeruginosa*	[238]
Temporin 1Tb + EDTA	Mature biofilm eradication	*S. epidermidis*	[232]
lin-SB056-1 + EDTA	Perturbation of membrane; eradication biofilm; chelation of divalent metal ions	*P. aeruginosa*	[239]
Bacteriophages			
Phages			
EFDG1	Mature biofilm eradication	*E. faecium, E. faecalis*	[240]
vB_EfaH_EF1TV	Mature biofilm eradication	*E. faecalis*	[241]
vB_PaeM_LS1	Disrupts and avoids dispersion of biofilms; inhibits biofilm growth	*P. aeruginosa*	[242]
vB_SauM_philPLA-RODI	Penetrates biofilms; inhibits biofilm formation	*S. aureus* *S. epidermidis*	[243]
Phage-derived Enzymes			
LysAB3	Degradation of bacterial wall peptidoglycan, biofilm eradication	*A. baumannii*	[244]
Dpo48	Degrades exopolysaccharide and eradicates biofilm	*A. baumannii*	[245]
Combined Phage Therapy			
Phage + amoxicillin	Biofilm eradication	*K. pneumoniae*	[246]
SAP-26 + rifampicin	Hydrolysis of bacterial wall; mature biofilm eradication; reduction of biofilm growth	*S. aureus*	[247]
Phage K + DRA88	Inhibits biofilm formation; disperses biofilms	*S. aureus*	[248]
Phage K + its derivatives (e.g., K.MS811)	Biofilm eradication	*S. aureus*	[249,250]
Phage M4 + E2005-24-39 + E2005-40-16 + W2005-24-39 + W2005-37-18-03	Biofilm eradication	*P. aeruginosa*	[251]
DL52 + DL54 + DL60 + DL62 + DL64 + DL68	Attachment to cell by binding to lipopolysaccharide; biofilm eradication	*P. aeruginosa*	[252]

Table 1. Cont.

Substance(s)	Mechanism of Action	Targets	References
Plant-Derived Natural Products			
Essential Oils or Principal Active Compounds			
Cinnamon (cinnamaldehyde)	Inhibits QS mechanism: regulates production of rhamnolipids, proteases, and alginate and swarming activity; disrupts synthesis of DNA, RNA, proteins, lipids, and polysaccharides; alters expression of genes related to biofilm formation (e.g., *icaA*)	*E. coli, P. aeruginosa, K. pneumoniae, A. baumannii, S. epidermidis, S. aureus,* MRSA, *S. enteridis, S.* Typhimurium	[253–257]
Clove	Disrupts QS communication: biofilm dispersal, inhibits AHL synthesis; downregulates *relA* gene	*E. coli, P. aeruginosa, K. pneumoniae, A. baumannii, S. aureus*	[253,257]
Thyme (thymol)	Downregulates *sarA* gene; increases membrane permeability; penetrates polysaccharide matrix: eradicates biofilms	*E. coli, P. aeruginosa, K. pneumoniae, A. baumannii, S. aureus, S. enteridis*	[257–259]
Tea tree oil	Alters expression of multiple genes related to biofilm formation (e.g., *sarA, cidA, igrA, ifrB*)	*S. aureus*	[260]
Oregano (carvacrol)	Increases membrane permeability; penetrates polysaccharide matrix; eradicates biofilms	*K. pneumoniae, P. aeruginosa, A. baumannii*	[258]
Halogenated furanones	QS inhibition; antagonist of LuxR	*E. coli* *P. aeruginosa*	[211,212]
Flavonoids (e.g., quercetin)	Represses exopolysaccharides production; inhibits *rpoS* gene expression; decreases swimming motility	*S. aureus, E. coli, P. aeruginosa, E. faecalis*	[261–264]
Combined Therapy			
Carvacrol + eugenol	Increases membrane permeability	*K. pneumoniae, P. aeruginosa, A. baumannii, S. aureus*	[258,265,266]
Cinnamaldehyde + eugenol	Membrane permeabilization	*S. epidermidis*	[267]
Curcumin + antibiotics (e.g., ciprofloxacin)	QS inhibition	*E. coli, K. pneumoniae, P. aeruginosa, S. aureus, E. faecalis*	[268]
Enzymes			
Dispersin B	Hydrolyses PNAG	*S. epidermidis, S. aureus, E. coli, A. pleuropneumoniae*	[38,269,270]
DNases	Hydrolyses DNA	*A. baumannii, K. pneumoniae, E. coli, P. aeruginosa, S. aureus*	[271–273]
Alginate lyase	Degrades alginate	*P. aeruginosa*	[274]
Lysozyme	Hydrolytic activity	*S. pneumoniae, Gardnerella vaginalis, S. aureus, P. aeruginosa*	[275–277]
Lysostaphin	Degrades cell wall	*S. aureus, S. epidermidis*	[278]
Proteases (e.g., SpeB)	Degrades cell wall	*Streptococcus* spp. *P. aeruginosa, S. aureus*	[279,280]
Paraoxonases (e.g., acylase I)	Inhibits QS	*A. hydrophila, P. putida, P. aeruginosa*	[216,281,282]
Lactonase	Inhibits QS	*P. aeruginosa*	[215,283]
Small molecules			
Small molecules (e.g., LP 3134, LP 3145, LP 4010)	Inhibition of diguanylate cyclase	*P. aeruginosa, A. baumannii*	[284]
Pilicides (FN075, BibC6, Ec240)	Blocks synthesis of curli and Type I pili, and inhibits chaperone-usher pathway for pili biogenesis	*E. coli*	[285,286]
Mannosides	Inhibits FimH of type I pili	*E. coli*	[287]
Ethyl pyruvate	Inhibits enzymes of the glycolytic pathway	*E. coli*	[288]

Table 1. Cont.

Substance(s)	Mechanism of Action	Targets	References
	Polysaccharides		
Psl, Pel	Disperses biofilm	*S. epidermidis*	[289]

OM: outer membrane; MRSA: methicillin-resistant *S. aureus*; QS: quorum sensing; SR: stringent response; STAMP: selectively targeted antimicrobial peptide; IM: inner membrane; EDTA: ethylenediaminetetraacetic acid; AHL: *N*-acyl-homoserine actones; PNAG: poly-(β-1,6)-*N*-acetylglucosamine; DNase: deoxyribonuclease; ECM: extracellular matrix.

ECM-disrupting enzymes are potentially also suitable inhibitors and dispersers of biofilms. Addition of exogenous enzymes such as Dispersin B or DNase I, which hydrolyze PNAG and eDNA, respectively, in combination with antibiotics eradicate biofilms of different species [290–292]. Other enzymes, such as alginate lyase [274], lysozyme [293], and lysostaphin [278], showed promising results in this respect. Additionally, proteases that cleave proteins of the ECM or proteins located at the bacterial cell surface with a function in biofilm formation disrupted streptococcal [279] and *S. aureus* biofilms [280]. Additionally, addition of exopolysaccharides of the ECM from biofilms of some bacteria can be used to inhibit biofilm formation of other microorganisms. For instance, Psl and Pel, which are produced in *Pseudomonas* biofilms, eradicate biofilms of *S. epidermidis* [289], and the polysaccharide A101 from *Vibrio* sp. QY101 disperses *Pseudomonas* biofilms [294]. Probably, these charged polysaccharides outcompete structures essential for biofilm integrity. Another molecule that destabilizes the ECM is ethyl pyruvate, which, in combination with the Ca^{2+}-chelator EDTA, inhibits biofilms of many microorganisms [288].

Molecules that inhibit the adhesion properties of bacteria prevent the initiation of biofilm formation. Mannosides are small molecules that inhibit FimH [287], a mannose-binding component of the Type I pili that facilitates adhesion of uropathogenic *E. coli*. Mannosides can be used in combination with antibacterial agents to prevent biofilms on catheters [295]. Similarly, pilicides, which are small ring-fused 2-pyridones, inhibit Type I piliation [286]. Small peptides, such as FN075 and BibC6, block the assembly of curli and pili by disrupting protein–protein interactions during assembly and thereby inhibit the formation of *E. coli* biofilms [285]. Overall, biofilm inhibitors and dispersers utilize different mechanisms that ultimately disrupt intermolecular interactions required for the biogenesis and establishment of biofilms or they degrade these components. As these activities do not affect bacterial viability, they must be provided in combination with antimicrobials for bacterial eradication.

4.2. Antimicrobial Substances

New antimicrobial substances, some of which exhibit good penetration in biofilms, have been proposed as alternatives to antibiotics. Among them, antimicrobial peptides, bacteriophages, and essential oils stand out as most promising and several examples are listed in Table 1. Antimicrobial peptides (AMPs) are small peptides of about 12–50 amino-acid residues, containing a considerable number of hydrophobic residues (≈50%) and positively charged residues [296]. They are produced by the innate immune system of animals, insects, plants, and humans to prevent bacterial, fungal, and viral infections [297,298]. They disrupt bacterial membranes through either one of three different mechanisms, (i) detergent-like membrane packing disruption, (ii) formation of pores in the barrel-stave model and (iii) toroidalpore model [299]. In addition, they can inhibit DNA, RNA, and protein synthesis. Hence, AMPs have a broad activity spectrum against microbes and, consequently, the probability of AMR development is relatively low compared to conventional antibiotics. Some AMPs from different sources have shown a good combination of antimicrobial and antibiofilm activities against superbugs (see examples in Table 1 and expanded in the AMP database: http://aps.unmc.edu/AP). An example is melittin, which is a major component of honeybee venom [300]. This cationic linear peptide of 26 amino-acid residues inserts into bacterial membranes forming short-lived pores and it also inhibits biofilm formation of several bacteria, including *P. aeruginosa* [221,223] and *K. pneumoniae* [222], among others (Table 1). However, natural AMPs exhibit drawbacks for their application in vivo, including low efficiency, low biostability due to enzymatic degradation, toxicity at the required concentrations, and inefficient delivery to the infection niche. In an effort to improve their utility, several strategies are being conducted, comprising the design of synthetic AMPs, combination with antibiotics, or conjugation to carriers (Table 1). As an example, cyclic derivatives of peptide1018 have been created to enhance the proteolytic stability and reduce aggregation of the peptide [301]. When 1018 was coadministrated with antibiotics, a high synergistic ability to prevent and eradicate biofilms of many bacteria was observed [219]. Some AMPs were encapsulated in vehicles such as polymers, nanoparticles, micelles, carbon nanotubes, and others [reviewed in 302]. The AMPs-carrying vehicles can diffuse through tissue layers and expose simultaneously a large number of peptides improving their effectivity while lowering toxicity and reducing degradation. One of the most commonly used delivery systems is gold nanoparticles (AuNPs) [302]. They have been proposed as conjugate to AMPs because they are of small size, high solubility, stability, and biocompatibility. Esculentin-1a conjugated to AuNPs [AuNPs@Esc(1–21)] exhibited about 15-fold higher activity than the peptide alone and, in contrast to the peptide, it was not toxic. In addition, it showed high resistance to proteases [238].

Phage therapy involves the use of lytic bacteriophages to kill bacteria [303]. It has some advantages compared with other antimicrobials, for example, their natural origin, lack of toxicity for humans or nontarget microbes, and their effectiveness against antibiotic-resistant bacteria. Moreover, they are self-replicating in the presence of host cells and disappear without host. As a disadvantage, phages are strain specific; hence, a successful treatment requires a full understanding of bacteriophage–host interactions, involving identification of the specific phage. Although the chance seems to be low, bacteria can acquire phage resistance at high frequency. A simple point mutation in the phage receptor on the bacterial cell surface already suffices for the bacteria to escape phage attack. In addition, bacteria have several broad strategies to escape from phage, e.g., CRISPR-Cas, restriction enzymes, O-antigen, etc. To overcome these limitations, a combination of phages (phage cocktails) is often recommended instead of a single phage. This therapy is already supported by authorities in certain countries where commercial products against bacteria, such as *Listeria monocytogenes*, *Salmonella enterica* and *E. coli*, as surface disinfectants or processing aids are available. Yet, while phage receptors are fully available in planktonic cells, their accessibility in biofilms is compromised. ECM structures can establish electrostatic interactions with phage particles preventing them from reaching the cell surface. However, some phages may carry polysaccharide-degrading enzymes and thus gain access to receptors on the bacterial cell wall. Additionally, the ECM contains released phage receptors from cell lysis that ultimately compete with cell-surface receptors. Enzymes contained in ECM, such as proteases, inactivate phages. On the other hand, the architecture of biofilms may limit phage diffusion. Biofilms with dense cell clusters established by tight cell–cell binding can limit the access of the phage to the entire community. Dormant cells within the biofilm are less susceptible to phages, as phage replication requires active bacterial metabolism [304,305]. Furthermore, biofilms can generate a state of hypermutability that stimulates the occurrence of phage resistance. Indeed, the emergence of phage-resistant populations among bacteria after phage therapy has been reported [251,306]. Overall, although lytic phages have bactericidal activities, only some hold some promise in the treatment biofilm infections (Table 1). For example, phage EFDG1 showed success in eliminating biofilms in vitro and preventing infection by *E. faecalis* and *E. faecium* [240], and bacteriophage vB_EfaH_EF1TV was recently shown to kill clinical *E. faecalis* strains and disrupt their biofilms [241]. Yet, to overcome phage-therapy limitations, different strategies are currently followed including combination with antimicrobials, phage cocktails, and genetically manipulated phages (Table 1). Examples of the latter include phages producing biofilm degrading enzymes such as dispersin B [307] or inhibiting enzymes or enzymes that that contribute to antibiotic penetration such as OmpF porin to enhance antibiotic penetration [308].

Essential oils extracted from plants comprise complex mixtures of volatile substances, including terpenes, terpenoids, and phenols, among others. Some of these compounds possess antimicrobial activity as they constitute part of the immune defense mechanism of plants against infectious agents. Several studies reported the antibiofilm activity of some essential oils against bacteria (Table 1). Many of them damage the bacterial membranes leading to the release of cytoplasm, although their mechanism of action is not uniquely caused by this route. Other essential oils also regulate the expression of genes involved in biofilm formation and biofilm dispersal. For example, essential oils from thyme, cinnamon, and clove exhibited a high antibiofilm activity against many bacteria, including ESKAPE bacteria [257]. Cinnamon oil was earlier proven to inhibit the production of rhamnolipids, proteases, and alginate as well as swarming motility in *P. aeruginosa* [256], which is consistent with inhibition of QS. Another essential oil, tea tree oil (TTO), has shown antibacterial and antibiofilm activity. TTO eradicates *S. aureus* biofilms by affecting the expression of 304 genes participating in many metabolic routes [260] and regulators such as SarA. The global regulator SarA positively controls expression of genes involved in biofilm formation. Additionally, the expression of *cidA* that encodes a murein-hydrolase regulator was downregulated whereas the expression of the *lgrA* and *B* operons, which inhibit autolysis, was upregulated. Together, this reduces the release of eDNA, which is a key component of the *S. aureus* ECM. Other studies have investigated the synergistic action of essential oils or their active principles with other antimicrobial molecules such as synthetic antimicrobial polymers (Table 1). Thus, these and other studies demonstrate that essential oils have a repertoire of killing activities and that they are promising as treatments against biofilms. Yet, their extraction is one of the most effort-requiring and time-consuming processes, which increases the costs of their application.

4.3. Alternative Methods

Physical methods hold promise for eradication and inhibition of biofilms. This is particularly important on surfaces such as chronic wounds [309,310], infected prosthetics, implants, and medical devices. Good examples of these methods include nanoparticles, sonication, irradiation (ultraviolet, visible, or infrared light), or biomaterials. Indeed, blue light, for example, was effective against biofilms formed by *A. baumannii*, *P. aeruginosa*, and *N. gonorrhoeae* although less so against biofilms of *E. coli* and *E. faecalis* [311]. In vivo studies in mouse burns showed that blue-light exposure could drastically reduce bacterial load and effectively protect mice from lethal infection with *P. aeruginosa* [312]. Blue light presumably exerts its effect on bacterial cells by exciting porphyrins which then generate ROS, as suggested by the resistance to blue light exhibited by a *P. aeruginosa* mutant defective in porphyrin biosynthetis [313]. Additionally, ultraviolet C light has been shown to efficiently eradicate *Pseudomonas* biofilms on precontaminated catheter-like tubes [314]. In general, irradiation has only an effect on superficial epidermal layers or the surface of materials because of poor accessibility of deeper tissues. On the other hand, nanoparticles, prepared from diverse materials, including both organic and inorganic materials, have a broad spectrum of antibacterial and antibiofilm activities, e.g., by disrupting bacterial membranes, interacting with proteins or DNA, or promoting the production of ROS [315]. Alternatively, different materials with topographic patterning have been developed to prevent biofilm formation. As the nature, hydrophobicity, and topology of the materials are relevant for substrate–bacteria interactions, these characteristics are conveniently modified in biomedical polymeric surfaces to generate catheters, implants, or devices with reduced bacteria-binding capacity [316,317]. Their effectivity is enhanced in combination with other antibacterial strategies, e.g., the use of nitric oxide-releasing materials, which, together, showed high synergic activity in the inhibition of bacterial growth and biofilm formation of *S. epidermidis* [318]. To summarize, compared with conventional antimicrobial agents, physical methods exhibit a broad-spectrum effectiveness under ambient conditions, are easy to operate at low cost, and low maintenance. Important disadvantages are long exposition times, and their application is mostly restricted to surfaces. Another interesting strategy for controlling biofilms is the use of probiotics, e.g., live microorganisms with demonstrated health benefits that inhibit pathogenic biofilms. Probiotics have been considered for human therapeutic applications, and even bacterial strains have been genetically modified to kill pathogenic strains and inhibit biofilm production. Probably the best example is the *E. coli* strain Nissle 1917 that has been extensively used for treatment of intestinal disorders [319]. This strain inhibits biofilm formation of pathogenic and nonpathogenic *E. coli*, *S. aureus*, and *S. epidermidis* [320]. In an attempt to improve its therapeutic potential, the strain was genetically modified to synthesize an antibiofilm enzyme, dispersin B, in response to the detection of autoinducers secreted by *P. aeruginosa*. The recombinant strain was active against *P. aeruginosa* gut infection in animal models [321].

5. Concluding Remarks

The capacity of microorganisms to evolve and adapt to environmental cues has led to a health crisis as they became resistant to most, or almost all, commercial antibiotics. Biofilm formation is an ancient form of bacterial adaptation that contributes substantially to the problem because of their recalcitrance to treatment. Indeed, biofilms are the origin of significant morbidity and mortality. As discussed here, biofilm recalcitrance integrates many mechanisms, including metabolic heterogeneity, stress responses, efflux pump regulation, entrapment and inactivation of antibiotics in the ECM, interbacterial communication, increased mutability, and exchange of genetic material. Many of these factors have been discovered particularly in strains of *P. aeruginosa*. However, the specificity and multifaceted nature of the described mechanisms indicate the necessity of studying them also in other bacteria. Even more challenging, but necessary, will be to study biofilms in natural infections, where heterogeneous bacterial populations are common, and many environmental factors, including host defenses or diffusion of antibiotics in tissues, are present.

The understanding of the mechanisms that mediate recalcitrance will definitely guide therapeutic strategies to successfully deal with biofilm infections. These should be accompanied with methodologies for rapid diagnosis of biofilm infections and characterization of the biofilm biology and composition in vivo. Additionally, the availability of a panel of substances to inhibit and disperse biofilms will contribute to the selection of adequate therapeutic strategies to deal with particular biofilm infections.

Author Contributions: Conceptualization, J.A.; Methodology, C.U., G.C.-E., J.T., R.C.M.-J., J.A. Writing—Original draft preparation, C.U., G.C.-E., R.C.M.-J., J.A.; Writing—Review and editing, R.C.M.-J., J.T., J.A.; Visualization, C.U., G.C.-E.; Supervision, J.A. All authors have read and agreed to the published version of the manuscript.

Funding: This research received no external funding.

Acknowledgments: We wish to thank Bridier Arnaud (Fougères Laboratory, ANSES, France) and Romain Briandet (Université Paris-Saclay, France) for kindly providing a high-resolution figure about the architecture of MDR biofilms.

Conflicts of Interest: The authors declare no conflict of interest.

References

1. O'Neill, J. Tackling Drug-Resistant Infections Globally: Final Report and Recommendations; the Review on Antimicrobial Resistance. 2016. Available online: https://amr-review.org/sites/default/files/160525_Final%20paper_with%20cover.pdf (accessed on 5 August 2020).
2. WHO (World Health Organization). High Levels of Antibiotic Resistance Found Worldwide, New Data Shows. 2018. Available online: https://www.who.int/news-room/detail/29-01-2018-high-levels-of-antibiotic-resistance-found-worldwide-new-data-shows (accessed on 8 August 2020).
3. EFSA (European Food Safety Authority); ECDC (European Centre for Disease Prevention and Control). The European Union summary report on antimicrobial resistance in zoonotic and indicator bacteria from humans, animals and food in 2017/2018. *EFSA J.* **2020**, *18*, e06007. [CrossRef]
4. Collignon, P. Fluoroquinolone use in food animals. *Emerg. Infect. Dis.* **2005**, *11*, 1789–1790. [CrossRef]
5. Landers, T.F.; Cohen, B.; Wittum, T.E.; Larson, E.L. A review of antibiotic use in food animals: Perspective, policy, and potential. *Public Health Rep.* **2012**, *127*, 4–22. [CrossRef] [PubMed]

6. Lebeaux, D.; Ghigo, J.; Beloin, C. Biofilm-related infections: Bridging the gap between clinical management and fundamental aspects of recalcitrance toward antibiotics. *Microbiol. Mol. Biol. Rev.* **2014**, *78*, 510–543. [CrossRef] [PubMed]
7. Ceri, H.; Olson, M.E.; Stremick, C.; Read, R.R.; Morck, D.; Buret, A. The calgary biofilm device: New technology for rapid determination of antibiotic susceptibilities of bacterial biofilms. *J. Clin. Microbiol.* **1999**, *37*, 1771–1776. [CrossRef] [PubMed]
8. Yassien, M.; Khardori, N.; Ahmedy, A.; Toama, M. Modulation of biofilms of *Pseudomonas aeruginosa* by quinolones. *Antimicrob. Agents Chemother.* **1995**, *39*, 2262–2268. [CrossRef] [PubMed]
9. Morck, D.W.; Lam, K.; McKay, S.G.; Olson, M.E.; Prosser, B.; Ellis, B.D.; Cleeland, R.; Costerton, J.W. Comparative evaluation of fleroxacin, ampicillin, trimethoprimsulfamethoxazole, and gentamicin as treatments of catheter-associated urinary tract infection in a rabbit model. *Int. J. Antimicrob. Agents* **1994**, *4*, S21–S27. [CrossRef]
10. Olsen, I. Biofilm-specific antibiotic tolerance and resistance. *Eur. J. Clin. Microbiol. Infect. Dis.* **2015**, *34*, 877–886. [CrossRef]
11. Davies, D. Understanding biofilm resistance to antibacterial agents. *Nat. Rev. Drug Discov.* **2003**, *2*, 114–122. [CrossRef]
12. Jamal, M.; Ahmad, W.; Andleeb, S.; Jalil, F.; Imran, M.; Nawaz, M.A.; Hussain, T.; Ali, M.; Rafiq, M.; Kamil, M.A. Bacterial biofilm and associated infections. *J. Chin. Med. Assoc.* **2018**, *81*, 7–11. [CrossRef]
13. Maurice, N.M.; Bedi, B.; Sadikot, R.T. *Pseudomonas aeruginosa* biofilms: Host response and clinical implications in lung infections. *Am. J. Resp. Cell Mol.* **2018**, *58*, 428–439. [CrossRef] [PubMed]
14. Longo, F.; Vuotto, C.; Donelli, G. Biofilm formation in *Acinetobacter baumannii*. *New Microbiol.* **2014**, *37*, 119–127. [PubMed]
15. Olivares, E.; Badel-Berchoux, S.; Provot, C.; Prévost, G.; Bernardi, T.; Jehl, F. Clinical impact of antibiotics for the treatment of *Pseudomonas aeruginosa* biofilm infections. *Front. Microbiol.* **2020**, *10*, 2894. [CrossRef] [PubMed]
16. Stickler, D.J. Bacterial biofilms in patients with indwelling urinary catheters. *Nat. Clin. Pract. Urol.* **2008**, *5*, 598–608. [CrossRef]
17. Donlan, R.M.; Costerton, J.W. Biofilms: Survival mechanisms of clinically relevant microorganisms. *Clin. Microbiol. Rev.* **2002**, *15*, 167–193. [CrossRef]
18. Falsetta, M.L.; Steichen, C.T.; McEwan, A.G.; Cho, C.; Ketterer, M.; Shao, J.; Hunt, J.; Jennings, M.P.; Apicella, M.A. The composition and metabolic phenotype of *Neisseria gonorrhoeae* biofilms. *Front. Microbiol.* **2011**, *2*, 75. [CrossRef]
19. WHO (World Health Organization). Global Priority List of Antibiotic-Resistant Bacteria to Guide Research, Discovery, and Development of New Antibiotics. 2017. Available online: https://www.who.int/medicines/publications/WHO-PPL-Short_Summary_25Feb-ET_NM_WHO.pdf (accessed on 5 August 2020).
20. López, D.; Vlamakis, H.; Kolter, R. Biofilms. *CSH Perspect. Biol.* **2010**, *2*, a000398. [CrossRef]
21. Davies, D.G.; Parsek, M.R.; Pearson, J.P.; Iglewski, B.H.; Costerton, J.W.; Greenberg, E.P. The involvement of cell-to-cell signals in the development of a bacterial biofilm. *Science* **1998**, *280*, 295–298. [CrossRef]
22. Prigent-Combaret, C.; Prensier, G.; Le Thi, T.T.; Vidal, O.; Lejeune, P.; Dorel, C. Developmental pathway for biofilm formation in curli-producing *Escherichia coli* strains: Role of flagella, curli and colanic acid. *Environ. Microbiol.* **2000**, *2*, 450–464. [CrossRef]
23. Tormo, M.A.; Knecht, E.; Götz, F.; Lasa, I.; Penades, J.R. Bap-dependent biofilm formation by pathogenic species of *Staphylococcus*: Evidence of horizontal gene transfer? *Microbiology* **2005**, *151*, 2465–2475. [CrossRef]
24. Borlee, B.R.; Goldman, A.D.; Murakami, K.; Samudrala, R.; Wozniak, D.J.; Parsek, M.R. *Pseudomonas aeruginosa* uses a cyclic-di-GMP-regulated adhesin to reinforce the biofilm extracellular matrix. *Mol. Microbiol.* **2010**, *75*, 827–842. [CrossRef] [PubMed]
25. Grijpstra, J.; Arenas, J.; Rutten, L.; Tommassen, J. Autotransporter secretion: Varying on a theme. *Res. Microbiol.* **2013**, *164*, 562–582. [CrossRef] [PubMed]
26. O'Toole, G.A.; Kolter, R. Flagellar and twitching motility are necessary for *Pseudomonas aeruginosa* biofilm development. *Mol. Microbiol.* **1998**, *30*, 295–304. [CrossRef] [PubMed]
27. Tommassen, J.; Arenas, J. Biological functions of the secretome of *Neisseria meningitidis*. *Front. Cell. Infect. Microbiol.* **2017**, *7*, 256. [CrossRef]
28. Muñoz-Egea, M.C.; García-Pedrazuela, M.; Mahillo-Fernandez, I.; Esteban, J. Effect of antibiotics and antibiofilm agents in the ultrastructure and development of biofilms developed by non pigmented rapidly growing *Mycobacteria*. *Microb. Drug Resist.* **2016**, *22*, 1–6. [CrossRef]
29. Flemming, H.C.; Wingender, J. The biofilm matrix. *Nat. Rev. Microbiol.* **2010**, *8*, 623–633. [CrossRef]
30. Das, T.; Sharma, P.K.; Busscher, H.J.; van der Mei, H.C. Role of extracellular DNA in initial bacterial adhesion and surface aggregation. *Appl. Environ. Microbiol.* **2010**, *76*, 3405–3408. [CrossRef]
31. Das, T.; Sharma, P.K.; Krom, B.P.; van der Mei, H.C.; Busscher, H.J. Role of eDNA on the adhesion forces between *Streptococcus mutans* and substratum surfaces: Influence of ionic strength and substratum hydrophobicity. *Langmuir* **2011**, *27*, 10113–10118. [CrossRef]
32. Qin, Z.; Ou, Y.; Yang, L.; Zhu, Y.; Tolker-Nielsen, T.; Molin, S.; Qu, D. Role of autolysin-mediated DNA release in biofilm formation of *Staphylococcus epidermidis*. *Microbiology* **2007**, *153*, 2083–2092. [CrossRef]
33. Arenas, J.; Nijland, R.; Rodriguez, F.J.; Bosma, T.N.; Tommassen, J. Involvement of three meningococcal surface-exposed proteins, the heparin-binding protein NhbA, the α-peptide of IgA protease and the autotransporter protease NalP, in initiation of biofilm formation. *Mol. Microbiol.* **2013**, *87*, 254–268. [CrossRef]
34. Whitchurch, C.B.; Tolker-Nielsen, T.; Ragas, P.C.; Mattick, J.S. Extracellular DNA required for bacterial biofilm formation. *Science* **2002**, *295*, 1487. [CrossRef] [PubMed]
35. Arenas, J.; Tommassen, J. Meningococcal biofilm formation: Let's stick together. *Trends Microbiol.* **2017**, *25*, 113–124. [CrossRef] [PubMed]

36. Castillo Pedraza, M.C.; Novais, T.F.; Faustoferri, R.C.; Quivey, R.G., Jr.; Terekhov, A.; Hamaker, B.R.; Klein, M.I. Extracellular DNA and lipoteichoic acids interact with exopolysaccharides in the extracellular matrix of *Streptococcus mutans* biofilms. *Biofouling* **2017**, *33*, 722–740. [CrossRef] [PubMed]
37. Wang, X.; Preston, J.F.; Romeo, T. The *pgaABCD* locus of *Escherichia coli* promotes the synthesis of a polysaccharide adhesin required for biofilm formation. *J. Bacteriol.* **2004**, *186*, 2724–2734. [CrossRef] [PubMed]
38. Izano, E.A.; Amarante, M.A.; Kher, W.B.; Kaplan, J.B. Differential roles of poly-*N*-acetylglucosamine surface polysaccharide and extracellular DNA in *Staphylococcus aureus* and *Staphylococcus epidermidis* biofilms. *Appl. Environ. Microbiol.* **2008**, *74*, 470–476. [CrossRef]
39. Da Re, S.; Ghigo, J.M. A CsgD-independent pathway for cellulose production and biofilm formation in *Escherichia coli*. *J. Bacteriol.* **2006**, *188*, 3073–3087. [CrossRef] [PubMed]
40. Solano, C.; García, B.; Valle, J.; Berasain, C.; Ghigo, J.M.; Gamazo, C.; Lasa, I. Genetic analysis of *Salmonella enteritidis* biofilm formation: Critical role of cellulose. *Mol. Microbiol.* **2002**, *43*, 793–808. [CrossRef]
41. Ude, S.; Arnold, D.L.; Moon, C.D.; Timms-Wilson, T.; Spiers, A.J. Biofilm formation and cellulose expression among diverse environmental *Pseudomonas* isolates. *Environ. Microbiol.* **2006**, *8*, 1997–2011. [CrossRef]
42. Stevenson, G.; Andrianopoulos, K.; Hobbs, M.; Reeves, P.R. Organization of the *Escherichia coli* K-12 gene cluster responsible for production of the extracellular polysaccharide colanic acid. *J. Bacteriol.* **1996**, *178*, 4885–4893. [CrossRef]
43. Lam, J.; Chan, R.; Lam, K.; Costerton, J.W. Production of mucoid microcolonies by *Pseudomonas aeruginosa* within infected lungs in cystic fibrosis. *Infect. Immun.* **1980**, *28*, 546–556.
44. Hentzer, M.; Teitzel, G.M.; Balzer, G.J.; Heydorn, A.; Molin, S.; Givskov, M.; Parsek, M.R. Alginate overproduction affects *Pseudomonas aeruginosa* biofilm structure and function. *J. Bacteriol.* **2001**, *183*, 5395–5401. [CrossRef] [PubMed]
45. Pulcrano, G.; Iula, D.V.; Raia, V.; Rossano, F.; Catania, M.R. Different mutations in *mucA* gene of *Pseudomonas aeruginosa* mucoid strains in cystic fibrosis patients and their effect on *algU* gene expression. *New Microbiol.* **2012**, *35*, 295–305. [PubMed]
46. Jennings, L.K.; Storek, K.M.; Ledvina, H.E.; Coulon, C.; Marmont, L.S.; Sadovskaya, I.; Secor, P.R.; Tseng, B.S.; Scian, M.; Filloux, A.; et al. Pel is a cationic exopolysaccharide that cross-links extracellular DNA in the *Pseudomonas aeruginosa* biofilm matrix. *Proc. Natl. Acad. Sci. USA* **2015**, *112*, 11353–11358. [CrossRef] [PubMed]
47. Byrd, M.S.; Sadovskaya, I.; Vinogradov, E.; Lu, H.; Sprinkle, A.B.; Richardson, S.H.; Ma, L.; Ralston, B.; Parsek, M.R.; Anderson, E.M.; et al. Genetic and biochemical analyses of the *Pseudomonas aeruginosa* Psl exopolysaccharide reveal overlapping roles for polysaccharide synthesis enzymes in Psl and LPS production. *Mol. Microbiol.* **2009**, *73*, 622–638. [CrossRef] [PubMed]
48. Ma, L.; Jackson, K.D.; Landry, R.M.; Parsek, M.R.; Wozniak, D.J. Analysis of *Pseudomonas aeruginosa* conditional Psl variants reveals roles for the Psl polysaccharide in adhesion and maintaining biofilm structure post attachment. *J. Bacteriol.* **2006**, *188*, 8213–8221. [CrossRef] [PubMed]
49. Lequette, Y.; Rollet, E.; Delangle, A.; Greenberg, E.P.; Bohin, J.P. Linear osmoregulated periplasmic glucans are encoded by the *opgGH* locus of *Pseudomonas aeruginosa*. *Microbiology* **2007**, *153*, 3255–3263. [CrossRef] [PubMed]
50. Coulon, C.; Vinogradov, E.; Filloux, A.; Sadovskaya, I. Chemical analysis of cellular and extracellular carbohydrates of a biofilm-forming strain *Pseudomonas aeruginosa* PA14. *PLoS ONE* **2010**, *5*, e14220. [CrossRef]
51. Bridier, A.; Dubois-Brissonnet, F.; Boubetra, A.; Thomas, V.; Briandet, R. The biofilm architecture of sixty opportunistic pathogens deciphered using a high throughput CLSM method. *J. Microbiol. Meth.* **2010**, *82*, 64–70. [CrossRef]
52. Arenas, J.; Cano, S.; Nijland, R.; van Dongen, V.; Rutten, L.; van der Ende, A.; Tommassen, J. The meningococcal autotransporter AutA is implicated in autoaggregation and biofilm formation. *Environ. Microbiol.* **2014**, *17*, 1321–1337. [CrossRef]
53. Arenas, J.; Paganelli, F.L.; Rodríguez-Castaño, P.; Cano-Crespo, S.; van der Ende, A.; van Putten, J.P.; Tommassen, J. Expression of the gene for autotransporter AutB of *Neisseria meningitidis* affects biofilm formation and epithelial transmigration. *Front. Cell. Infect. Microbiol.* **2016**, *6*, 162. [CrossRef]
54. Stewart, P.S.; Peyton, B.M.; Drury, W.J.; Murga, R. Quantitative observations of heterogeneities in *Pseudomonas aeruginosa* biofilms. *Appl. Environ. Microbiol.* **1993**, *59*, 327–329. [CrossRef] [PubMed]
55. Brauner, A.; Fridman, O.; Gefen, O.; Balaban, N.Q. Distinguishing between resistance, tolerance and persistence to antibiotic treatment. *Nat. Rev. Microbiol.* **2016**, *14*, 320–330. [CrossRef] [PubMed]
56. Zgurskaya, H.I.; Weeks, J.W.; Ntreh, A.T.; Nickels, L.M.; Wolloscheck, D. Mechanism of coupling drug transport reactions located in two different membranes. *Front. Microbiol.* **2015**, *6*, 100. [CrossRef] [PubMed]
57. Arzanlou, M.; Chai, W.C.; Venter, H. Intrinsic, adaptive and acquired antimicrobial resistance in Gram-negative bacteria. *Essays Biochem.* **2017**, *61*, 49–59. [CrossRef] [PubMed]
58. Hernando-Amado, S.; Sanz-Garcia, F.; Blanco, P.; Martinez, J.L. Fitness costs associated with the acquisition of antibiotic resistance. *Essays Biochem.* **2017**, *61*, 37–48. [CrossRef] [PubMed]
59. Fernández, L.; Breidenstein, E.B.; Hancock, R.E. Creeping baselines and adaptive resistance to antibiotics. *Drug Resist. Update* **2011**, *14*, 1–21. [CrossRef]
60. El-Halfawy, O.M.; Valvano, M.A. Antimicrobial heteroresistance: An emerging field in need of clarity. *Clin. Microbiol. Rev.* **2015**, *28*, 191–207. [CrossRef]
61. Andersson, D.I.; Nicoloff, H.; Hjort, K. Mechanisms and clinical relevance of bacterial heteroresistance. *Nat. Rev. Microbiol.* **2019**, *17*, 479–496. [CrossRef]

62. Band, V.I.; Crispell, E.K.; Napier, B.A.; Herrera, C.M.; Tharp, G.K.; Vavikolanu, K.; Pohl, J.; Read, T.D.; Bosinger, S.E.; Trent, M.S.; et al. Antibiotic failure mediated by a resistant subpopulation in *Enterobacter cloacae*. *Nat. Microbiol.* **2016**, *1*, 1–9. [CrossRef]
63. Hall, C.W.; Mah, T.F. Molecular mechanisms of biofilm-based antibiotic resistance and tolerance in pathogenic bacteria. *FEMS Microbiol. Rev.* **2017**, *41*, 276–301. [CrossRef]
64. Balaban, N.Q.; Helaine, S.; Lewis, K.; Ackermann, M.; Aldridge, B.; Andersson, D.I.; Brynildsen, M.P.; Bumann, D.; Camilli, A.; Collins, J.J.; et al. Definitions and guidelines for research on antibiotic persistence. *Nat. Rev. Microbiol.* **2019**, *17*, 441–448. [CrossRef] [PubMed]
65. Lewis, K. Persister cellules, la dormance et les maladies infectieuses. *Nat. Rev. Microbiol.* **2007**, *5*, 48–56. [CrossRef] [PubMed]
66. Wilmaerts, D.; Windels, E.M.; Verstraeten, N.; Michiels, J. General mechanisms leading to persister formation and awakening. *Trends Genet.* **2019**, *35*, 401–411. [CrossRef] [PubMed]
67. De Beer, D.; Stoodley, P.; Lewandowski, Z. Liquid flow in heterogeneous biofilms. *Biotechnol. Bioeng.* **1994**, *44*, 636–641. [CrossRef] [PubMed]
68. Stewart, P.S. Diffusion in biofilms. *J. Bacteriol.* **2003**, *185*, 1485–1491. [CrossRef] [PubMed]
69. Sadovskaya, I.; Vinogradov, E.; Li, J.; Hachani, A.; Kowalska, K.; Filloux, A. High-level antibiotic resistance in *Pseudomonas aeruginosa* biofilm: The *ndvB* gene is involved in the production of highly glycerol-phosphorylated β-(1-3)-glucans, which bind aminoglycosides. *Glycobiology* **2010**, *20*, 895–904. [CrossRef] [PubMed]
70. Colvin, K.M.; Gordon, V.D.; Murakami, K.; Borlee, B.R.; Wozniak, D.J.; Wong, G.C.; Parsek, M.R. The Pel polysaccharide can serve a structural and protective role in the biofilm matrix of *Pseudomonas aeruginosa*. *PLoS Pathog.* **2011**, *7*, e1001264. [CrossRef]
71. Wang, S.; Liu, X.; Liu, H.; Zhang, L.; Guo, Y.; Yu, S.; Wozniak, D.J.; Ma, L.Z. The exopolysaccharide Psl–eDNA interaction enables the formation of a biofilm skeleton in *Pseudomonas aeruginosa*. *Environ. Microbiol. Rep.* **2015**, *7*, 330–340. [CrossRef]
72. Billings, N.; Millan, M.R.; Caldara, M.; Rusconi, R.; Tarasova, Y.; Stocker, R.; Ribbeck, K. The extracellular matrix component Psl provides fast-acting antibiotic defense in *Pseudomonas aeruginosa* biofilms. *PLoS Pathog.* **2013**, *9*, e1003526. [CrossRef]
73. Mulcahy, H.; Charron-Mazenod, L.; Lewenza, S. Extracellular DNA chelates cations and induces antibiotic resistance in *Pseudomonas aeruginosa* biofilms. *PLoS Pathog.* **2008**, *4*, e1000213. [CrossRef]
74. Wilton, M.; Charron-Mazenod, L.; Moore, R.; Lewenza, S. Extracellular DNA acidifies biofilms and induces aminoglycoside resistance in *Pseudomonas aeruginosa*. *Antimicrob. Agents Chemother.* **2016**, *60*, 544–553. [CrossRef] [PubMed]
75. Doroshenko, N.; Tseng, B.S.; Howlin, R.P.; Deacon, J.; Wharton, J.A.; Thurner, P.J.; Gilmore, B.F.; Parsek, M.R.; Stoodley, P. Extracellular DNA impedes the transport of vancomycin in *Staphylococcus epidermidis* biofilms preexposed to subinhibitory concentrations of vancomycin. *Antimicrob. Agents Chemother.* **2014**, *58*, 7273–7282. [CrossRef] [PubMed]
76. Johnson, L.; Horsman, S.R.; Charron-Mazenod, L.; Turnbull, A.L.; Mulcahy, H.; Surette, M.G.; Lewenza, S. Extracellular DNA-induced antimicrobial peptide resistance in *Salmonella enterica* serovar Typhimurium. *BMC Microbiol.* **2013**, *13*, 115. [CrossRef] [PubMed]
77. Davis, B.D. Mechanism of bactericidal action of aminoglycosides. *Microbiol. Rev.* **1987**, *51*, 341–350. [CrossRef]
78. Taber, H.W.; Mueller, J.P.; Miller, P.F.; Arrow, A.S. Bacterial uptake of aminoglycoside antibiotics. *Microbiol. Rev.* **1987**, *51*, 439–457. [CrossRef] [PubMed]
79. Ramirez, M.S.; Tolmasky, M.E. Aminoglycoside modifying enzymes. *Drug Resist. Updat.* **2010**, *13*, 151–171. [CrossRef] [PubMed]
80. Hancock, R.E. Alterations in outer membrane permeability. *Annu. Rev. Microbiol.* **1984**, *38*, 237–264. [CrossRef] [PubMed]
81. Perez, A.C.; Pang, B.; King, L.B.; Tan, L.; Murrah, K.A.; Reimche, J.L.; Wren, J.T.; Richardson, S.H.; Ghandi, U.; Swords, W.E. Residence of *Streptococcus pneumoniae* and *Moraxella catarrhalis* within polymicrobial biofilm promotes antibiotic resistance and bacterial persistence in vivo. *Pathog. Dis.* **2014**, *70*, 280–288. [CrossRef]
82. Armbruster, C.E.; Hong, W.; Pang, B.; Weimer, K.E.; Juneau, R.A.; Turner, J.; Swords, W.E. Indirect pathogenicity of *Haemophilus influenzae* and *Moraxella catarrhalis* in polymicrobial otitis media occurs via interspecies quorum signaling. *mBio* **2010**, *1*, e00102-10. [CrossRef]
83. Flemming, H.C.; Wingender, J.; Szewzyk, U.; Steinberg, P.; Rice, S.A.; Kjelleberg, S. Biofilms: An emergent form of bacterial life. *Nat. Rev. Microbiol.* **2016**, *14*, 563–575. [CrossRef]
84. Stewart, P.S.; Franklin, M.J. Physiological heterogeneity in biofilms. *Nat. Rev. Microbiol.* **2008**, *6*, 199–210. [CrossRef] [PubMed]
85. Borriello, G.; Richards, L.; Ehrlich, G.D.; Stewart, P.S. Arginine or nitrate enhances antibiotic susceptibility of *Pseudomonas aeruginosa* in biofilms. *Antimicrob. Agents Chemother.* **2006**, *50*, 382–384. [CrossRef] [PubMed]
86. Haagensen, J.A.; Klausen, M.; Ernst, R.K.; Miller, S.I.; Folkesson, A.; Tolker-Nielsen, T.; Molin, S. Differentiation and distribution of colistin-and sodium dodecyl sulfate-tolerant cells in *Pseudomonas aeruginosa* biofilms. *J. Bacteriol.* **2007**, *189*, 28–37. [CrossRef] [PubMed]
87. Kushwaha, G.S.; Oyeyemi, B.F.; Bhavesh, N.S. Stringent response protein as a potential target to intervene persistent bacterial infection. *Biochimie* **2019**, *165*, 67–75. [CrossRef] [PubMed]
88. Kusser, W.; Ishiguro, E.E. Suppression of mutations conferring penicillin tolerance by interference with the stringent control mechanism of *Escherichia coli*. *J. Bacteriol.* **1987**, *169*, 4396–4398. [CrossRef] [PubMed]
89. Tuomanen, E.; Tomasz, A. Induction of autolysis in nongrowing *Escherichia coli*. *J. Bacteriol.* **1986**, *167*, 1077–1080. [CrossRef]
90. Wu, N.; He, L.; Cui, P.; Wang, W.; Yuan, Y.; Liu, S.; Xu, T.; Zhang, S.; Wu, J.; Zhang, W.; et al. Ranking of persister genes in the same *Escherichia coli* genetic background demonstrates varying importance of individual persister genes in tolerance to different antibiotics. *Front. Microbiol.* **2015**, *6*, 1003. [CrossRef]

91. Bernier, S.P.; Lebeaux, D.; DeFrancesco, A.S.; Valomon, A.; Soubigou, G.; Coppée, J.Y.; Ghigo, J.M.; Beloin, C. Starvation, together with the SOS response, mediates high biofilm-specific tolerance to the fluoroquinolone ofloxacin. *PLoS Genet.* **2013**, *9*, e1003144. [CrossRef]
92. Nguyen, D.; Joshi-Datar, A.; Lepine, F.; Bauerle, E.; Olakanmi, O.; Beer, K.; McKay, G.; Siehnel, R.; Schafhauser, J.; Wang, Y.; et al Active starvation responses mediate antibiotic tolerance in biofilms and nutrient-limited bacteria. *Science* **2011**, *334*, 982–986. [CrossRef]
93. Khakimova, M.; Ahlgren, H.G.; Harrison, J.J.; English, A.M.; Nguyen, D. The stringent response controls catalases in *Pseudomonas aeruginosa* and is required for hydrogen peroxide and antibiotic tolerance. *J. Bacteriol.* **2013**, *195*, 2011–2020. [CrossRef]
94. Martins, D.; McKay, G.; Sampathkumar, G.; Khakimova, M.; English, A.M.; Nguyen, D. Superoxide dismutase activity confers (p) ppGpp-mediated antibiotic tolerance to stationary-phase *Pseudomonas aeruginosa*. *Proc. Natl. Acad. Sci. USA* **2018**, *115*, 9797–9802. [CrossRef] [PubMed]
95. Viducic, D.; Ono, T.; Murakami, K.; Susilowati, H.; Kayama, S.; Hirota, K.; Miyake, Y. Functional analysis of *spoT*, *relA* and *dksA* genes on quinolone tolerance in *Pseudomonas aeruginosa* under nongrowing condition. *Microbiol. Immunol.* **2006**, *50*, 349–357. [CrossRef] [PubMed]
96. Geiger, T.; Kästle, B.; Gratani, F.L.; Goerke, C.; Wolz, C. Two small (p) ppGpp synthases in *Staphylococcus aureus* mediate tolerance against cell envelope stress conditions. *J. Bacteriol.* **2014**, *196*, 894–902. [CrossRef] [PubMed]
97. Maslowska, K.H.; Makiela-Dzbenska, K.; Fijalkowska, I.J. The SOS system: A complex and tightly regulated response to DNA damage. *Environ. Mol. Mutagen.* **2019**, *60*, 368–384. [CrossRef]
98. Dörr, T.; Lewis, K.; Vulić, M. SOS response induces persistence to fluoroquinolones in *Escherichia coli*. *PLoS Genet.* **2009**, *5*, e1000760. [CrossRef]
99. Baharoglu, Z.; Mazel, D. SOS, the formidable strategy of bacteria against aggressions. *FEMS Microbiol. Rev.* **2014**, *38*, 1126–1145. [CrossRef]
100. Gerdes, K.; Maisonneuve, E. Bacterial persistence and toxin-antitoxin loci. *Annu. Rev. Microbiol.* **2012**, *66*, 103–123. [CrossRef]
101. Keren, I.; Shah, D.; Spoering, A.; Kaldalu, N.; Lewis, K. Specialized persister cells and the mechanism of multidrug tolerance in *Escherichia coli*. *J. Bacteriol.* **2004**, *186*, 8172–8180. [CrossRef]
102. Shah, D.; Zhang, Z.; Khodursky, A.; Kaldalu, N.; Kurg, K.; Lewis, K. Persisters: A distinct physiological state of *E. coli*. *BMC Microbiol.* **2006**, *6*, 53. [CrossRef]
103. González Barrios, A.F.; Zuo, R.; Hashimoto, Y.; Yang, L.; Bentley, W.E.; Wood, T.K. Autoinducer 2 controls biofilm formation in *Escherichia coli* through a novel motility quorum-sensing regulator (MqsR, B3022). *J. Bacteriol.* **2006**, *188*, 305–316. [CrossRef]
104. Wang, X.; Wood, T.K. Toxin-antitoxin systems influence biofilm and persister cell formation and the general stress response. *Appl. Environ. Microbiol.* **2011**, *77*, 5577–5583. [CrossRef] [PubMed]
105. Fraikin, N.; Rousseau, C.J.; Goeders, N.; Van Melderen, L. Reassessing the role of the type II MqsRA toxin-antitoxin system in stress response and biofilm formation: *mqsA* is transcriptionally uncoupled from *mqsR*. *mBio* **2019**, *10*, e02678-19. [CrossRef] [PubMed]
106. Engelberg-Kulka, H.; Amitai, S.; Kolodkin-Gal, I.; Hazan, R. Bacterial programmed cell death and multicellular behavior in bacteria. *PLoS Genet.* **2006**, *2*, e135. [CrossRef] [PubMed]
107. Wozniak, R.A.F.; Waldor, M.K. A toxin–antitoxin system promotes the maintenance of an integrative conjugative element. *PLoS Genet.* **2009**, *5*, e1000439. [CrossRef] [PubMed]
108. Soucy, S.M.; Huang, J.; Gogarten, J.P. Horizontal gene transfer: Building the web of life. *Nat. Rev. Genet.* **2015**, *16*, 472–482. [CrossRef] [PubMed]
109. Deng, Y.; Bao, X.; Ji, L.; Chen, L.; Liu, J.; Miao, J.; Chen, D.; Bian, H.; Li, Y.; Yu, G. Resistance integrons: Class 1, 2 and 3 integrons. *Ann. Clin. Microbiol. Antimicrob.* **2015**, *14*, 45. [CrossRef] [PubMed]
110. Gillings, M.R. Integrons: Past, present, and future. *Microbiol. Mol. Biol. Rev.* **2014**, *78*, 257–277. [CrossRef]
111. Strugeon, E.; Tilloy, V.; Ploy, M.C.; Da Re, S. The stringent response promotes antibiotic resistance dissemination by regulating integron integrase expression in biofilms. *mBio* **2016**, *7*, e00868-16. [CrossRef]
112. Borriello, G.; Werner, E.; Roe, F.; Kim, A.M.; Ehrlich, G.D.; Stewart, P.S. Oxygen limitation contributes to antibiotic tolerance of *Pseudomonas aeruginosa* in biofilms. *Antimicrob. Agents Chemother.* **2004**, *48*, 2659–2664. [CrossRef]
113. James, G.A.; Ge Zhao, A.; Usui, M.; Underwood, R.A.; Nguyen, H.; Beyenal, H.; DeLancey, E.; Hunt, A.A.; Bernstein, H.C.; Fleckman, P.; et al. Microsensor and transcriptomic signatures of oxygen depletion in biofilms associated with chronic wounds. *Wound Repair Regen.* **2016**, *24*, 373–383. [CrossRef]
114. Kiamco, M.M.; Atci, E.; Mohamed, A.; Call, D.R.; Beyenal, H. Hyperosmotic agents and antibiotics affect dissolved oxygen and pH concentration gradients in *Staphylococcus aureus* biofilms. *Appl. Environ. Microbiol.* **2017**, *83*, e02783-16. [CrossRef] [PubMed]
115. Rivera, K.R.; Pozdin, V.A.; Young, A.T.; Erb, P.D.; Wisniewski, N.A.; Magness, S.T.; Daniele, M. Integrated phosphorescence-based photonic biosensor (iPOB) for monitoring oxygen levels in 3D cell culture systems. *Biosens. Bioelectron.* **2019**, *123*, 131–140. [CrossRef] [PubMed]
116. Kolpen, M.; Kühl, M.; Bjarnsholt, T.; Moser, C.; Hansen, C.R.; Liengaard, L.; Kharazmi, A.; Pressler, T.; Høiby, N.; Jensen, P.Ø. Nitrous oxide production in sputum from cystic fibrosis patients with chronic *Pseudomonas aeruginosa* lung infection. *PLoS ONE* **2014**, *9*, e84353. [CrossRef] [PubMed]

117. Tack, K.J.; Sabath, L.D. Increased minimum inhibitory concentrations with anaerobiasis for tobramycin, gentamicin, and amikacin, compared to latamoxef, piperacillin, chloramphenicol, and clindamycin. *Chemotherapy* **1985**, *31*, 204–210. [CrossRef] [PubMed]
118. Stewart, P.S.; Franklin, M.J.; Williamson, K.S.; Folsom, J.P.; Boegli, L.; James, G.A. Contribution of stress responses to antibiotic tolerance in *Pseudomonas aeruginosa* biofilms. *Antimicrob. Agents Chemother.* **2015**, *59*, 3838–3847. [CrossRef] [PubMed]
119. Dwyer, D.J.; Collins, J.J.; Walker, G.C. Unraveling the physiological complexities of antibiotic lethality. *Annu. Rev. Pharmacol. Toxicol.* **2015**, *55*, 313–332. [CrossRef] [PubMed]
120. Kohanski, M.A.; Dwyer, D.J.; Hayete, B.; Lawrence, C.A.; Collins, J.J. A common mechanism of cellular death induced by bactericidal antibiotics. *Cell* **2007**, *130*, 797–810. [CrossRef]
121. Imlay, J.A. The molecular mechanisms and physiological consequences of oxidative stress: Lessons from a model bacterium. *Nat. Rev. Microbiol.* **2013**, *11*, 443–454. [CrossRef]
122. Jensen, P.Ø.; Briales, A.; Brochmann, R.P.; Wang, H.; Kragh, K.N.; Kolpen, M.; Hempel, C.; Bjarnsholt, T.; Høiby, N.; Ciofu, O. Formation of hydroxyl radicals contributes to the bactericidal activity of ciprofloxacin against *Pseudomonas aeruginosa* biofilms. *Pathog. Dis.* **2014**, *70*, 440–443. [CrossRef]
123. Du, D.; Wang-Kan, X.; Neuberger, A.; van Veen, H.W.; Pos, K.M.; Piddock, L.J.; Luisi, B.F. Multidrug efflux pumps: Structure, function and regulation. *Nat. Rev. Microbiol.* **2018**, *16*, 523–539. [CrossRef]
124. Du, D.; van Veen, H.W.; Murakami, S.; Pos, K.M.; Luisi, B.F. Structure, mechanism and cooperation of bacterial multidrug transporters. *Curr. Opin. Struc. Biol.* **2015**, *33*, 76–91. [CrossRef] [PubMed]
125. Kuroda, T.; Tsuchiya, T. Multidrug efflux transporters in the MATE family. *Biochim. Biophys. Acta* **2009**, *1794*, 763–768. [CrossRef] [PubMed]
126. Morita, Y.; Kodama, K.; Shiota, S.; Mine, T.; Kataoka, A.; Mizushima, T.; Tsuchiya, T. NorM, a putative multidrug efflux protein, of *Vibrio parahaemolyticus* and its homolog in *Escherichia coli*. *Antimicrob. Agents Chemother.* **1998**, *42*, 1778–1782. [CrossRef] [PubMed]
127. He, G.X.; Kuroda, T.; Mima, T.; Morita, Y.; Mizushima, T.; Tsuchiya, T. An H^+-coupled multidrug efflux pump, PmpM, a member of the MATE family of transporters, from *Pseudomonas aeruginosa*. *J. Bacteriol.* **2004**, *186*, 262–265. [CrossRef] [PubMed]
128. Su, X.Z.; Chen, J.; Mizushima, T.; Kuroda, T.; Tsuchiya, T. AbeM, an H^+-coupled *Acinetobacter baumannii* multidrug efflux pump belonging to the MATE family of transporters. *Antimicrob. Agents Chemother.* **2005**, *49*, 4362–4364. [CrossRef] [PubMed]
129. Saleh, M.; Bay, D.C.; Turner, R.J. Few Conserved amino acids in the small multidrug resistance transporter EmrE influence drug polyselectivity. *Antimicrob. Agents Chemother.* **2018**, *62*, e00461-18. [CrossRef] [PubMed]
130. Paulsen, I.T.; Brown, M.H.; Dunstan, S.J.; Skurray, R.A. Molecular characterization of the staphylococcal multidrug resistance export protein QacC. *J. Bacteriol.* **1995**, *177*, 2827–2833. [CrossRef] [PubMed]
131. Mousa, J.J.; Bruner, S.D. Structural and mechanistic diversity of multidrug transporters. *Nat. Prod. Rep.* **2016**, *33*, 1255–1267. [CrossRef]
132. Schindler, B.D.; Kaatz, G.W. Multidrug efflux pumps of Gram-positive bacteria. *Drug Resist. Updat.* **2016**, *27*, 1–13. [CrossRef]
133. Costa, S.S.; Viveiros, M.; Amaral, L.; Couto, I. Multidrug efflux pumps in *Staphylococcus aureus*: An update. *Open Microbiol. J.* **2013**, *7*, 59–71. [CrossRef]
134. Kobayashi, N.; Nishino, K.; Yamaguchi, A. Novel macrolide-specific ABC-type efflux transporter in *Escherichia coli*. *J. Bacteriol.* **2001**, *183*, 5639–5644. [CrossRef] [PubMed]
135. Hassan, K.A.; Liu, Q.; Henderson, P.J.; Paulsen, I.T. Homologs of the *Acinetobacter baumannii* AceI transporter represent a new family of bacterial multidrug efflux systems. *mBio* **2015**, *6*, e01982-14. [CrossRef] [PubMed]
136. Shi, X.; Chen, M.; Yu, Z.; Bell, J.M.; Wang, H.; Forrester, I.; Villareal, H.; Jakana, J.; Du, D.; Luisi, B.F.; et al. In situ structure and assembly of the multidrug efflux pump AcrAB-TolC. *Nat. Commun.* **2019**, *10*, 2635. [CrossRef]
137. Tsutsumi, K.; Yonehara, R.; Ishizaka-Ikeda, E.; Miyazaki, N.; Maeda, S.; Iwasaki, K.; Nakagawa, A.; Yamashita, E. Structures of the wild-type MexAB-OprM tripartite pump reveal its complex formation and drug efflux mechanism. *Nat. Commun.* **2019**, *10*, 1520. [CrossRef] [PubMed]
138. Wieczorek, P.; Sacha, P.; Hauschild, T.; Zórawski, M.; Krawczyk, M.; Tryniszewska, E. Multidrug resistant *Acinetobacter baumannii*—the role of AdeABC (RND family) efflux pump in resistance to antibiotics. *Folia Histochem. Cytobiol.* **2008**, *46*, 257–267. [CrossRef] [PubMed]
139. Zhang, Y.; Xiao, M.; Horiyama, T.; Zhang, Y.; Li, X.; Nishino, K.; Yan, A. The multidrug efflux pump MdtEF protects against nitrosative damage during the anaerobic respiration in *Escherichia coli*. *J. Biol. Chem.* **2011**, *286*, 26576–26584. [CrossRef] [PubMed]
140. Zou, Y.; Woo, J.; Ahn, J. Cellular and molecular responses of *Salmonella* Typhimurium to antimicrobial-induced stresses during the planktonic-to-biofilm transition. *Lett. Appl. Microbiol.* **2012**, *55*, 274–282. [CrossRef] [PubMed]
141. Kvist, M.; Hancock, V.; Klemm, P. Inactivation of efflux pumps abolishes bacterial biofilm formation. *Appl. Environ. Microbiol.* **2008**, *74*, 7376–7382. [CrossRef]
142. Ikonomidis, A.; Tsakris, A.; Kanellopoulou, M.; Maniatis, A.N.; Pournaras, S. Effect of the proton motive force inhibitor carbonyl cyanide-m-chlorophenylhydrazone (CCCP) on *Pseudomonas aeruginosa* biofilm development. *Lett. Appl. Microbiol.* **2008**, *47*, 298–302. [CrossRef]
143. Baugh, S.; Phillips, C.R.; Ekanayaka, A.S.; Piddock, L.J.; Webber, M.A. Inhibition of multidrug efflux as a strategy to prevent biofilm formation. *J. Antimicrob. Chemother.* **2014**, *69*, 673–681. [CrossRef]
144. Gillis, R.J.; White, K.G.; Choi, K.H.; Wagner, V.E.; Schweizer, H.P.; Iglewski, B.H. Molecular basis of azithromycin-resistant *Pseudomonas aeruginosa* biofilms. *Antimicrob. Agents Chemother.* **2005**, *49*, 3858–3867. [CrossRef] [PubMed]

145. Pamp, S.J.; Gjermansen, M.; Johansen, H.K.; Tolker-Nielsen, T. Tolerance to the antimicrobial peptide colistin in *Pseudomonas aeruginosa* biofilms is linked to metabolically active cells, and depends on the *pmr* and *mexAB-oprM* genes. *Mol. Microbiol.* **2008**, *68*, 223–240. [CrossRef] [PubMed]
146. Zhang, L.; Mah, T.F. Involvement of a novel efflux system in biofilm-specific resistance to antibiotics. *J. Bacteriol.* **2008**, *190*, 4447–4452. [CrossRef] [PubMed]
147. Bay, D.C.; Stremick, C.A.; Slipski, C.J.; Turner, R.J. Secondary multidrug efflux pump mutants alter *Escherichia coli* biofilm growth in the presence of cationic antimicrobial compounds. *Res. Microbiol.* **2017**, *168*, 208–221. [CrossRef] [PubMed]
148. Masi, M.; Winterhalter, M.; Pagès, J.M. Outer membrane porins. *Subcell. Biochem.* **2019**, *92*, 79–123. [CrossRef] [PubMed]
149. Davin-Regli, A.; Bolla, J.M.; James, C.E.; Lavigne, J.P.; Chevalier, J.; Garnotel, E.; Molitor, A. Membrane permeability and regulation of drug "influx and efflux" in enterobacterial pathogens. *Curr. Drug Targets* **2008**, *9*, 750–759. [CrossRef]
150. Van Boxtel, R.; Wattel, A.A.; Arenas, J.; Goessens, W.H.; Tommassen, J. Acquisition of carbapenem resistance by plasmid-encoded-AmpC-expressing *Escherichia coli*. *Antimicrob. Agents Chemother.* **2016**, *61*, e01413-16. [CrossRef]
151. Gaddy, J.A.; Tomaras, A.P.; Actis, L.A. The *Acinetobacter baumannii* 19606 OmpA protein plays a role in biofilm formation on abiotic surfaces and in the interaction of this pathogen with eukaryotic cells. *Infect. Immun.* **2009**, *77*, 3150–3160. [CrossRef]
152. Vuotto, C.; Longo, F.; Pascolini, C.; Donelli, G.; Balice, M.P.; Libori, M.F.; Tiracchia, V.; Salvia, A.; Varaldo, P.E. Biofilm formation and antibiotic resistance in *Klebsiella pneumoniae* urinary strains. *J. Appl. Microbiol.* **2017**, *123*, 1003–1018. [CrossRef]
153. Edgar, R.; Bibi, E. MdfA, an *Escherichia coli* multidrug resistance protein with an extraordinarily broad spectrum of drug recognition. *J. Bacteriol.* **1997**, *179*, 2274–2280. [CrossRef]
154. Bohn, C.; Bouloc, P. The *Escherichia coli cmlA* gene encodes the multidrug efflux pump Cmr/MdfA and is responsible for isopropyl-beta-D-thiogalactopyranoside exclusion and spectinomycin sensitivity. *J. Bacteriol.* **1998**, *180*, 6072–6075. [CrossRef] [PubMed]
155. Li, X.Z.; Plésiat, P.; Nikaido, H. The challenge of efflux-mediated antibiotic resistance in Gram-negative bacteria. *Clin. Microbiol. Rev.* **2015**, *28*, 337–418. [CrossRef] [PubMed]
156. Ma, D.; Alberti, M.; Lynch, C.; Nikaido, H.; Hearst, J.E. The local repressor AcrR plays a modulating role in the regulation of *acrAB* genes of *Escherichia coli* by global stress signals. *Mol. Microbiol.* **1996**, *19*, 101–112. [CrossRef] [PubMed]
157. Hirakawa, H.; Takumi-Kobayashi, A.; Theisen, U.; Hirata, T.; Nishino, K.; Yamaguchi, A. AcrS/EnvR represses expression of the *acrAB* multidrug efflux genes in *Escherichia coli*. *J. Bacteriol.* **2008**, *190*, 6276–6279. [CrossRef] [PubMed]
158. Nishino, K.; Yamaguchi, A. Role of histone-like protein H-NS in multidrug resistance of *Escherichia coli*. *J. Bacteriol.* **2004**, *186*, 1423–1429. [CrossRef] [PubMed]
159. Eguchi, Y.; Oshima, T.; Mori, H.; Aono, R.; Yamamoto, K.; Ishihama, A.; Utsumi, R. Transcriptional regulation of drug efflux genes by EvgAS, a two-component system in *Escherichia coli*. *Microbiology* **2003**, *149*, 2819–2828. [CrossRef] [PubMed]
160. Rahmati, S.; Yang, S.; Davidson, A.L.; Zechiedrich, E.L. Control of the AcrAB multidrug efflux pump by quorum-sensing regulator SdiA. *Mol. Microbiol.* **2002**, *43*, 677–685. [CrossRef] [PubMed]
161. Kettles, R.A.; Tschowri, N.; Lyons, K.J.; Sharma, P.; Hengge, R.; Webber, M.A.; Grainger, D.C. The *Escherichia coli* MarA protein regulates the ycgZ-ymgABC operon to inhibit biofilm formation. *Mol. Microbiol.* **2019**, *112*, 1609–1625. [CrossRef]
162. Heacock-Kang, Y.; Sun, Z.; Zarzycki-Siek, J.; Poonsuk, K.; McMillan, I.A.; Chuanchuen, R.; Hoang, T.T. Two regulators, PA3898 and PA2100, modulate the *Pseudomonas aeruginosa* multidrug resistance MexAB-OprM and EmrAB efflux pumps and biofilm formation. *Antimicrob. Agents Chemother.* **2018**, *62*, e01459-18. [CrossRef]
163. Di Cagno, R.; De Angelis, M.; Calasso, M.; Gobbetti, M. Proteomics of the bacterial cross-talk by quorum sensing. *J. Proteomics.* **2011**, *74*, 19–34. [CrossRef]
164. Arevalo-Ferro, C.; Hentzer, M.; Reil, G.; Görg, A.; Kjelleberg, S.; Givskov, M.; Riedel, K.; Eberl, L. Identification of quorum-sensing regulated proteins in the opportunistic pathogen *Pseudomonas aeruginosa* by proteomics. *Environ. Microbiol.* **2003**, *5*, 1350–1369. [CrossRef] [PubMed]
165. Bjarnsholt, T.; Jensen, P.Ø.; Burmølle, M.; Hentzer, M.; Haagensen, J.A.; Hougen, H.P.; Calum, H.; Madsen, K.F.; Moser, C.; Molin, S.; et al. *Pseudomonas aeruginosa* tolerance to tobramycin, hydrogen peroxide and polymorphonuclear leukocytes is quorum-sensing dependent. *Microbiology* **2005**, *151*, 373–383. [CrossRef] [PubMed]
166. Popat, R.; Crusz, S.A.; Messina, M.; Williams, P.; West, S.A.; Diggle, S.P. Quorum-sensing and cheating in bacterial biofilms. *Proc. Biol. Sci.* **2012**, *279*, 4765–4771. [CrossRef] [PubMed]
167. Yarwood, J.M.; Bartels, D.J.; Volper, E.M.; Greenberg, E.P. Quorum sensing in *Staphylococcus aureus* biofilms. *J. Bacteriol.* **2004**, *186*, 1838–1850. [CrossRef] [PubMed]
168. Dale, J.L.; Cagnazzo, J.; Phan, C.Q.; Barnes, A.M.; Dunny, G.M. Multiple roles for *Enterococcus faecalis* glycosyltransferases in biofilm-associated antibiotic resistance, cell envelope integrity, and conjugative transfer. *Antimicrob. Agents Chemother.* **2015**, *59*, 4094–4105. [CrossRef] [PubMed]
169. Hazan, R.; Que, Y.A.; Maura, D.; Strobel, B.; Majcherczyk, P.A.; Hopper, L.R.; Wilbur, D.J.; Hreha, T.N.; Barquera, B.; Rahme, L.G. Auto poisoning of the respiratory chain by a quorum-sensing-regulated molecule favors biofilm formation and antibiotic tolerance. *Curr. Biol.* **2016**, *26*, 195–206. [CrossRef]
170. Hoffman, L.R.; Déziel, E.; d'Argenio, D.A.; Lépine, F.; Emerson, J.; McNamara, S.; Gibson, R.L.; Ramsey, B.W.; Miller, S.I. Selection for *Staphylococcus aureus* small-colony variants due to growth in the presence of *Pseudomonas aeruginosa*. *Proc. Natl. Acad. Sci. USA* **2006**, *103*, 19890–19895. [CrossRef]

171. Orazi, G.; O'Toole, G.A. *Pseudomonas aeruginosa* alters *Staphylococcus aureus* sensitivity to vancomycin in a biofilm model of cystic fibrosis infection. *mBio* **2017**, *8*, e00873-17. [CrossRef]
172. Ryan, R.P.; Fouhy, Y.; Garcia, B.F.; Watt, S.A.; Niehaus, K.; Yang, L.; Tolker-Nielsen, T.; Dow, J.M. Interspecies signalling via the *Stenotrophomonas maltophilia* diffusible signal factor influences biofilm formation and polymyxin tolerance in *Pseudomonas aeruginosa*. *Mol. Microbiol.* **2008**, *68*, 75–86. [CrossRef]
173. Guérin, J.; Bigot, S.; Schneider, R.; Buchanan, S.K.; Jacob-Dubuisson, F. Two-partner secretion: Combining efficiency and simplicity in the secretion of large proteins for bacteria-host and bacteria-bacteria interactions. *Front. Cell. Infect. Microbiol.* **2017**, *7*, 148. [CrossRef]
174. Pérez, A.; Merino, M.; Rumbo-Feal, S.; Álvarez-Fraga, L.; Vallejo, J.A.; Beceiro, A.; Ohneck, E.J.; Mateos, J.; Fernández-Puente, P.; Actis, L.A.; et al. The FhaB/FhaC two-partner secretion system is involved in adhesion of *Acinetobacter baumannii* AbH12O-A2 strain. *Virulence* **2017**, *8*, 959–974. [CrossRef] [PubMed]
175. Neil, R.B.; Apicella, M.A. Role of HrpA in biofilm formation of *Neisseria meningitidis* and regulation of the *hrpBAS* transcripts. *Infect. Immun.* **2009**, *77*, 2285–2293. [CrossRef] [PubMed]
176. Aoki, S.K.; Diner, E.J.; de Roodenbeke, C.T.K.; Burgess, B.R.; Poole, S.J.; Braaten, B.A.; Jones, A.M.; Webb, J.S.; Hayes, C.S.; Cotter, P.A.; et al. A widespread family of polymorphic contact-dependent toxin delivery systems in bacteria. *Nature* **2010**, *468*, 439–442. [CrossRef] [PubMed]
177. Arenas, J.; Schipper, K.; van Ulsen, P.; van der Ende, A.; Tommassen, J. Domain exchange at the 3′end of the gene encoding the fratricide meningococcal two-partner secretion protein A. *BMC Genet.* **2013**, *14*, 622. [CrossRef] [PubMed]
178. Garcia, E.C.; Perault, A.I.; Marlatt, S.A.; Cotter, P.A. Interbacterial signaling via *Burkholderia* contact-dependent growth inhibition system proteins. *Proc. Natl. Acad. Sci. USA* **2016**, *113*, 8296–8301. [CrossRef] [PubMed]
179. Ghosh, A.; Baltekin, Ö.; Wäneskog, M.; Elkhalifa, D.; Hammarlöf, D.L.; Elf, J.; Koskiniemi, S. Contact-dependent growth inhibition induces high levels of antibiotic-tolerant persister cells in clonal bacterial populations. *EMBO J.* **2018**, *37*, e98026. [CrossRef] [PubMed]
180. Arenas, J.; de Maat, V.; Catón, L.; Krekorian, M.; Herrero, J.C.; Ferrara, F.; Tommassen, J. Fratricide activity of MafB protein of *N. meningitidis* strain B16B6. *BMC Microbiol.* **2015**, *15*, 156. [CrossRef] [PubMed]
181. Arenas, J.; Catón, L.; van den Houven, T.; de Maat, V.; Cruz herrero, J.; Tommassen, J. The outer-membrane protein MafA of *Neisseria meningitidis* constitutes a novel protein secretion pathway specific for the fratricide protein MafB. *Virulence* **2020**, *11*, 1701–1715. [CrossRef]
182. Hausner, M.; Wuertz, S. High rates of conjugation in bacterial biofilms as determined by quantitative in situ analysis. *Appl. Environ. Microbiol.* **1999**, *65*, 3710–3713. [CrossRef]
183. Molin, S.; Tolker-Nielsen, T. Gene transfer occurs with enhanced efficiency in biofilms and induces enhanced stabilisation of the biofilm structure. *Cur. Opin. Biotechnol.* **2003**, *14*, 255–261. [CrossRef]
184. Hathroubi, S.; Mekni, M.A.; Domenico, P.; Nguyen, D.; Jacques, M. Biofilms: Microbial shelters against antibiotics. *Microb. Drug Resist.* **2017**, *23*, 147–156. [CrossRef] [PubMed]
185. Savage, V.J.; Chopra, I.; O'Neill, A.J. *Staphylococcus aureus* biofilms promote horizontal transfer of antibiotic resistance. *Antimicrob. Agents Chemother.* **2013**, *57*, 1968–1970. [CrossRef] [PubMed]
186. Tanner, W.D.; Atkinson, R.M.; Goel, R.K.; Toleman, M.A.; Benson, L.S.; Porucznik, C.A.; VanDerslice, J.A. Horizontal transfer of the bla_{NDM-1} gene to *Pseudomonas aeruginosa* and *Acinetobacter baumannii* in biofilms. *FEMS Microbiol. Lett.* **2017**, *364*, fnx048. [CrossRef] [PubMed]
187. Dubey, G.P.; Ben-Yehuda, S. Intercellular nanotubes mediate bacterial communication. *Cell* **2011**, *144*, 590–600. [CrossRef] [PubMed]
188. Pande, S.; Shitut, S.; Freund, L.; Westermann, M.; Bertels, F.; Colesie, C.; Bischofs, I.B.; Kost, C. Metabolic cross-feeding via intercellular nanotubes among bacteria. *Nat. Commun.* **2015**, *6*, 1–13. [CrossRef]
189. Kouzel, N.; Oldewurtel, E.R.; Maier, B. Gene transfer efficiency in gonococcal biofilms: Role of biofilm age, architecture, and pilin antigenic variation. *J. Bacteriol.* **2015**, *197*, 2422–2431. [CrossRef]
190. Hannan, S.; Ready, D.; Jasni, A.S.; Rogers, M.; Pratten, J.; Roberts, A.P. Transfer of antibiotic resistance by transformation with eDNA within oral biofilms. *FEMS Immunol. Med. Microbiol.* **2010**, *59*, 345–349. [CrossRef]
191. Solheim, H.T.; Sekse, C.; Urdahl, A.M.; Wasteson, Y.; Nesse, L.L. Biofilm as an environment for dissemination of *stx* genes by transduction. *Appl. Environ. Microbiol.* **2013**, *79*, 896–900. [CrossRef]
192. Rumbo, C.; Fernández-Moreira, E.; Merino, M.; Poza, M.; Mendez, J.A.; Soares, N.C.; Mosquera, A.; Chaves, F.; Bou, G. Horizontal transfer of the OXA-24 carbapenemase gene via outer membrane vesicles: A new mechanism of dissemination of carbapenem resistance genes in *Acinetobacter baumannii*. *Antimicrob. Agents Chemother.* **2011**, *55*, 3084–3090. [CrossRef]
193. Woodford, N.; Ellington, M.J. The emergence of antibiotic resistance by mutation. *Clin. Microbiol. Infect.* **2007**, *13*, 5–18. [CrossRef]
194. Schroeder, J.W.; Yeesin, P.; Simmons, L.A.; Wang, J.D. Sources of spontaneous mutagenesis in bacteria. *Crit. Rev. Biochem. Mol. Biol.* **2018**, *53*, 29–48. [CrossRef] [PubMed]
195. Van Acker, H.; Coenye, T. The role of reactive oxygen species in antibiotic-mediated killing of bacteria. *Trends Microbiol.* **2017**, *25*, 456–466. [CrossRef] [PubMed]
196. Leong, P.M.; Hsia, H.C.; Miller, J.H. Analysis of spontaneous base substitutions generated in mismatch-repair-deficient strains of *Escherichia coli*. *J. Bacteriol.* **1986**, *168*, 412–416. [CrossRef] [PubMed]

197. Schaaper, R.M.; Dunn, R.L. Spectra of spontaneous mutations in *Escherichia coli* strains defective in mismatch correction: The nature of in vivo DNA replication errors. *Proc. Natl. Acad. Sci. USA* **1987**, *84*, 6220–6224. [CrossRef] [PubMed]
198. Eliopoulos, G.M.; Blázquez, J. Hypermutation as a factor contributing to the acquisition of antimicrobial resistance. *Clin. Infect. Dis.* **2003**, *37*, 1201–1209. [CrossRef] [PubMed]
199. Maciá, M.D.; Blanquer, D.; Togores, B.; Sauleda, J.; Pérez, J.L.; Oliver, A. Hypermutation is a key factor in development of multiple-antimicrobial resistance in *Pseudomonas aeruginosa* strains causing chronic lung infections. *Antimicrob. Agents Chemother.* **2005**, *49*, 3382–3386. [CrossRef]
200. Driffield, K.; Miller, K.; Bostock, J.M.; O'Neill, A.J.; Chopra, I. Increased mutability of *Pseudomonas aeruginosa* in biofilms. *J. Antimicrob. Chemother.* **2008**, *61*, 1053–1056. [CrossRef]
201. Prunier, A.L.; Malbruny, B.; Laurans, M.; Brouard, J.; Duhamel, J.F.; Leclercq, R. High rate of macrolide resistance in *Staphylococcus aureus* strains from patients with cystic fibrosis reveals high proportions of hypermutable strains. *J. Infect. Dis.* **2003**, *187*, 1709–1716. [CrossRef]
202. Román, F.; Cantón, R.; Pérez-Vázquez, M.; Baquero, F.; Campos, J. Dynamics of long-term colonization of respiratory tract by *Haemophilus influenzae* in cystic fibrosis patients shows a marked increase in hypermutable strains. *J. Clin. Microbiol.* **2004**, *42*, 1450–1459. [CrossRef]
203. Kovacs, B.; Le Gall-David, S.; Vincent, P.; Le Bars, H.; Buffet-Bataillon, S.; Bonnaure-Mallet, M.; Jolivet-Gougeon, A. Is biofilm formation related to the hypermutator phenotype in clinical *Enterobacteriaceae* isolates? *FEMS Microbiol. Lett.* **2013**, *347*, 116–122. [CrossRef]
204. Ninio, J. Transient mutators: A semiquantitative analysis of the influence of translation and transcription errors on mutation rates. *Genetics* **1991**, *129*, 957–962. [PubMed]
205. Springer, B.; Kidan, Y.G.; Prammananan, T.; Ellrott, K.; Böttger, E.C.; Sander, P. Mechanisms of streptomycin resistance: Selection of mutations in the 16S rRNA gene conferring resistance. *Antimicrob. Agents Chemother.* **2001**, *45*, 2877–2884. [CrossRef] [PubMed]
206. Guénard, S.; Muller, C.; Monlezun, L.; Benas, P.; Broutin, I.; Jeannot, K.; Plésiat, P. Multiple mutations lead to MexXY-OprM-dependent aminoglycoside resistance in clinical strains of *Pseudomonas aeruginosa*. *Antimicrob. Agents Chemother.* **2014**, *58*, 221–228. [CrossRef] [PubMed]
207. Moskowitz, S.M.; Ernst, R.K.; Miller, S.I. PmrAB, a two-component regulatory system of *Pseudomonas aeruginosa* that modulates resistance to cationic antimicrobial peptides and addition of aminoarabinose to lipid A. *J. Bacteriol.* **2004**, *186*, 575–579. [CrossRef] [PubMed]
208. Paltansing, S.; Kraakman, M.; van Boxtel, R.; Kors, I.; Wessels, E.; Goessens, W.; Tommassen, J.; Bernards, A. Increased expression levels of chromosomal AmpC β-lactamase in clinical *Escherichia coli* isolates and their effect on susceptibility to extended-spectrum cephalosporins. *Microb. Drug Resist.* **2015**, *21*, 7–16. [CrossRef] [PubMed]
209. Walther-Rasmussen, J.; Høiby, N. Class A carbapenemases. *J. Antimicrob. Chemother.* **2007**, *60*, 470–482. [CrossRef] [PubMed]
210. Ghafourian, S.; Sadeghifard, N.; Soheili, S.; Sekawi, Z. Extended spectrum beta-lactamases: Definition, classification and epidemiology. *Curr. Issues Mol. Biol.* **2015**, *17*, 11–21. [CrossRef]
211. Hentzer, M.; Riedel, K.; Rasmussen, T.B.; Heydorn, A.; Andersen, J.B.; Parsek, M.R.; Rice, S.A.; Eberl, L.; Molin, S.; Høiby, N.; et al. Inhibition of quorum sensing in *Pseudomonas aeruginosa* biofilm bacteria by a halogenated furanone compound. *Microbiology* **2002**, *148*, 87–102. [CrossRef]
212. Manefield, M.; Rasmussen, T.B.; Henzter, M.; Andersen, J.B.; Steinberg, P.; Kjelleberg, S.; Givskov, M. Halogenated furanones inhibit quorum sensing through accelerated LuxR turnover. *Microbiology* **2002**, *148*, 1119–1127. [CrossRef]
213. Lee, J.H.; Park, J.H.; Cho, H.S.; Joo, S.W.; Cho, M.H.; Lee, J. Anti-biofilm activities of quercetin and tannic acid against *Staphylococcus aureus*. *Biofouling* **2013**, *29*, 491–499. [CrossRef]
214. Manner, S.; Skogman, M.; Goeres, D.; Vuorela, P.; Fallarero, A. Systematic exploration of natural and synthetic flavonoids for the inhibition of *Staphylococcus aureus* biofilms. *Int. J. Mol. Sci.* **2013**, *14*, 19434–19451. [CrossRef] [PubMed]
215. Rémy, B.; Mion, S.; Plener, L.; Elias, M.; Chabrière, E.; Daudé, D. Interference in bacterial quorum sensing: A biopharmaceutical perspective. *Front. Pharmacol.* **2018**, *9*, 203. [CrossRef] [PubMed]
216. Kalia, V.C.; Patel, S.K.; Kang, Y.C.; Lee, J.K. Quorum sensing inhibitors as antipathogens: Biotechnological applications. *Biotechnol. Adv.* **2019**, *37*, 68–90. [CrossRef] [PubMed]
217. Andresen, L.; Tenson, T.; Hauryliuk, V. Cationic bactericidal peptide 1018 does not specifically target the stringent response alarmone (p) ppGpp. *Sci. Rep.* **2016**, *6*, 1–6. [CrossRef] [PubMed]
218. De la Fuente-Núñez, C.; Reffuveille, F.; Haney, E.F.; Straus, S.K.; Hancock, R.E. Broad-spectrum anti-biofilm peptide that targets a cellular stress response. *PLoS Pathog.* **2014**, *10*, e1004152. [CrossRef]
219. Reffuveille, F.; de la Fuente-Núñz, C.; Mansour, S.; Hancock, R.E. A broad-spectrum antibiofilm peptide enhances antibiotic action against bacterial biofilms. *Antimicrob. Agents Chemother.* **2014**, *58*, 5363–5371. [CrossRef] [PubMed]
220. Adil, M.; Singh, K.; Verma, P.K.; Khan, A.U. Eugenol-induced suppression of biofilm-forming genes in *Streptococcus mutans*: An approach to inhibit biofilms. *J. Glob. Antimicrob. Resist.* **2014**, *2*, 286–292. [CrossRef]
221. Gopal, R.; Lee, J.H.; Kim, Y.G.; Kim, M.S.; Seo, C.H.; Park, Y. Anti-microbial, anti-biofilm activities and cell selectivity of the NRC-16 peptide derived from witch flounder, *Glyptocephalus cynoglossus*. *Mar. Drugs* **2013**, *11*, 1836–1852. [CrossRef]
222. Dosler, S.; Karaaslan, E.; Alev Gerceker, A. Antibacterial and anti-biofilm activities of melittin and colistin, alone and in combination with antibiotics against Gram-negative bacteria. *J. Chemother.* **2016**, *28*, 95–103. [CrossRef]

223. Picoli, T.; Peter, C.M.; Zani, J.L.; Waller, S.B.; Lopes, M.G.; Boesche, K.N.; Vargas, G.D.; Hübner, S.O.; Fischer, G. Melittin and its potential in the destruction and inhibition of the biofilm formation by *Staphylococcus aureus*, *Escherichia coli* and *Pseudomonas aeruginosa* isolated from bovine milk. *Microb. Pathog.* **2017**, *112*, 57–62. [CrossRef]
224. Bardbari, A.M.; Arabestani, M.R.; Karami, M.; Keramat, F.; Aghazadeh, H.; Alikhani, M.Y.; Bagheri, K.P. Highly synergistic activity of melittin with imipenem and colistin in biofilm inhibition against multidrug-resistant strong biofilm producer strains of *Acinetobacter baumannii*. *Eur. J. Clin. Microbiol.* **2018**, *37*, 443–454. [CrossRef] [PubMed]
225. Yuan, Y.; Zai, Y.; Xi, X.; Ma, C.; Wang, L.; Zhou, M.; Shaw, C.; Chen, T. A novel membrane-disruptive antimicrobial peptide from frog skin secretion against cystic fibrosis isolates and evaluation of anti-MRSA effect using *Galleria mellonella* model. *Biochim. Biophys. Acta* **2019**, *1863*, 849–856. [CrossRef] [PubMed]
226. Yüksel, E.; Karakeçili, A. Antibacterial activity on electrospun poly (lactide-co-glycolide) based membranes via magainin II grafting. *Mater. Sci. Eng. C* **2014**, *45*, 510–518. [CrossRef] [PubMed]
227. Kim, M.K.; Kang, N.H.; Ko, S.J.; Park, J.; Park, E.; Shin, D.W.; Kim, S.H.; Lee, S.A.; Lee, J.I.; Lee, S.H.; et al. Antibacterial and antibiofilm activity and mode of action of magainin 2 against drug-resistant *Acinetobacter baumannii*. *Int. J. Mol. Sci.* **2018**, *19*, 3041. [CrossRef] [PubMed]
228. Shtreimer Kandiyote, N.; Mohanraj, G.; Mao, C.; Kasher, R.; Arnusch, C.J. Synergy on surfaces: Anti-biofouling interfaces using surface-attached antimicrobial peptides PGLa and magainin-2. *Langmuir* **2018**, *34*, 11147–11155. [CrossRef] [PubMed]
229. Overhage, J.; Campisano, A.; Bains, M.; Torfs, E.C.; Rehm, B.H.; Hancock, R.E. Human host defense peptide LL-37 prevents bacterial biofilm formation. *Infect. Immun.* **2008**, *76*, 4176–4182. [CrossRef]
230. Feng, X.; Sambanthamoorthy, K.; Palys, T.; Paranavitana, C. The human antimicrobial peptide LL-37 and its fragments possess both antimicrobial and antibiofilm activities against multidrug-resistant *Acinetobacter baumannii*. *Peptides* **2013**, *49*, 131–137. [CrossRef]
231. Kang, J.; Dietz, M.J.; Li, B. Antimicrobial peptide LL-37 is bactericidal against *Staphylococcus aureus* biofilms. *PLoS ONE* **2019**, *14*, e0216676. [CrossRef]
232. Maisetta, G.; Grassi, L.; Di Luca, M.; Bombardelli, S.; Medici, C.; Brancatisano, F.L.; Esin, S.; Batoni, G. Anti-biofilm properties of the antimicrobial peptide temporin 1Tb and its ability, in combination with EDTA, to eradicate *Staphylococcus epidermidis* biofilms on silicone catheters. *Biofouling* **2016**, *32*, 787–800. [CrossRef]
233. Grassi, L.; Maisetta, G.; Maccari, G.; Esin, S.; Batoni, G. Analogs of the frog-skin antimicrobial peptide temporin 1Tb exhibit a wider spectrum of activity and a stronger antibiofilm potential as compared to the parental peptide. *Front. Chem.* **2017**, *5*, 24. [CrossRef]
234. Luca, V.; Stringaro, A.; Colone, M.; Pini, A.; Mangoni, M.L. Esculentin(1-21), an amphibian skin membrane-active peptide with potent activity on both planktonic and biofilm cells of the bacterial pathogen *Pseudomonas aeruginosa*. *Cell. Mol. Life Sci.* **2013**, *70*, 2773–2786. [CrossRef] [PubMed]
235. Beljantseva, J.; Kudrin, P.; Jimmy, S.; Ehn, M.; Pohl, R.; Varik, V.; Tozawa, Y.; Shingler, V.; Tenson, T.; Rejman, D.; et al. Molecular mutagenesis of ppGpp: Turning a RelA activator into an inhibitor. *Sci. Rep.* **2017**, *7*, 1–10. [CrossRef] [PubMed]
236. Eckert, R.; Brady, K.M.; Greenberg, E.P.; Qi, F.; Yarbrough, D.K.; He, J.; McHardy, I.; Anderson, M.H.; Shi, W. Enhancement of antimicrobial activity against *Pseudomonas aeruginosa* by coadministration of G10KHc and tobramycin. *Antimicrob. Agents Chemother.* **2006**, *50*, 3833–3838. [CrossRef] [PubMed]
237. Molhoek, E.M.; van Dijk, A.; Veldhuizen, E.J.; Haagsman, H.P.; Bikker, F.J. A cathelicidin-2-derived peptide effectively impairs *Staphylococcus epidermidis* biofilms. *Int. J. Antimicrob. Agents* **2011**, *37*, 476–479. [CrossRef] [PubMed]
238. Casciaro, B.; Moros, M.; Rivera-Fernández, S.; Bellelli, A.; Jesús, M.; Mangoni, M.L. Gold-nanoparticles coated with the antimicrobial peptide esculentin-1a(1-21)NH2 as a reliable strategy for antipseudomonal drugs. *Acta Biomater.* **2017**, *47*, 170–181. [CrossRef] [PubMed]
239. Maisetta, G.; Grassi, L.; Esin, S.; Serra, I.; Scorciapino, M.A.; Rinaldi, A.C.; Batoni, G. The semi-synthetic peptide lin-SB056-1 in combination with EDTA exerts strong antimicrobial and antibiofilm activity against *Pseudomonas aeruginosa* in conditions mimicking cystic fibrosis sputum. *Int. J. Mol. Sci.* **2017**, *18*, 1994. [CrossRef]
240. Khalifa, L.; Brosh, Y.; Gelman, D.; Coppenhagen-Glazer, S.; Beyth, S.; Poradosu-Cohen, R.; Que, Y.A.; Beyth, N.; Hazan, R. Targeting *Enterococcus faecalis* biofilms with phage therapy. *Appl. Environ. Microbiol.* **2015**, *81*, 2696–2705. [CrossRef]
241. D'Andrea, M.M.; Frezza, D.; Romano, E.; Marmo, P.; De Angelis, L.H.; Perini, N.; Thaller, M.C.; Di Lallo, G. The lytic bacteriophage vB_EfaH_EF1TV, a new member of the *Herelleviridae* family, disrupts biofilm produced by *Enterococcus faecalis* clinical strains. *J. Glob. Antimicrob. Resist.* **2020**, *21*, 68–75. [CrossRef]
242. Yuan, Y.; Qu, K.; Tan, D.; Li, X.; Wang, L.; Cong, C.; Xiu, Z.; Xu, Y. Isolation and characterization of a bacteriophage and its potential to disrupt multi-drug resistant *Pseudomonas aeruginosa* biofilms. *Microb. Pathog.* **2019**, *128*, 329–336. [CrossRef]
243. Gutiérrez, D.; Vandenheuvel, D.; Martínez, B.; Rodríguez, A.; Lavigne, R.; García, P. Two phages, phiIPLA-RODI and phiIPLA-C1C, lyse mono- and dual-species staphylococcal biofilms. *Appl. Environ. Microbiol.* **2015**, *81*, 3336–3348. [CrossRef]
244. Zhang, J.; Xu, L.L.; Gan, D.; Zhang, X. In vitro study of bacteriophage AB3 endolysin LysAB3 activity against *Acinetobacter baumannii* biofilm and biofilm-bound *A. baumannii*. *Clin. Lab.* **2018**, *64*, 1021–1030. [CrossRef]
245. Liu, Y.; Mi, Z.; Mi, L.; Huang, Y.; Li, P.; Liu, H.; Yuan, X.; Niu, W.; Jiang, N.; Bai, C.; et al. Identification and characterization of capsule depolymerase Dpo48 from *Acinetobacter baumannii* phage IME200. *PeerJ* **2019**, *7*, e6173. [CrossRef] [PubMed]

246. Bedi, M.S.; Verma, V.; Chhibber, S. Amoxicillin and specific bacteriophage can be used together for eradication of biofilm of *Klebsiella pneumoniae* B5055. *World J. Microbiol. Biot.* **2009**, *25*, 1145. [CrossRef]
247. Rahman, M.; Kim, S.; Kim, S.M.; Seol, S.Y.; Kim, J. Characterization of induced *Staphylococcus aureus* bacteriophage SAP-26 and its anti-biofilm activity with rifampicin. *Biofouling* **2011**, *27*, 1087–1093. [CrossRef] [PubMed]
248. Alves, D.R.; Gaudion, A.; Bean, J.E.; Esteban, P.P.; Arnot, T.C.; Harper, D.R.; Kot, W.; Hanser, L.H.; Enright, M.C.; Jenkins, A.T.A. Combined use of bacteriophage K and a novel bacteriophage to reduce *Staphylococcus aureus* biofilm formation. *Appl. Environ. Microbiol.* **2014**, *80*, 6694–6703. [CrossRef] [PubMed]
249. Kelly, D.; McAuliffe, O.; O'Mahony, J.; Coffey, A. Development of a broad-host-range phage cocktail for biocontrol. *Bioeng. Bugs.* **2011**, *2*, 31–37. [CrossRef]
250. Kelly, D.; McAuliffe, O.; Ross, R.P.; Coffey, A. Prevention of *Staphylococcus aureus* biofilm formation and reduction in established biofilm density using a combination of phage K and modified derivatives. *Lett. Appl. Microbiol.* **2012**, *54*, 286–291. [CrossRef]
251. Fu, W.; Forster, T.; Mayer, O.; Curtin, J.J.; Lehman, S.M.; Donlan, R.M. Bacteriophage cocktail for the prevention of biofilm formation by *Pseudomonas aeruginosa* on catheters in an in vitro model system. *Antimicrob. Agents Chemother.* **2010**, *54*, 397–404. [CrossRef]
252. Alves, D.R.; Perez-Esteban, P.; Kot, W.; Bean, J.E.; Arnot, T.; Hansen, L.H.; Enright, M.C.; Jenkins, A.T.A. A novel bacteriophage cocktail reduces and disperses *Pseudomonas aeruginosa* biofilms under static and flow conditions. *Microb. Biotechnol.* **2016**, *9*, 61–74. [CrossRef] [PubMed]
253. Khan, M.S.A.; Zahin, M.; Hasan, S.; Husain, F.M.; Ahmad, I. Inhibition of quorum sensing regulated bacterial functions by plant essential oils with special reference to clove oil. *Lett. Appl. Microbiol.* **2009**, *49*, 354–360. [CrossRef]
254. Nuryastuti, T.; van der Mei, H.C.; Busscher, H.J.; Iravati, S.; Aman, A.T.; Krom, B.P. Effect of cinnamon oil on *icaA* expression and biofilm formation by *Staphylococcus epidermidis*. *Appl. Environ. Microbiol.* **2009**, *75*, 6850–6855. [CrossRef] [PubMed]
255. De Jesus Pimentel-Filho, N.; de Freitas Martins, M.C.; Nogueira, G.B.; Mantovani, H.C.; Vanetti, M.C.D. Bovicin HC5 and nisin reduce *Staphylococcus aureus* adhesion to polystyrene and change the hydrophobicity profile and Gibbs free energy of adhesion. *Int. J. Food Microbiol.* **2014**, *190*, 1–8. [CrossRef] [PubMed]
256. Kalia, M.; Yadav, V.K.; Singh, P.K.; Sharma, D.; Pandey, H.; Narvi, S.S.; Agarwal, V. Effect of cinnamon oil on quorum sensing-controlled virulence factors and biofilm formation in *Pseudomonas aeruginosa*. *PLoS ONE.* **2015**, *10*, e0135495. [CrossRef] [PubMed]
257. Alibi, S.; Ben Selma, W.; Ramos-Vivas, J.; Smach, M.A.; Touati, R.; Boukadida, J.; Navas, J.; Mansour, H.B. Anti-oxidant, antibacterial, anti-biofilm, and anti-quorum sensing activities of four essential oils against multidrug-resistant bacterial clinical isolates. *Curr. Res. Transl. Med.* **2020**, *68*, 59–66. [CrossRef] [PubMed]
258. Raei, P.; Pourlak, T.; Memar, M.Y.; Alizadeh, N.; Aghamali, M.; Zeinalzadeh, E.; Asgharzadeh, M.; Kafil, H.S. Thymol and carvacrol strongly inhibit biofilm formation and growth of carbapenemase-producing Gram negative bacilli. *Cell. Mol. Biol.* **2017**, *63*, 108–112. [CrossRef] [PubMed]
259. Valliammai, A.; Selvaraj, A.; Yuvashree, U.; Aravindraja, C.; Karutha Pandian, S. *sarA*-dependent antibiofilm activity of thymol enhances the antibacterial efficacy of rifampicin against *Staphylococcus aureus*. *Front. Microbiol.* **2020**, *11*, 1744. [CrossRef]
260. Zhao, X.; Liu, Z.; Liu, Z.; Meng, R.; Shi, C.; Chen, X.; Bu, X.; Guo, N. Phenotype and RNA-seq-based transcriptome profiling of *Staphylococcus aureus* biofilms in response to tea tree oil. *Microb. Pathog.* **2018**, *123*, 304–313. [CrossRef]
261. Samoilova, Z.; Muzyka, N.; Lepekhina, E.; Oktyabrsky, O.; Smirnova, G. Medicinal plant extracts can variously modify biofilm formation in *Escherichia coli*. *Antonie Van Leeuwenhoek* **2014**, *105*, 709–722. [CrossRef]
262. Da Costa Júnior, S.D.; de Oliveira Santos, J.V.; de Almeida Campos, L.A.; Pereira, M.A.; Magalhães, N.S.S.; Cavalcanti, I.M.F. Antibacterial and antibiofilm activities of quercetin against clinical isolates of *Staphyloccocus aureus* and *Staphylococcus saprophyticus* with resistance profile. *IJEAB* **2018**, *3*, 266213. [CrossRef]
263. Ouyang, J.; Sun, F.; Feng, W.; Sn, Y.; Qiu, X.; Xiong, L.; Liu, T.; Chen, Y. Quercetin is an effective inhibitor of quorum sensing, biofilm formation and virulence factors in *Pseudomonas aeruginosa*. *J. Appl. Microbiol.* **2016**, *120*, 966–974. [CrossRef]
264. Qayyum, S.; Sharma, D.; Bisht, D.; Khan, A.U. Identification of factors involved in *Enterococcus faecalis* biofilm under quercetin stress. *Microb. Pathog.* **2019**, *126*, 205–211. [CrossRef] [PubMed]
265. Lambert, R.J.W.; Skandamis, P.N.; Coote, P.J.; Nychas, G.J. A study of the minimum inhibitory concentration and mode of action of oregano essential oil, thymol and carvacrol. *J. Appl. Microbiol.* **2001**, *91*, 453–462. [CrossRef] [PubMed]
266. Namivandi-Zangeneh, R.; Yang, Y.; Xu, S.; Wong, E.H.; Boyer, C. Antibiofilm platform based on the combination of antimicrobial polymers and essential oils. *Biomacromolecules* **2020**, *21*, 262–272. [CrossRef] [PubMed]
267. Sharma, G.; Raturi, K.; Dang, S.; Gupta, S.; Gabrani, R. Inhibitory effect of cinnamaldehyde alone and in combination with thymol, eugenol and thymoquinone against *Staphylococcus epidermidis*. *J. Herb. Med.* **2017**, *9*, 68–73. [CrossRef]
268. Kali, A.; Bhuvaneshwar, D.; Charles, P.M.V.; Seetha, K.S. Antibacterial synergy of curcumin with antibiotics against biofilm producing clinical bacterial isolates. *J. Basic Clin. Pharm.* **2016**, *7*, 93–96. [CrossRef] [PubMed]
269. Burton, E.; Yakandawala, N.; LoVetri, K.; Madhyastha, M.S. A microplate spectrofluorometric assay for bacterial biofilms. *J. Ind. Microbiol. Biotchnol.* **2007**, *34*, 1–4. [CrossRef] [PubMed]
270. Izano, E.A.; Sadovskaya, I.; Wang, H.; Vinogradov, E.; Ragunath, C.; Ramasubbu, N.; Jabbouri, S.; Perru, M.B.; Kaplan, J.B. Poly-N-acetylglucosamine mediates biofilm formation and detergent resistance in *Aggregatibacter actinomycetemcomitans*. *Microb. Pathog.* **2007**, *44*, 52–60. [CrossRef]

271. Seidl, K.; Goerke, C.; Wolz, C.; Mack, D.; Berger-Bächi, B.; Bischoff, M. *Staphylococcus aureus* CcpA affects biofilm formation. *Infect. Immun.* **2008**, *76*, 2044–2050. [CrossRef]
272. Tetz, G.V.; Artemenko, N.K.; Tetz, V.V. Effect of DNase and antibiotics on biofilm characteristics. *Antimicrob. Agents Chemother.* **2009**, *53*, 1204–1209. [CrossRef]
273. Parks, Q.M.; Young, R.L.; Poch, K.R.; Malcolm, K.C.; Vasil, M.L.; Nick, J.A. Neutrophil enhancement of *Pseudomonas aeruginosa* biofilm development: Human F-actin and DNA as targets for therapy. *J. Med. Microbiol.* **2009**, *58*, 492–502. [CrossRef]
274. Ramsey, D.M.; Wozniak, D.J. Understanding the control of *Pseudomonas aeruginosa* alginate synthesis and the prospects for management of chronic infections in cystic fibrosis. *Mol. Microbiol.* **2005**, *56*, 309–322. [CrossRef] [PubMed]
275. Vollmer, W.; Tomasz, A. The *pgdA* gene encodes for a peptidoglycan N-acetylglucosamine deacetylase in *Streptococcus pneumoniae*. *J. Biol. Chem.* **2000**, *275*, 20496–20501. [CrossRef] [PubMed]
276. Hukić, M.; Seljmo, D.; Ramovic, A.; Ibrišimović, M.A.; Dogan, S.; Hukic, J.; Bojic, E.F. The effect of lysozyme on reducing biofilms by *Staphylococcus aureus, Pseudomonas aeruginosa*, and *Gardnerella vaginalis*: An *in vitro* examination. *Microb. Drug Resist.* **2018**, *24*, 353–358. [CrossRef] [PubMed]
277. Eladawy, M.; El-Mowafy, M.; El-Sokkary, M.M.A.; Barwa, R. Effects of lysozyme, proteinase K, and cephalosporins on biofilm formation by clinical isolates of *Pseudomonas aeruginosa*. *Interdiscip. Perspect. Infect. Dis.* **2020**, *2020*, 6156720. [CrossRef] [PubMed]
278. Bastos, M.C.F.; Coutinho, B.G.; Coelho, M.L.V. Lysostaphin: A staphylococcal bacteriolysin with potential clinical applications. *Pharmaceuticals* **2010**, *3*, 1139–1161. [CrossRef] [PubMed]
279. Connolly, K.L.; Roberts, A.L.; Holder, R.C.; Reid, S.D. Dispersal of Group A streptococcal biofilms by the cysteine protease SpeB leads to increased disease severity in a murine model. *PLoS ONE* **2011**, *6*, e18974. [CrossRef] [PubMed]
280. Park, J.H.; Lee, J.H.; Cho, M.H.; Herzberg, M.; Lee, J. Acceleration of protease effect on *Staphylococcus aureus* biofilm dispersal. *FEMS Microbiol. Lett.* **2012**, *335*, 31–38. [CrossRef]
281. Yang, F.; Wang, L.H.; Wang, J.; Dong, Y.H.; Hu, J.Y.; Zhang, L.H. Quorum quenching enzyme activity is widely conserved in the sera of mammalian species. *FEBS Lett.* **2005**, *579*, 3713–3717. [CrossRef]
282. Paul, D.; Kim, Y.S.; Ponnusamy, K.; Kweon, J.H. Application of quorum quenching to inhibit biofilm formation. *Environm. Eng. Sci.* **2009**, *26*, 1319–1324. [CrossRef]
283. Gupta, P.; Chhibber, S.; Harjai, K. Efficacy of purified lactonase and ciprofloxacin in preventing systemic spread of *Pseudomonas aeruginosa* in murine burn wound model. *Burns* **2015**, *41*, 153–162. [CrossRef]
284. Sambanthamoorthy, K.; Luo, C.; Pattabiraman, N.; Feng, X.; Koestler, B.; Waters, C.M.; Palys, T.J. Identification of small molecules inhibiting diguanylate cyclases to control bacterial biofilm development. *Biofouling* **2014**, *30*, 17–28. [CrossRef] [PubMed]
285. Cegelski, L.; Pinkner, J.S.; Hammer, N.D.; Cusumano, C.K.; Hung, C.S.; Chorell, E.; Åberg, V.; Walker, J.N.; Seed, P.C.; Almqvist, F.; et al. Small-molecule inhibitors target *Escherichia coli* amyloid biogenesis and biofilm formation. *Nat. Chem. Biol.* **2009**, *5*, 913–919. [CrossRef] [PubMed]
286. Greene, S.E.; Pinkner, J.S.; Chorell, E.; Dodson, K.W.; Shaffer, C.L.; Conover, M.S.; Livny, J.; Hadjifrangiskou, M.; Almqvist, F.; Hultgren, S.J. Pilicide ec240 disrupts virulence circuits in uropathogenic *Escherichia coli*. *mBio* **2014**, *5*, e02038. [PubMed]
287. Cusumano, C.K.; Pinkner, J.S.; Han, Z.; Greene, S.E.; Ford, B.A.; Crowley, J.R.; Henderson, J.R.; Jenetka, J.W.; Hultgren, S.J. Treatment and prevention of urinary tract infection with orally active FimH inhibitors. *Sci. Transl. Med.* **2011**, *3*, 109ra115. [CrossRef]
288. Debebe, T.; Krüger, M.; Huse, K.; Kacza, J.; Mühlberg, K.; König, B.; Birkenmeier, G. Ethyl pyruvate: An anti-microbial agent that selectively targets pathobionts and biofilms. *PLoS ONE* **2016**, *11*, e0162919. [CrossRef] [PubMed]
289. Qin, Z.; Yang, L.; Qu, D.; Molin, S.; Tolker-Nielsen, T. *Pseudomonas aeruginosa* extracellular products inhibit staphylococcal growth, and disrupt established biofilms produced by *Staphylococcus epidermidis*. *Microbiology* **2009**, *155*, 2148–2156. [CrossRef] [PubMed]
290. Donelli, G.; Francolini, I.; Romoli, D.; Guaglianone, E.; Piozzi, A.; Ragunath, C.; Kaplan, J.B. Synergistic activity of dispersin B and cefamandole nafate in inhibition of staphylococcal biofilm growth on polyurethanes. *Antimicrob. Agents Chemother.* **2007**, *51*, 2733–2740. [CrossRef] [PubMed]
291. Kaplan, J.B. Therapeutic potential of biofilm-dispersing enzymes. *Int. J. Artif. Organs.* **2009**, *32*, 545–554. [CrossRef]
292. Darouiche, R.O.; Mansouri, M.D.; Gawande, P.V.; Madhyastha, S. Antimicrobial and antibiofilm efficacy of triclosan and DispersinB®combination. *J. Antimicrob. Chemother.* **2009**, *64*, 88–93. [CrossRef]
293. Ragland, S.A.; Criss, A.K. From bacterial killing to immune modulation: Recent insights into the functions of lysozyme. *PLoS Pathog.* **2017**, *13*, e1006512. [CrossRef]
294. Jiang, P.; Li, J.; Han, F.; Duan, G.; Lu, X.; Gu, Y.; Yu, W. Antibiofilm activity of an exopolysaccharide from marine bacterium *Vibrio* sp. QY101. *PLoS ONE* **2011**, *6*, e18514. [CrossRef] [PubMed]
295. Siddiq, D.M.; Darouiche, R.O. New strategies to prevent catheter-associated urinary tract infections. *Nat. Rev. Urol.* **2012**, *9*, 305–314. [CrossRef] [PubMed]
296. Brogden, K.A. Antimicrobial peptides: Pore formers or metabolic inhibitors in bacteria? *Nat. Rev. Microbiol.* **2005**, *3*, 238–250. [CrossRef] [PubMed]
297. Zhang, L.J.; Gallo, R.L. Antimicrobial peptides. *Curr. Biol.* **2016**, *26*, R14–R19. [CrossRef]
298. Galdiero, E.; Lombardi, L.; Falanga, A.; Libralato, G.; Guida, M.; Carotenuto, R. Biofilms: Novel strategies based on antimicrobial peptides. *Pharmaceutics* **2019**, *11*, 322. [CrossRef]

299. Malmsten, M. Antimicrobial peptides. *Upsala J. Med. Sci.* **2014**, *119*, 199–204. [CrossRef]
300. Memariani, H.; Memariani, M.; Shahidi-Dadras, M.; Nasiri, S.; Akhavan, M.M.; Moravvej, H. Melittin: From honeybees to superbugs. *Appl. Microbiol. Biotech.* **2019**, *103*, 3265–3276. [CrossRef]
301. Etayash, H.; Pletzer, D.; Kumar, P.; Straus, S.K.; Hancock, R.E.W. A cyclic derivative of host-defence peptide IDR-1018 improves proteolytic stability, suppresses inflammation, and enhances *in vivo* activity. *J. Med. Chem.* **2020**, *63*, 9228–9236. [CrossRef]
302. Martin-Serrano, Á.; Gómez, R.; Ortega, P.; de la Mata, F.J. Nanosystems as vehicles for the delivery of antimicrobial peptides (AMPs). *Pharmaceutics* **2019**, *11*, 448. [CrossRef]
303. Pires, D.P.; Melo, L.D.; Boas, D.V.; Sillankorva, S.; Azeredo, J. Phage therapy as an alternative or complementary strategy to prevent and control biofilm-related infections. *Curr. Opin. Microbiol.* **2017**, *39*, 48–56. [CrossRef]
304. Sillankorva, S.; Oliveira, R.; Vieira, M.J.; Sutherland, I.; Azeredo, J. *Pseudomonas fluorescens* infection by bacteriophage ΦS1: The influence of temperature, host growth phase and media. *FEMS Microbiol. Lett.* **2004**, *241*, 13–20. [CrossRef] [PubMed]
305. Jamal, M.; Hussain, T.; Das, C.R.; Andleeb, S. Characterization of Siphoviridae phage Z and studying its efficacy against multidrug-resistant *Klebsiella pneumoniae* planktonic cells and biofilm. *J. Med. Microbiol.* **2015**, *64*, 454–462. [CrossRef] [PubMed]
306. Le, S.; Yao, X.; Lu, S.; Tan, Y.; Rao, X.; Li, M.; Jin, X.; Wang, J.; Zhao, Y.; Wu, N.C.; et al. Chromosomal DNA deletion confers phage resistance to *Pseudomonas aeruginosa*. *Sci. Rep.* **2014**, *4*, 4738. [CrossRef] [PubMed]
307. Lu, T.K.; Collins, J.J. Engineered bacteriophage targeting gene networks as adjuvants for antibiotic therapy. *Proc. Natl. Acad. Sci. USA* **2009**, *106*, 4629–4634. [CrossRef] [PubMed]
308. Lu, T.K.; Collins, J.J. Dispersing biofilms with engineered enzymatic bacteriophage. *Proc. Natl. Acad. Sci. USA* **2007**, *104*, 11197–11202. [CrossRef]
309. Wu, Y.K.; Cheng, N.C.; Cheng, C.M. Biofilms in chronic wounds: Pathogenesis and diagnosis. *Trends Biotechnol.* **2019**, *37*, 505–517. [CrossRef]
310. LuTheryn, G.; Glynne-Jones, P.; Webb, J.S.; Carugo, D. Ultrasound-mediated therapies for the treatment of biofilms in chronic wounds: A review of present knowledge. *Microb. Biotechnol.* **2020**, *13*, 613–628. [CrossRef]
311. Ferrer-Espada, R.; Wang, Y.; Goh, X.S.; Dai, T. Antimicrobial blue light inactivation of microbial isolates in biofilms. *Lasers Surg. Med.* **2020**, *52*, 472–478. [CrossRef]
312. Dai, T.; Gupta, A.; Huang, Y.Y.; Yin, R.; Murray, C.K.; Vrahas, M.S.; Sherwood, M.E.; Tegos, G.P.; Hamblin, M.R. Blue light rescues mice from potentially fatal *Pseudomonas aeruginosa* burn infection: Efficacy, safety, and mechanism of action. *Antimicrob. Agents Chemother.* **2013**, *57*, 1238–1245. [CrossRef]
313. Rupel, K.; Zupin, L.; Ottaviani, G.; Bertani, I.; Martinelli, V.; Porrelli, D.; Vodret, S.; Vuerich, R.; da Silva, D.P.; Bussani, R.; et al. Blue laser light inhibits biofilm formation *in vitro* and *in vivo* by inducing oxidative stress. *NPJ Biofilms Microb.* **2019**, *5*, 1–11. [CrossRef]
314. Bak, J.; Ladefoged, S.D.; Tvede, M.; Begovic, T.; Gregersen, A. Disinfection of *Pseudomonas aeruginosa* biofilm contaminated tube lumens with ultraviolet C light emitting diodes. *Biofouling* **2010**, *26*, 31–38. [CrossRef] [PubMed]
315. Reshma, V.G.; Syama, S.; Sruthi, S.; Reshma, S.C.; Remya, N.S.; Mohanan, P.V. Engineered nanoparticles with antimicrobial property. *Curr. Drug Metab.* **2017**, *18*, 1040–1054. [CrossRef] [PubMed]
316. Xu, L.C.; Siedlecki, C.A. Submicron-textured biomaterial surface reduces staphylococcal bacterial adhesion and biofilm formation. *Acta Biomater.* **2012**, *8*, 72–81. [CrossRef] [PubMed]
317. Meng, J.; Zhang, P.; Wang, S. Recent progress in biointerfaces with controlled bacterial adhesion by using chemical and physical methods. *Chem. Asian J.* **2014**, *9*, 2004–2016. [CrossRef] [PubMed]
318. Xu, L.C.; Wo, Y.; Meyerhoff, M.E.; Siedlecki, C.A. Inhibition of bacterial adhesion and biofilm formation by dual functional textured and nitric oxide releasing surfaces. *Acta Biomater.* **2017**, *51*, 53–65. [CrossRef]
319. Różańska, D.; Regulska-Ilow, B.; Choroszy-Król, I.; Ilow, R. [The role of *Escherichia coli* strain Nissle 1917 in the gastro-intestinal diseases]. *Postepy Hig. Med. Dosw. Online* **2014**, *6*, 1251–1256. [CrossRef]
320. Fang, K.; Jin, X.; Hong, S.H. Probiotic *Escherichia coli* inhibits biofilm formation of pathogenic *E. coli* via extracellular activity of DegP. *Sci. Rep.* **2018**, *8*, 4339. [CrossRef]
321. Hwang, I.Y.; Koh, E.; Wong, A.; March, J.C.; Bentley, W.E.; Lee, Y.S.; Chang, M.W. Engineered probiotic *Escherichia coli* can eliminate and prevent *Pseudomonas aeruginosa* gut infection in animal models. *Nat. Commun.* **2017**, *8*, 15028. [CrossRef]

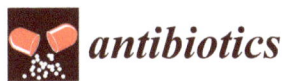

Article

Biofilm-Induced Antibiotic Resistance in Clinical *Acinetobacter baumannii* Isolates

Abebe Mekuria Shenkutie [1], **Mian Zhi Yao** [1], **Gilman Kit-hang Siu** [1], **Barry Kin Chung Wong** [2] and **Polly Hang-mei Leung** [1,*]

[1] Department of Health Technology and Informatics, the Hong Kong Polytechnic University, Hong Kong, China; abebe-mekuria.shenkutie@connect.polyu.hk (A.M.S.); mian-zhi.yao@connect.polyu.hk (M.Z.Y.); gilman.siu@polyu.edu.hk (G.K.-h.S.)
[2] Department of Pathology, United Christian Hospital, Hong Kong, China; wongkc@ha.org.hk
* Correspondence: polly.hm.leung@polyu.edu.hk; Tel.: +852-34008570

Received: 22 October 2020; Accepted: 14 November 2020; Published: 17 November 2020

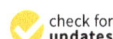

Abstract: In order to understand the role of biofilm in the emergence of antibiotic resistance, a total of 104 clinical *Acinetobacter baumannii* strains were investigated for their biofilm-forming capacities and genes associated with biofilm formation. Selected biofilm-formers were tested for antibiotic susceptibilities when grown in biofilm phase. Reversibility of antibiotic susceptibility in planktonic cells regrown from biofilm were investigated. We found 59.6% of the strains were biofilm-formers, among which, 66.1% were non-multidrug resistant (MDR) strains. Presence of virulence genes *bap*, *csuE*, and *abaI* was significantly associated with biofilm-forming capacities. When strains were grown in biofilm state, the minimum biofilm eradication concentrations were 44, 407, and 364 times higher than the minimum bactericidal concentrations (MBC) for colistin, ciprofloxacin, and imipenem, respectively. Persisters were detected after treating the biofilm at 32–256 times the MBC of planktonic cells. Reversibility test for antibiotic susceptibility showed that biofilm formation induced reversible antibiotic tolerance in the non-MDR strains but a higher level of irreversible resistance in the extensively drug-resistant (XDR) strain. In summary, we showed that the non-MDR strains were strong biofilm-formers. Presence of persisters in biofilm contributed to the reduced antibiotic susceptibilities. Biofilm-grown *Acinetobacter baumannii* has induced antibiotic tolerance in non-MDR strains and increased resistance levels in XDR strains. To address the regulatory mechanisms of biofilm-specific resistance, thorough investigations at genome and transcription levels are warranted.

Keywords: *Acinetobacter baumannii*; biofilm; antibiotic resistance; antibiotic tolerance; persister

1. Introduction

A. baumannii is a significant opportunistic pathogen responsible for a high proportion of healthcare-associated infections [1]. Due to the critical impact of the multidrug-resistant *A. baumannii* on public health, the World Health Organization has categorized this organism as a priority I pathogen among the antibiotic-resistant microorganisms [2–6]. Recent reports have shown that the environmental reservoir is the major source of multidrug-resistant *A. baumannii* outbreaks in hospital environments [7]. The ability of *A. baumannii* to form biofilm facilitates its survival and persistence in the hospital environments [8,9], this in turn contributes to the extensive spread of this pathogen across the globe [10].

Biofilm is a multilayer of highly coordinated microorganisms attached to surfaces in the presence of moisture. Bacterial cells within the biofilm are highly coordinated and undergo phenotype switch to produce a community that is resistant to the adverse external environment. Such phenotype switch also promotes the emergence of antibiotic resistance through the expression of the antibiotic-resistance genes, genetic mutation, or transfer of genes associated with antibiotic-resistance [11].

Virulence genes associated with biofilm formation in *A. baumannii* include *bap*, *csu* locus, *adeFGH*, *ompA*, and *abaI* [10]. *bap* encodes a large bacterial surface protein consisting of 8621 amino acids [11]. The predicted structure of Bap was similar to bacterial adhesins of the immunoglobulin-like fold superfamily and may function as an intercellular adhesin that supports the development of the mature biofilm structure [12]. *csuE* belongs to the *csu* operon, which encodes the chaperone-usher pili assembly system as production of pili is required in the early steps of biofilm formation on abiotic surfaces [13]. *ompA* encodes a porin protein that is involved in adhesion to the epithelial cell, antibiotic resistance, and biofilm formation [8]. *adeFGH* encodes a resistance–nodulation–cell division antibiotics efflux system, which is involved in the synthesis and transportation of autoinducer molecules during biofilm formation [14]. *abaI* encodes an autoinducer synthase, which is an enzyme involved in quorum sensing. Mutation of *abaI* fails to produce acyl-homoserine lactone signals and impairs biofilm maturation [5]. Certain biofilm-associated genes influence the expression of antibiotic resistance, suggesting the link between biofilm formation and antibiotic resistance.

In the past decade, most of the published studies on antimicrobial resistance of *A. baumannii* focused on the planktonic states of the pathogen [5,15,16]. However, biofilm of *A. baumannii* is responsible for various types of catheter-related infections, antimicrobial resistance performed using planktonic cells may not be representative for biofilms. In order to understand the virulence potential and the influence of biofilm growth on antibiotic susceptibility, we characterized the biofilm-producing capacities of the *A. baumannii* strains isolated from clinical specimens and to examine the responses of biofilm cells to antimicrobial agents. It has been documented that antibiotic-resistant strains of *A. baumannii* were strong biofilm formers [10], such properties are beneficial to the survival and dissemination of the resistant strains. However, antibiotic-sensitive strains are vulnerable to antibiotic challenges, in order to protect themselves from antibiotics present in the surrounding environments, the sensitive strains may have the abilities to form biofilm. Therefore, the study investigated the relationship between antibiotic susceptibility and biofilm-forming ability. The results obtained from the phenotypic characterization of the biofilm-producing capacity and biofilm susceptibility tests may offer valuable insights into the development of preventive strategies for biofilm-associated infections in hospital environments.

2. Materials and Methods

2.1. Clinical Isolates

A total of 104 archived and nonduplicate *Acinetobacter species* isolates were collected from different hospitals in Hong Kong. All strains of *Acinetobacter* species were collected from sputum, blood, urine, soft tissue, and hospital environments. The collected isolates were kept in Luria-Bertani (Oxoid Ltd., Basingstoke, UK) broth containing 20% glycerol at −80 °C until use. The reference strains *A. baumannii* ATCC 19606 and *E. coli* ATCC 25922 were used as control strains in the biofilm assay or antibiotic susceptibility tests.

2.2. Confirmation of Bacterial Identities

Identities of the *A. baumannii* isolates were confirmed using a multiplex PCR assay. Three pairs of primers targeting *recA*, *gyrB*, and ITS were used [17]. PCR was performed in a final reaction volume of 40 µL containing 5X Phusion HF Buffer, 10 mM dNTP, and Phusion DNA Polymerase (all from New England BioLabs, MA, USA), and 0.5 µM of each primer using a Veriti thermocycler (Applied Biosystems, Foster City, CA, USA) under the following conditions: initial denaturation at 98 °C for 5 min; 35 cycles of denaturation (95 °C, 30 s), annealing (54 °C, 30 s) and extension (72 °C, 1 min); a final extension step at 72 °C for 10 min. PCR products were separated by 1.5% agarose gel electrophoresis the gel was stained with 0.5 µg/mL RedSafe nucleic acid staining solution (iNtRON biotechnology, Gyeonggi, Korea). The stained gel was visualized using a Gel Doc System XR (Bio-Rad Laboratories, Richmond, CA, USA).

2.3. Multilocus Sequence Typing (MLST)

The Oxford scheme of MLST targeting seven chromosomal housekeeping genes was performed according to the method described in the MLST database (http://pubmlst.org/abaumannii). The seven housekeeping genes (*gltA, gyrB, ghdB, recA, cpn60, gpi,* and *rpoD*) of 104 *A. baumannii* isolates were amplified and sequenced according to the method described by Bartual et al. [18]. The allele number of each gene was obtained by comparing its sequence with the reference sequences in the database. The sequence type of a given isolate was identified by matching the seven locus numbers obtained. If a sequence did not match with any reference sequences in the database, it was designated as a new allele. In addition, if the seven loci did not match with any existing allele combinations in the database, the isolates were regarded as new sequence types.

2.4. Biofilm Formation

Biofilm-forming capacities of the isolates were evaluated with a Calgary Biofilm Device (CBD) with slight modifications of the procedures described by Ceri et al. [19] and the manufacturer (Innovotech, Edmonton, AB, Canada). Briefly, 3–5 colonies were picked from an overnight LB agar plate and inoculated into 10 mL Maximum Recovery Diluent to a turbidity equivalent to 0.5 McFarland standard. The inoculum was mixed 1:1 with LB broth. For each *A. baumannii* strain, 150 μL of bacterial suspension was inoculated into the well of a 96-well microtiter plate. The plate was then covered with a plastic lid with 96 pegs (Innovotech). The microtiter plate was incubated at 37 °C for 48 h on a platform shaker set at 110 rpm. After incubation, planktonic cells were aspirated from the wells and discarded; the wells were washed three times with Maximum Recovery Diluent. Both the plates and lids with pegs were inverted and allowed to dry for 2 h at room temperature. Biofilm mass quantification was performed in octuplicate, and each assay was repeated on three separate days.

2.5. Quantification of Biofilm Mass

Biofilm masses formed on the 96-well microtiter plate was quantified using the crystal violet staining method. After drying of the microtiter plate and the lid with pegs, 200 μL of 0.1% aqueous crystal violet solution was added into each well of the microtiter plate, which was covered with the lid with pegs. The set up was incubated at room temperature for 15 min. After staining, the wells and the pegs were washed three times with Maximum Recovery Diluent to remove the excess stain and air-dried. After drying, 200 μL of 33% (*v/v*) acetic acid was added to each well of the microtiter plate to extract the crystal violet bound to the biofilm. Absorbance was measured at 570 nm using a microplate spectrophotometer (BIO-RAD). The average optical density (OD) for each *A. baumannii* isolate was calculated, and the biofilm-forming capacity was interpreted according to the guideline described by Stepanović et al. [20]. The cut-off OD (ODc) was defined as three standard deviations above the mean OD of the uninoculated control. Classification criteria are shown in Table 1.

Table 1. Classification of biofilm-forming capacity based on optical density (OD) value.

Classification	OD Range		
Non-biofilm producer		OD	≤ODc
Weak biofilm producer	ODc	<OD	≤2 × ODc
Moderate biofilm producer	2 × ODc	<OD	≤4 × ODc
Strong biofilm producer		OD	>4 × ODc

2.6. Detection of Biofilm-Associated Genes

PCR detection of biofilm-associated genes (*bap, csuE, ompA, adeFGH, abaI*) was performed on a Veriti thermocycler (Applied Biosystems) using sets of primers shown in Table S1. PCR was performed in a 20-µL reaction consisting of 1 µL extracted genomic DNA, 10 µL Luna Universal qPCR Master Mix (New England Biolabs, USA), 1 µL (10 µM) of each primer. The reaction condition was initial denaturation at 95 °C for 7 min, followed by 35 cycles of denaturation at 95 °C for 30 s, annealing at 60 °C for 1 min and extension at 72 °C for 30 s, and a final extension of 72 °C for 10 min. PCR products were separated by 1.5% agarose gel electrophoresis the gel was stained with 0.5 µg/mL RedSafe nucleic acid staining solution (iNtRON Biotechnology, Korea). The stained gel was visualized using a Gel Doc System XR (Bio-Rad Laboratories).

2.7. Determination of Minimal Inhibitory Concentration (MIC) and Minimum Bactericidal Concentration (MBC)

Antimicrobial susceptibility testing was determined by broth microdilution techniques according to the procedures described in the CLSI guidelines [21]. Interpretation of susceptible, intermediate, and resistant was based on CLSI guidelines. Ten antimicrobials covering seven categories of antimicrobials used for the treatment of *A. baumannii* infections were included in the determination of MIC and MBC. These included penicillin-β-lactamase inhibitor (ampicillin-sulbactam), cephalosporin (cefotaxime, ceftazidime), a carbapenem (imipenem, meropenem), aminoglycoside (gentamycin), a fluoroquinolone (ciprofloxacin, levofloxacin), tetracycline (tetracycline), lipopeptide (colistin) were included in the study. *E. coli* ATCC 25922 and *A. baumannii* ATCC 19606 (*A. baumannii* ST1861) were used as control strains. The strains were regarded as multidrug-resistant (MDR) if they were resistant to at least three classes of antimicrobial agents, including penicillin and cephalosporin (including inhibitor combinations), fluoroquinolones, and aminoglycosides. MDR strains that were resistant to carbapenem were regarded as extensively drug-resistant (XDR) [22]. XDR strains were resistant to colistin, and all other classes of antibiotics were regarded as pan drug-resistant (PDR).

After MIC determination, 10 µL aliquots from the wells that showed no visible bacterial growth were inoculated onto LB agar plates and incubated at 37 °C for 24 h. The MBC was the lowest concentration of antibiotic that killed 99.9% of the initial bacterial population.

2.8. Determination of Minimal Biofilm Inhibitory Concentration (MBIC) and Minimum Biofilm Eradication Concentration (MBEC) Assay

The antibiotic susceptibility test for biofilm was performed according to the procedures described by Moskowitz et al. [23]. After the biofilm was formed on the CBD pegs, the pegs were rinsed three times in a 96-well plate containing 150 µL of Maximum Recovery Diluent. The lid with pegs was then transferred to the new a standard 96-well plate with wells containing 150 µL Mueller–Hinton broth with antibiotics diluted two-fold serially (ranged from 2 to 1024 µg/mL). The 96-well plate was incubated overnight at 37 °C. Following incubation, turbidity in each well was examined visually. MBIC was defined as the minimal antibiotic concentration at which no bacterial growth was observed, which meant the minimal antibiotic concentration that inhibited the release of planktonic bacteria from the biofilm.

Following the MBIC examination, MBEC was determined. The lid with pegs was removed and rinsed three times in a 96-well plate containing 150 µL of Maximum Recovery Diluent to remove the planktonic cells. The lid was then placed in a second 96-well plate containing 150 µL Mueller–Hinton broth. The plate was shaken at a speed of 180 rpm for 10 min to detach the biofilm cells from the pegs into the Mueller–Hinton broth. The viability of the biofilm was determined by plate count after 24 h of incubation at 37 °C. MBEC was defined as the minimal antibiotic concentration required to eradicate the biofilm.

2.9. Confocal Laser Scanning Microscopy Imaging of Biofilm

Confocal laser scanning microscopy (CLSM) was performed to estimate the proportion of viable cells in the biofilm formed on the pegs. After the formation of biofilm, the pegs were separated from the lid using sterilized pliers and washed three times with Maximum Recovery Diluent to remove the planktonic cells [19]. Biofilm cells on the pegs were dual stained with a mixture of 3.35 µM SYTO-9 and 20 µM propidium iodide according to the instructions of the Film Tracer Live/Dead Biofilm Viability Kit (Cat no: L10316 Invitrogen). CLSM images were acquired using a Leica TCS SPE Confocal Microscope (Leica) with a 63x objective lens. The live and dead cells embedded in subpopulations of biofilm cells were estimated using a software BioFilmAnalyzer [24].

3. Reversibility of Antibiotic Resistance of the Biofilm Cells

A study was performed to evaluate the antibiotic susceptibility profile after the biofilm cells were grown in the planktonic state. Two hyper-biofilm forming *A. baumannii* (ST1894 and ST373) and one weak biofilm former (ST195) were selected for this part of the study. ST1894 and ST373 were non-MDR strains; ST195 was an XDR strain. The biofilm cells of these three *A. baumannii* strains were subcultured on LB agar. MBICs of three antibiotics (colistin, imipenem, and ciprofloxacin) for the biofilm cells and MICs for the resumed planktonic cells were determined according to the procedures described above.

3.1. Enumeration of Persister Cells from Planktonic and Biofilm Populations

Persister cells in the planktonic and biofilm populations were enumerated according to the procedures described by Marques [25] with slight modification. A hyper-biofilm-producing and non-MDR *A. baumannii* ST1894 strain were selected for the isolation of persister cells. The strain was streaked onto a LB agar plate and incubated at 37 °C for 24 h. One to two colonies were inoculated into 5 mL LB broth, which was incubated at 37 °C with agitation (180 rpm) for 12 h. After incubation, the broth culture was diluted to 1% in 20 mL of fresh LB broth and incubated at 37 °C with agitation (180 rpm) for 24 h.

To enumerate persister cells in the planktonic population, 10 mL of overnight LB broth culture of ST1894 was collected by centrifugation at 8000 rpm for 10 min at 4 °C and resuspended in 10 mL of saline at 4 °C. The washing step was repeated one more time. Cell density was adjusted to an absorbance of 0.8 at 600 nm. A duplicated set of bacterial cell suspension was prepared in the same way. Ninty-eight microliters of 2048 µg/mL ciprofloxacin (20× MIC) or 98 µL saline containing 0.1% acetic acid was added to the 10 mL bacterial cell suspension and incubated at 37 °C with agitation at 180 rpm for 24 h. Viable bacterial cells were enumerated using the plate count method. One hundred microliters of the experiment and control samples were inoculated onto the LB agar plate containing 1% $MgCl_2.7H_2O$ to neutralize the ciprofloxacin. Plate count was performed in triplicate at time points 0, 1, 3, 5, 7, 9, 12, 15, and 24 h after incubation. The number of persister cells present in the planktonic population was determined according to the formula shown below:

$$\text{The number of persisters in planktonic cells/mL} = \frac{\text{Number of colonies} \times \text{dilution factor}}{\text{Volume plated}}$$

To enumerate persister cells in the biofilm population, an overnight LB broth culture of ST1894 was used to grow biofilm using a CBD according to the procedures described elsewhere in this article. After incubation for 48 h, the pegs were removed from the CBD using pliers and each peg was placed in a centrifuge tube with 1 mL Maximum Recovery Diluent. The biofilm cells formed on the pegs were detached by centrifuging at 18,000 rpm for 10 min and were resuspended in 10 mL saline at 4 °C. Cell density was adjusted to an absorbance of 0.8 at 600 nm. Ninty-eight microliters of 2048 µg/mL ciprofloxacin (20 × MIC) or 98 µL saline containing 0.1% acetic acid was added to the 10 mL bacterial cell suspension and incubated at 37 °C with agitation at 180 rpm for 24 h. The number of viable biofilm cells for each treated and nontreated sample was counted according to the steps as described for planktonic cells. The number of persister cells isolated from the biofilm population was determined according to the formula shown below:

$$\text{Number of persisters in biofilm/mL} = \frac{\text{Number of colonies} \times \text{dilution factor} \times \text{total sample volume}}{\text{Volume plated} \times \text{surface area of peg}}$$

3.2. Statistical Analysis

The association between biofilm-forming abilities and biofilm-associated genes was analyzed using chi-squared tests. SPSS version 24 (IBM Corporation, Armonk, NY, USA) was used for statistical analysis. p-value ≤ 0.05 was considered as statistically significant for the data analyzed in this study.

4. Results

4.1. Antibiotic Susceptibility Profiles of the A. baumannii Strains

The MICs for 10 antibiotics (listed in Table 2) covering seven major antibiotic classes were determined for the 104 *A. baumannii* isolates. The antibiotic susceptibility profiles of the isolates are summarized in Table 2. The results showed that 79.8% (82/104) of the isolates were susceptible to colistin, but only 4.8% (5/104) of the isolates were susceptible to ampicillin-sulbactam. There were 29.8% (31/104) to 52.9% (55/104) of isolates susceptible to the remaining eight antibiotics. Among the 104 isolates, 46.2% (48/104) of strains were non-MDR strains, 30.8% (32/104) were XDR strains, and 23.1% (24/104) were PDR strains (Table 3 and Figure S1).

Table 2. Antimicrobials susceptibility profiles the *Acinetobacter baumannii* isolates (n=104). S, I, and R represent susceptible, intermediate, and resistant, respectively.

Antimicrobials	MIC Breakpoints (µg/mL)			Susceptible (%)	Intermediate (%)	Resistant (%)
	Susceptible	Intermediate	Resistant			
Colistin	≤2	-	≥4	79.8	-	20.2
Imipenem	≤2	4	≥8	48.1	-	51.9
Meropenem	≤2	4	≥8	48.1	-	51.9
Cefotaxime	≤8	16–32	≥64	29.8	13.5	56.7
Ceftazidime	≤8	16	≥32	39.4	-	60.6
Ciprofloxacin	≤1	2	≥4	48.1	-	51.9
Levofloxacin	≤1	2	≥4	48.1	-	51.9
Gentamycin	≤2	4	≥8	52.9	-	47.1
Tetracycline	≤4	8	≥16	48.1	-	51.9
Ampicillin-sulbactam	≤4	8	≥16	4.8	3.8	91.3

Table 3. The relationship among biofilm-producing ability of *A. baumannii* with antibiotic resistance.

Biofilm-Producing Ability	% of Isolates	% of Isolates with Different Antibiotic Susceptibility Profiles		
		Non-MDR 46.2% (48/104)	XDR 30.8% (32/104)	PDR 23.1% (24/104)
Biofilm-forming	>59.6% (62/104)	>66.1% (41/62)	>17.7% (11/62)	>16.1% (10/62)
Strong	25% (26/104)	92.3% (24/26)	7.7% (2/26)	0% (0/26)
Moderate	14.4% (15/104)	66.7% (10/15)	26.7% (4/15)	6.7% (1/15)
Weak	20.2% (21/104)	33.3% (7/21)	23.8% (5/21)	42.9% (9/21)
Non-biofilm-forming	40.4% (42/104)	16.7% (7/42)	50% (21/42)	33.3% (14/42)

4.2. Biofilm-Forming Capacities of the A. baumannii Isolates

Among the 104 *A. baumannii* isolates studied, 59.6% were biofilm formers, of which 25% were strong biofilm producers, 14.4% were moderate biofilm producers, and 20.2% were weak biofilm. The biofilm control strain *A. baumannii* ATCC19606 was a strong biofilm former. Table 3 summarizes the distribution of biofilm-forming abilities of isolates with various antibiotic susceptibility and biofilm-associated gene profiles. As shown in Table 3, the result reveals that 66.1% of the biofilm-forming isolates were non-MDR strains. In addition, 83.3% of the non-biofilm formers were resistant to multiple antibiotic classes. Overall, these results indicated that the more antibiotic susceptible *A. baumannii* isolates were able to form biofilm than the resistant isolates ($p = 3 \times 10^{-6}$).

The biofilm-forming capacities of each sequence type are also summarized in Figure S1. The results showed that the isolates with the same sequence type had different biofilm-producing capacities, as in the case of ST2028, ST1417, ST195, ST1860, and ST2037.

4.3. Distribution of Biofilm-Associated Virulence Genes in the Clinical A. baumannii Strains

The percentages of *A. baumannii* strains carrying *bap*, *csuE*, *adeFGH*, *ompA*, and *abaI* were 9.6%, 85.6%, 95.2%, 89.4%, and 82.7%, respectively. The relationship between the presence of biofilm-associated genes and biofilm-forming capacities are presented in Table 4. The presence of *bap*, *csuE*, and *abaI* was significantly associated with biofilm-forming capacities of the isolates (*p*-values ranging from 0.005 to 0.033). The results showed that 100% of *bap*-positive isolates were biofilm formers. On the other hand, 55.3% of biofilm formers were *bap*-negative. Based on the results, the presence of *Bap* indicates the strains are biofilm-formers but the reverse is not true. Over 80% of the *csuE*-negative and *abaI*-negative isolates were biofilm formers, but more than 50% biofilm formers carried these two genes. Similar patterns were observed in *adeFGH* and *ompA* but were not statistically significant (*p*-values = 0.07 and 0.193, respectively).

Table 4. Relationship between the presence of biofilm-associated genes and biofilm-forming capacities among the *A. baumannii* isolates.

Biofilm-Associated Gene	Biofilm-Forming No. (%)	Non-Biofilm-Forming No. (%)	*p*-Value
bap			0.005
Positive	10 (100)	0 (0)	
Negative	52 (55.3)	42 (44.7)	
csuE			0.02
Positive	49 (55.1)	40 (44.9)	
Negative	13 (86.7)	2 (13.3)	
adeFGH			0.07
Positive	57 (57.6)	42 (42.4)	
Negative	5 (100.0)	0 (0)	
ompA			0.193
Positive	53 (57)	40 (43)	
Negative	9 (81.8)	2 (18.2)	
abaI			0.033
Positive	47 (54.7)	39 (45.3)	
Negative	15 (83.3)	3 (16.7)	

4.4. Comparison of MIC and MBIC

The MICs and MBICs for colistin, ciprofloxacin, and imipenem were tested against nine different sequence types. These strains were biofilm-forming and susceptible to the three antibiotics being investigated. Antibiotic resistance profiles for biofilm compared to counter-plankton cells are summarized in Table 5. The MBICs increased drastically when compared to those of the planktonic cells. The fold-increase ranged from 2 to 32 fold for colistin, 4 to 64 fold for ciprofloxacin, and 4 to

2048 fold for imipenem. When compared between MICs and MBICs, the average fold-increase was 21, 31, and 386 for colistin, ciprofloxacin, and imipenem, respectively. The susceptibility profiles of most of the strains changed from sensitive to resistant when grown in biofilm state. However, the biofilm formed by ST1990 and ST1417 remained sensitive to ciprofloxacin and imipenem, and biofilm formed by ST1855 remained sensitive to colistin.

Table 5. Antibiotic susceptibility profiles of selected sequence types of *A. baumannii* planktonic and biofilm cells.

MLST	Colistin			Ciprofloxacin			Imipenem		
	MIC for Planktonic Cells (μg/mL)	MBIC for Biofilm Cells (μg/mL)	Fold Change	MIC for planktonic Cells (μg/mL)	MBIC for Biofilm Cells (μg/mL)	Fold Change	MIC for Planktonic Cells (μg/mL)	MBIC for Biofilm Cells (μg/mL)	Fold Change
ST1894	0.5	16	32	1	64	64	0.125	256	2048
ST1990	0.5	8	16	0.5	2	4	0.125	2	16
ST1417	0.25	8	32	0.5	2	4	0.25	4	16
ST1992	2	4	2	0.5	4	8	0.25	32	128
ST373	1	32	32	0.5	16	32	0.25	32	128
ST1862	1	4	4	1	8	8	0.015	8	533.3
ST1964	0.5	16	32	1	64	64	4	16	4
ST1855	0.5	2	4	0.5	16	32	0.015	8	533.3
ST1861 *	0.5	16	32	1	64	64	0.5	32	64

* This strain is *Acinetobacter baumannii* ATCC 19606, the control strain for biofilm assay.

4.5. Comparison of MBC and MBEC

Following the determination of MICs and MBICs, we evaluated the MBCs and MBECs of nine *A. baumannii* isolates. The results showed that the MBECs of the nine isolates have increased. Up to 64-fold increase in the concentration of colistin and up to a 1024-fold increase in the concentration of ciprofloxacin and imipenem was required to eradicate *A. baumannii* biofilm compared to the planktonic cells (Table 6). Although the three strains, ST1990, ST1417, and ST1855, had MBICs falling within the sensitive ranges, the MBECs were much higher than the MBICs (Table 5). When compared between MBCs and MBECs, the average fold-increase was 44, 407, and 364 for colistin, ciprofloxacin, and imipenem, respectively. To visualize the viability of biofilm cells after antibiotic treatment, biofilm preparations of a hyper-biofilm-producing strain ST1894 were treated with antibiotics, stained with a LIVE/DEAD BacLight bacterial viability kit and examined using CLSM. The results showed that viable cells in the biofilm can still be detected even after treating with antibiotics at 32–256 times the MBC (Figure 1). The findings of this study suggest that biofilm-producing strains *A. baumannii* cannot be eradicated with the same concentration of antimicrobials required to eradicate planktonic cells.

Table 6. Comparison of MBC and MBEC of *A. baumannii* of different MLSTs.

MLST	Colistin			Ciprofloxacin			Imipenem		
	MBC for Planktonic Cells (μg/mL)	MBEC for Biofilm Cells (μg/mL)	Fold Change	MBC for Planktonic Cells (μg/mL)	MBEC for Biofilm Cells (μg/mL)	Fold Change	MBC for Planktonic Cells (μg/mL)	MBEC for Biofilm Cells (μg/mL)	Fold Change
ST1894	4	256	64	8	1024	128	4	1024	256
ST1990	0.5	32	64	1	1024	1024	1	64	64
ST1417	1	32	32	2	64	32	0.5	64	128
ST1992	2	8	4	1	1024	1024	1	1024	1024
ST373	4	128	32	32	1024	32	4	32	8
ST1862	2	128	64	2	512	256	1	1024	1024
ST1964	4	256	64	2	32	16	4	512	128
ST1855	0.5	32	64	1	1024	1024	2	1024	512
ST1861 *	4	16	4	8	1024	128	1	128	128

* This strain is *Acinetobacter baumannii* ATCC 19606, the control strain for biofilm assay.

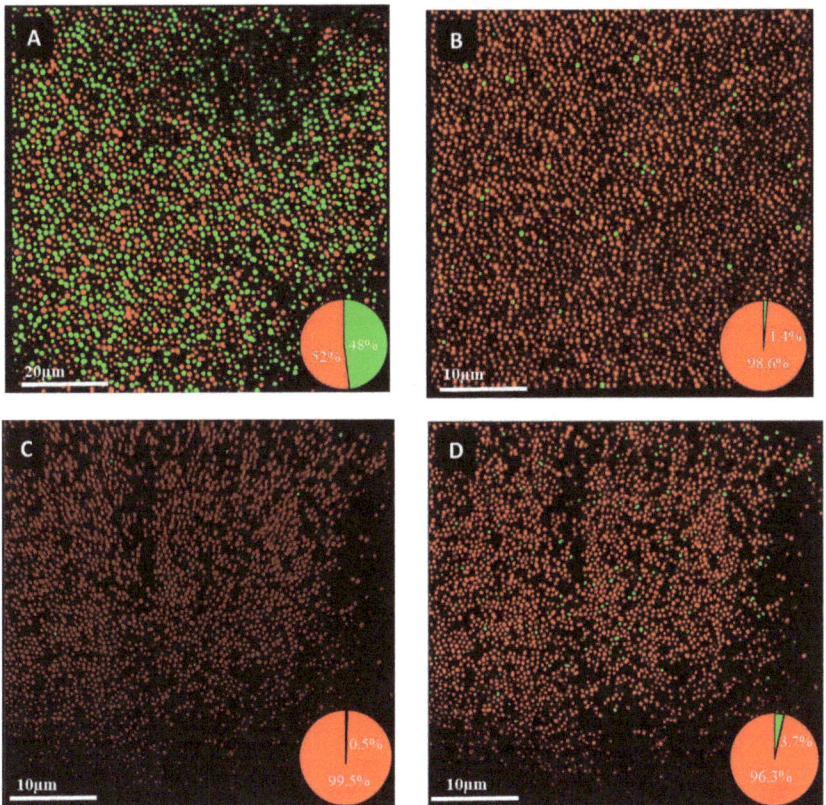

Figure 1. CLSM images of *A. baumannii* ST1894 biofilm treated with bactericidal antibiotics. (**A**) Untreated biofilm cells, (**B**) biofilm treated with 512 μg/mL imipenem, (**C**) biofilm treated with 128 μg/mL colistin, (**D**) biofilm treated with 512 μg/mL ciprofloxacin. Biofilm was incubated with antibiotics at 37 °C for 48 h, which was followed by costaining with propidium iodide (PI) and SYTO 9, and examined under CLSM. Dead cells were stained with PI and appeared red. Viable cells were stained with SYTO 9 and appeared green in color.

4.6. Reversibility of Antibiotic Susceptibility in Planktonic Cells Regrown from Biofilm

Reversibility of antibiotic resistance was analyzed for two non-MDR strains *A. baumannii* ST1894, ST373, and one XDR strain *A. baumannii* ST195. Biofilm cells of the three strains were regrown into the planktonic phase and then treated with colistin, imipenem, and ciprofloxacin. The MIC, MBIC, and MIC of the reverted planktonic cells are summarized in Table 7. The results showed that biofilm cells of *A. baumannii* ST1894 reverted to sensitive phenotype when the strain was regrown into planktonic cells. For *A. baumannii* ST373, reversion to sensitive phenotype occurred in colistin and imipenem but not in ciprofloxacin. This suggests that biofilm cells of that strain might have developed mutation associated with ciprofloxacin resistance. Besides, other mechanisms might be involved, such as mutations in the efflux pumps or regulators of efflux pumps could also lead to ciprofloxacin resistance. *A. baumannii* ST195 was resistant to ciprofloxacin and imipenem but sensitive to colistin. The MICs of the reverted planktonic cells were the same as the MBICs for the three antibiotics. The results showed that the antibiotic susceptibility of the strain did not revert to the original pattern. The level of resistance to ciprofloxacin and imipenem has increased, and the strain did not revert to its sensitive phenotype for colistin. Together the results showed that biofilm formation in *A. baumannii* promotes either antibiotic tolerance that is reversible or the emergence of antibiotics resistance that is irreversible.

Table 7. Reversibility of antibiotic resistance of biofilm cells.

Strain	Biofilm Forming	Colistin			Ciprofloxacin			Imipenem			Reason for Reduced Susceptibility in Biofilm
		MIC	MBIC	MIC of Reverted Planktonic Cells	MIC	MBIC	MIC of Reverted Planktonic Cells	MIC	MBIC	MIC of Reverted Planktonic Cells	
ST1894 Non-MDR	Strong	0.5	16	0.5	1	64	1	0.125	256	0.125	Tolerance
ST373 Non-MDR	Strong	1	32	1	0.5	16	16	0.25	32	0.25	Tolerance or resistant mutant for ciprofloxacin
ST195 XDR	Weak	1	16	16	4	64	64	8	32	32	Resistant mutant

4.7. Isolation of Persister Cells in Planktonic and Biofilm Cells

When *A. baumannii* ST1894 was treated with ciprofloxacin at a concentration equaled 20 times of its MIC, all planktonic cells were eradicated after 16 h of exposure to the antibiotic (Figure 2). However, 100 ± 30 CFU/peg biofilm cells survived after 24-h exposure to ciprofloxacin, which supports our hypothesis that persister cells in the biofilm was one of the reasons for the reduced susceptibility to antibiotics. Besides, these persister cells were responsible for the regrowth of biofilm cells after the cells were treated with antibiotic. Further examination of biofilm using CLSM demonstrated the presence of 1.9% persister cells when the biofilm was treated with ciprofloxacin at concentration of 1024 times of its MIC (Figure 3). Hence, the presence of persister cells in biofilm could be the reason for multidrug tolerance to different classes of antibiotics.

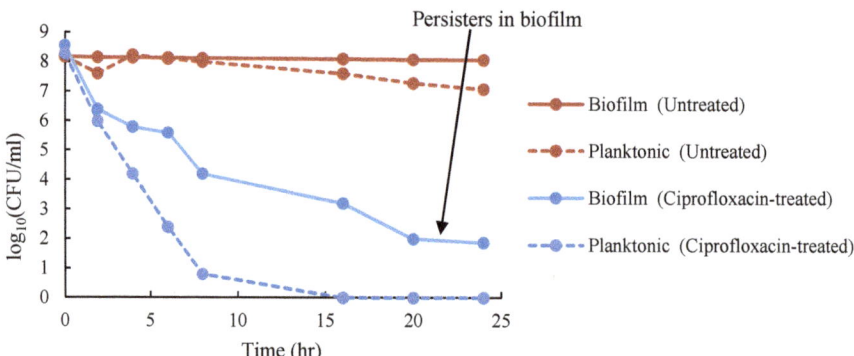

Figure 2. Detection of persisters from biofilm and planktonic cells of *A. baumannii* ST 1894. The number of viable biofilm and planktonic cells at different time points after treatment with 2048 µg/mL ciprofloxacin. Red solid and dotted lines represent untreated biofilm and planktonic cells, respectively. Blue solid and dotted lines represent biofilm and planktonic cells treated with ciprofloxacin, respectively.

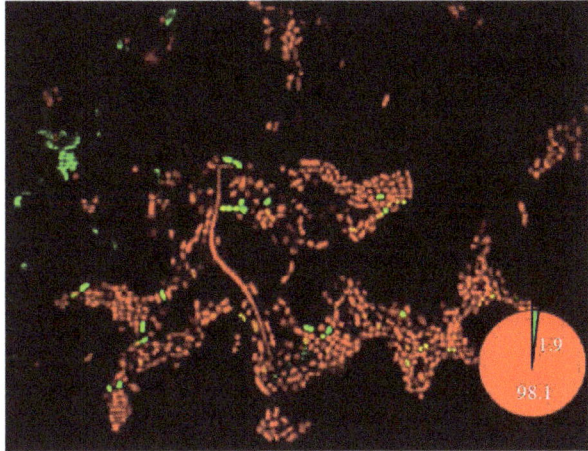

Figure 3. CLSM image of *A. baumannii* ST1894 biofilm treated with ciprofloxacin at 1024 × MIC. Viable bacterial cells in the biofilm was detected by a Live/Dead Biofilm Viability Kit. Persister cells appear green in color, dead cells appear red in color.

5. Discussion

The ability of *A. baumannii* to produce biofilm enhances its survival in adverse environments and increases the risk of healthcare-associated infections. The present study evaluated the biofilm-formation abilities of the clinical *A. baumannii* strains and the role of biofilm production for reduced susceptibility to antibiotics. The result showed that 59.6% of the clinical *A. baumannii* isolates were able to form a biofilm. This result is similar to the findings reported by Anghel et al. that about 63% of *A. baumannii* clinical strains were biofilm producers [26]. Our results showed that the strains with the same sequence types might have different biofilm-producing capacities, as in the case of ST2028, ST1417, ST195, ST1860, and ST2037.

Previous studies have documented that biofilm-forming strains were more resistant to antibiotics than the non-biofilm-forming strains [10,27]. However, in this study, we found that a significantly higher proportion of biofilm-forming isolates were non-MDR strains. Our results indicated an inverse relation between antibiotic resistance and biofilm-forming ability of the isolates. This finding is also in line with other studies that biofilm-forming *A. baumannii* was more susceptible to antibiotics [28,29]. A possible explanation for this might be that biofilm formation ensures the survival of the susceptible strains when exposed to antibiotics. However, the variations in methodologies involved in assessing biofilm formation may lead to different observations among different research groups. A standardized biofilm assay is needed for more objective comparison between different studies.

In this study, we observed that the majority of XDR and PDR *A. baumannii* isolates were weak or non-biofilm producers. The results are in accordance with the recent findings that biofilm-forming isolates exhibited lower rates of carbapenem resistance than the non-biofilm-forming isolates [30,31]. This result may be explained by the fact that energy required for expressing the carbapenemase and β-lactamases might reduce the biofilm formation in the isolates harboring those genes.

We also evaluated the relationship between biofilm-associated virulence genes and biofilm-forming abilities of the *A. baumannii* strains. *bap* was detected in a small proportion of strains tested, and all *bap*-positive strains were biofilm-formers, indicating the role of *Bap* in biofilm formation. It has been documented that *Bap* protein is necessary for mature biofilm formation on various abiotic surfaces; disruption of *Bap* resulted in a reduction of biofilm mass [32]. *csuE*, *adeFGH*, *ompA*, and *abaI* were detected in 82.7–95.2% of the *A. baumannii* strains; almost 50% of these strains were non-biofilm-forming strains. It is, therefore, necessary to compare the expression levels of the biofilm-associated genes in the biofilm producers and non-biofilm producers.

To examine the emergence of antibiotic resistance during biofilm formation, MIC, MBIC, MBC, and MBEC of colistin, ciprofloxacin, and imipenem against nine selected *A. baumannii* strains were studied. These nine strains were non-MDR and strong biofilm formers. The results showed that biofilm cells of the nine strains developed a high-level of antibiotic resistance and required as high as 2048 times the MIC to inhibit the release of planktonic bacterial cells from biofilm or as high as 1024 times the MBC to eradicate the biofilm cells. Among the three antibiotics tested, imipenem had a high average fold-increase in both MBIC (386-fold) and MBEC (364-fold). As imipenem is uncharged and can penetrate the negatively charged biofilm matrix, thus, the high level of imipenem resistance was unlikely due to poor penetration. Resistance could be a result of the expression of β-lactamase, as a previous study reported that the activity of the β-lactamase promoter was elevated in biofilm cells of *Pseudomonas aeruginosa* [33]. Other possibilities for the emergence of imipenem resistance in the biofilm include the expression of the drug efflux system *adeFGH*, which is involved in the synthesis and transportation of autoinducer molecules during biofilm formation [14].

Ciprofloxacin had much higher fold-increase in MBEC than that in MBIC (407-fold vs. 31-fold), as ciprofloxacin is actively against metabolically active bacterial cells [34], it will be more difficult to eradicate persister cells developed in the biofilm, which are metabolically dormant. Colistin had the lowest average fold-increase in MBIC (21-fold) and MBEC (44-fold) compared to imipenem and ciprofloxacin. Studies also showed that colistin is effective against the metabolically inactive bacterial population in the biofilm [34]. Another study also showed that the bactericidal activity of colistin increased under anaerobic conditions, as the bactericidal action of the antibiotic was independent of the hydroxyl radical formed during aerobic respiration [34]. Overall, *A. baumannii* developed antibiotic resistance during biofilm formation, and the level of biofilm-specific resistance varied according to the induced responses of the biofilm population and the action mechanisms of the antibiotics.

CLSM images of a non-MDR *A. baumannii* ST1984 strain showed that 0.5%–3.7% of biofilm cells were viable after treatment with colistin, ciprofloxacin, and imipenem at 256–4096 times the MICs of these antibiotics. It is possible that the percentages of viable cells were higher because the presence of extracellular DNA in the biofilm might be stained by the propidium iodide stain and lead to an overestimation of dead cell proportions. The presence of persister cells is worrisome since colistin is the last resort for treatment of MDR *A. baumannii*, the emergence of biofilm-specific resistance makes the pathogen untreatable with the conventional antibiotics.

Although Qi et al. have reported the enhancement of antibiotic resistance by biofilm formation [28], our study investigated the reversibility of antibiotic resistance developed in the biofilm. We re-grew the biofilm cells to planktonic state and assessed the changes in MICs in three *A. baumannii* strains. Our novel findings demonstrated that reversion from resistant to susceptible occurred in two non-MDR strains but not in the XDR strain. Such a transient increase in antibiotic resistance in the non-MDR strains was due to the tolerance of antibiotics by the biofilm cells. There are multiple mechanisms involved in the development of antibiotic tolerance in biofilm. The reduced metabolic activity of biofilm and induction of stress responses due to the limitation of nutrients in the biofilm environment triggers antibiotic tolerance [35]. The presence of persister cells in the biofilm population activates the toxin/antitoxin systems, which leads to inhibition of protein translation, initiation of dormancy, and tolerance to antibiotics [36]. In this study, we demonstrated the presence of persister cells in *A. baumannii* strain ST1894, one of the two non-MDR strains, using CLSM imaging and persister cell isolation after treating with a high concentration of ciprofloxacin. The presence of persister cells made the pathogen extremely multidrug tolerant and could eventually lead to the emergence of antibiotic resistance. For the XDR strain (*A. baumannii* ST195), the planktonic cells regrown from biofilm cells exhibited a higher level of antibiotic resistance. This could be caused by mutations of drug targets upon exposure to high antibiotic concentrations. There are two noteworthy issues regarding this XDR strain. First, irreversible colistin resistance was developed during biofilm formation, making the physicians barehanded to treat the infected patients. Second, although the strain was a weak biofilm former, high-level of irreversible antibiotic resistance was enhanced during biofilm formation. Detailed investigation at the genetic level is needed to understand the underlying regulatory mechanisms involved in the emergence of biofilm-mediated antibiotic resistance.

6. Conclusions

We showed a negative relationship between biofilm-forming capacity and antibiotic susceptibility, in which the strong biofilm-formers were non-MDR strains. We also demonstrated the presence of persisters in the biofilm cells, which accounted for reduced susceptibilities of the *A. baumannii* strains. Another important finding was that growth in biofilm induced reversible antibiotic tolerance in the non-MDR strains but a higher level of irreversible resistance in the XDR strain, including the conversion from colistin sensitive to resistant. To address the regulatory mechanisms of biofilm-specific resistance, research should be undertaken to investigate the alterations at the genome and transcription levels of *A. baumannii* grown in biofilm status. A thorough understanding of the various contributing factors facilitates the design of new therapeutics that target biofilm-specific resistance.

Supplementary Materials: The following are available online at http://www.mdpi.com/2079-6382/9/11/817/s1, Figure S1: Biofilm-producing abilities and antibiotic susceptibility profiles of *A. baumannii* strains with different MLSTs, Table S1: Primers used for amplification of biofilm-associated genes.

Author Contributions: Conceptualization, A.M.S. and P.H.-m.L.; methodology, A.M.S. and M.Z.Y.; validation, A.M.S.; formal analysis, A.M.S.; investigation, A.M.S. and M.Z.Y.; resources, G.K.-h.S. and B.K.C.W.; writing—original draft preparation, A.M.S.; writing—review and editing, P.H.-m.L.; visualization, A.M.S. and P.H.-m.L.; supervision, P.H.-m.L.; project administration, P.H.-m.L.; funding acquisition, P.H.-m.L. All authors have read and agreed to the published version of the manuscript.

Funding: A.M. Shenkutie is supported by the Hong Kong Fellowship Scheme PH16-01625.

Acknowledgments: The CLSM imaging was performed at the Hong Kong Polytechnic University Research Facility in Life Sciences with the support of Clara H.L. Hung.

Conflicts of Interest: The authors declare no conflict of interest.

References

1. Fournier, P.E.; Richet, H.; Weinstein, R.A. The epidemiology and control of *Acinetobacter baumannii* in health care facilities. *Clin. Infect. Dis.* **2006**, *42*, 692–699. [CrossRef] [PubMed]
2. World Health Organization. WHO Priority Pathogens List for R&D of New Antibiotics. Available online: https://www.who.int/en/news-room/detail/27-02-2017-who-publishes-list-of-bacteria-forwhich-new-antibiotics-are-urgently-needed (accessed on 10 August 2020).
3. Piperaki, E.T.; Tzouvelekis, L.; Miriagou, V.; Daikos, G. Carbapenem-resistant *Acinetobacter baumannii*: In pursuit of an effective treatment. *Clin. Microbiol. Infect.* **2019**, *25*, 951–957. [CrossRef] [PubMed]
4. Ho, P.L.; Wu, T.C.; Chao, D.V.K.; Hung, I.F.N.; Liu, L.; Lung, D.C. *Reducing Bacterial Resistance with IMPACT*, 5th ed.; Centre for Health Protection: Hong Kong, China, 2017.
5. Niu, T.; Guo, L.; Luo, Q.; Zhou, K.; Yu, W.; Chen, Y.; Huang, C.; Xiao, Y. Wza gene knockout decreases *Acinetobacter baumannii* virulence and affects *wzy*-dependent capsular polysaccharide synthesis. *Virulence* **2020**, *11*, 1–13. [CrossRef] [PubMed]
6. Leung, E.C.M.; Leung, P.H.M.; Lai, R.W. Emergence of carbapenem-resistant *Acinetobacter baumannii* ST195 harboring bla_{Oxa-23} isolated from bacteremia in Hong Kong. *Microb. Drug Resist.* **2019**, *25*, 1199–1203. [CrossRef] [PubMed]
7. Cheng, V.C.; Wong, S.; Chen, J.H.; So, S.Y.; Wong, S.C.; Ho, P.L.; Yuen, K.Y. Control of multidrug-resistant *Acinetobacter baumannii* in Hong Kong: Role of environmental surveillance in communal areas after a hospital outbreak. *Am. J. Infect. Control* **2018**, *46*, 60–66. [CrossRef]
8. Gaddy, J.A.; Tomaras, A.P.; Actis, L.A. The *Acinetobacter baumannii* 19606 OmpA protein plays a role in biofilm formation on abiotic surfaces and in the interaction of this pathogen with eukaryotic cells. *Infect. Immun.* **2009**, *77*, 3150–3160. [CrossRef]

9. Donlan, R.M.; Costerton, J.W. Biofilms: Survival mechanisms of clinically relevant microorganisms. *Clin. Microbiol. Rev.* **2002**, *15*, 167–193. [CrossRef]
10. Yang, C.H.; Su, P.W.; Moi, S.H.; Chuang, L.Y. Biofilm formation in *Acinetobacter baumannii*: Genotype-phenotype correlation. *Molecules* **2019**, *24*, 1849. [CrossRef]
11. Burmølle, M.; Webb, J.S.; Rao, D.; Hansen, L.H.; Sørensen, S.J.; Kjelleberg, S. Enhanced biofilm formation and increased resistance to antimicrobial agents and bacterial invasion are caused by synergistic interactions in multispecies biofilms. *Appl. Environ. Microbiol.* **2006**, *72*, 3916–3923. [CrossRef]
12. Loehfelm, T.W.; Luke, N.R.; Campagnari, A.A. Identification and characterization of an *Acinetobacter baumannii* biofilm-associated protein. *J. Bacteriol.* **2008**, *190*, 1036–1044. [CrossRef]
13. Tomaras, A.P.; Dorsey, C.W.; Edelmann, R.E.; Actis, L.A. Attachment to and biofilm formation on abiotic surfaces by *Acinetobacter baumannii*: Involvement of a novel chaperone-usher pili assembly system. *Microbiology* **2003**, *149*, 3473–3484. [CrossRef] [PubMed]
14. He, X.; Lu, F.; Yuan, F.; Jiang, D.; Zhao, P.; Zhu, J.; Cheng, H.; Cao, J.; Lu, G. Biofilm formation caused by clinical *Acinetobacter baumannii* isolates is associated with overexpression of the *adeFGH* efflux pump. *Antimicrob. Agents Chemother.* **2015**, *59*, 4817–4825. [CrossRef] [PubMed]
15. Peleg, A.Y.; Seifert, H.; Paterson, D.L. *Acinetobacter baumannii*: Emergence of a successful pathogen. *Clin. Microbiol. Rev.* **2008**, *21*, 538–582. [CrossRef] [PubMed]
16. Visca, P.; Seifert, H.; Towner, K.J. *Acinetobacter* infection–an emerging threat to human health. *IUBMB Life* **2011**, *63*, 1048–1054. [CrossRef]
17. Chen, T.L.; Lee, Y.T.; Kuo, S.C.; Yang, S.P.; Fung, C.P.; Lee, S.D. Rapid identification of *Acinetobacter baumannii*, *Acinetobacter nosocomialis* and *Acinetobacter pittii* with a multiplex PCR assay. *J. Med. Microbiol.* **2014**, *63*, 1154–1159. [CrossRef]
18. Bartual, S.G.; Seifert, H.; Hippler, C.; Luzon, M.A.D.; Wisplinghoff, H.; Rodríguez-Valera, F. Development of a multilocus sequence typing scheme for characterization of clinical isolates of *Acinetobacter baumannii*. *J. Clin. Microbiol.* **2005**, *43*, 4382–4390. [CrossRef]
19. Ceri, H.; Olson, M.; Stremick, C.; Read, R.; Morck, D.; Buret, A. The Calgary biofilm device: New technology for rapid determination of antibiotic susceptibilities of bacterial biofilms. *J. Clin. Microbiol.* **1999**, *37*, 1771–1776. [CrossRef]
20. Stepanović, S.; Vuković, D.; Dakić, I.; Savić, B.; Švabić-Vlahović, M. A Modified microtiter-plate test for quantification of staphylococcal biofilm formation. *J. Microbiol. Methods* **2000**, *40*, 175–179. [CrossRef]
21. CLSI. *Performance Standards for Antimicrobial Susceptibility Testing*, 27th ed.; Clinical and Laboratory Standards Institute: Wayne, PA, USA, 2019.
22. Manchanda, V.; Sanchaita, S.; Singh, N. Multidrug resistant *Acinetobacter*. *J. Glob. Infect. Dis.* **2010**, *2*, 291. [CrossRef]
23. Moskowitz, S.M.; Foster, J.M.; Emerson, J.; Burns, J.L. Clinically feasible biofilm susceptibility assay for isolates of *Pseudomonas aeruginosa* from patients with cystic fibrosis. *J. Clin. Microbiol.* **2004**, *42*, 1915–1922. [CrossRef]
24. Bogachev, M.I.; Volkov, V.Y.; Markelov, O.A.; Trizna, E.Y.; Baydamshina, D.R.; Melnikov, V.; Murtazina, R.R.; Zelenikhin, P.V.; Sharafutdinov, I.S.; Kayumov, A.R. Fast and simple tool for the quantification of biofilm-embedded cells sub-populations from fluorescent microscopic images. *PLoS ONE* **2018**, *13*, e0193267. [CrossRef] [PubMed]
25. Marques, C.N. Isolation of persister cells from biofilm and planktonic populations of *Pseudomonas aeruginosa*. *Bio-Protocol* **2015**, *5*, e1590. [CrossRef]
26. Anghel, I.; Chifiriuc, M.C.; Anghel, G.A. Pathogenic features and therapeutical implications of biofilm development ability in microbial strains isolated from rhinologic chronic infections. *Farmacia* **2011**, *59*, 770–783.
27. Babapour, E.; Haddadi, A.; Mirnejad, R.; Angaji, S.A.; Amirmozafari, N. Biofilm formation in clinical isolates of nosocomial *Acinetobacter baumannii* and its relationship with multidrug resistance. *Asian Pac. J. Trop. Biomed.* **2016**, *6*, 528–533. [CrossRef]
28. Qi, L.; Li, H.; Zhang, C.; Liang, B.; Li, J.; Wang, L.; Du, X.; Liu, X.; Qiu, S.; Song, H. Relationship between antibiotic resistance, biofilm formation, and biofilm-specific resistance in *Acinetobacter baumannii*. *Front. Microbiol.* **2016**, *7*, 483. [CrossRef] [PubMed]

29. Rodríguez-Baño, J.; Marti, S.; Soto, S.; Fernández-Cuenca, F.; Cisneros, J.M.; Pachón, J.; Pascual, A.; Martínez-Martínez, L.; McQueary, C.; Actis, L. Biofilm formation in *Acinetobacter baumannii*: Associated features and clinical implications. *Clin. Microbiol. Infect.* **2008**, *14*, 276–278. [CrossRef]
30. Wang, Y.C.; Huang, T.W.; Yang, Y.S.; Kuo, S.C.; Chen, C.T.; Liu, C.P.; Liu, Y.M.; Chen, T.L.; Chang, F.Y.; Wu, S.H. Biofilm formation is not associated with worse outcome in *Acinetobacter baumannii* bacteraemic pneumonia. *Sci. Rep.* **2018**, *8*, 7289. [CrossRef]
31. Perez, L.R.R. *Acinetobacter baumannii* displays inverse relationship between meropenem resistance and biofilm production. *J. Chemother.* **2015**, *27*, 13–16. [CrossRef]
32. Brossard, K.A.; Campagnari, A.A. The *Acinetobacter baumannii* biofilm-associated protein plays a role in adherence to human epithelial cells. *Infect. Immun.* **2012**, *80*, 228–233. [CrossRef]
33. Bagge, N.; Hentzer, M.; Andersen, J.B.; Ciofu, O.; Givskov, M.; Høiby, N. Dynamics and spatial distribution of β-lactamase expression in *Pseudomonas aeruginosa* biofilms. *Antimicrob. Agents. Chemother.* **2004**, *48*, 1168–1174. [CrossRef]
34. Pamp, S.J.; Gjermansen, M.; Johansen, H.K.; Tolker-Nielsen, T. Tolerance to the antimicrobial peptide colistin in *Pseudomonas aeruginosa* biofilms is linked to metabolically active cells, and depends on the pmr and *mexAB-oprM* genes. *Mol. Microbiol.* **2008**, *68*, 223–240. [CrossRef] [PubMed]
35. Bernier, S.P.; Lebeaux, D.; DeFrancesco, A.S.; Valomon, A.; Soubigou, G.; Coppée, J.Y.; Ghigo, J.M.; Beloin, C. Starvation, together with the sos response, mediates high biofilm-specific tolerance to the fluoroquinolone ofloxacin. *PLoS Genet.* **2013**, *9*, e1003144. [CrossRef] [PubMed]
36. Page, R.; Peti, W. Toxin-antitoxin systems in bacterial growth arrest and persistence. *Nat. Chem. Biol.* **2016**, *12*, 208–214. [CrossRef] [PubMed]

Publisher's Note: MDPI stays neutral with regard to jurisdictional claims in published maps and institutional affiliations.

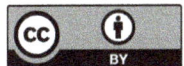

© 2020 by the authors. Licensee MDPI, Basel, Switzerland. This article is an open access article distributed under the terms and conditions of the Creative Commons Attribution (CC BY) license (http://creativecommons.org/licenses/by/4.0/).

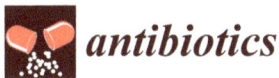

Article

Increased Intraspecies Diversity in *Escherichia coli* Biofilms Promotes Cellular Growth at the Expense of Matrix Production

Andreia S. Azevedo [1,2,3,4,*,†], Gislaine P. Gerola [1,†], João Baptista [1,†], Carina Almeida [1,2,5], Joana Peres [1], Filipe J. Mergulhão [1] and Nuno F. Azevedo [1]

1. LEPABE-Laboratory for Process Engineering, Environment, Biotechnology and Energy, Faculty of Engineering, University of Porto, 4200-465 Porto, Portugal; gislainepassarela@hotmail.com (G.P.G.); joaobaptista11023@gmail.com (J.B.); carina.almeida@iniav.pt (C.A.); jperes@fe.up.pt (J.P.); filipem@fe.up.pt (F.J.M.); nazevedo@fe.up.pt (N.F.A.)
2. Laboratório de Investigação em Biofilmes Rosário Oliveira, Centre of Biological Engineering, University of Minho Braga, 4710-057 Braga, Portugal
3. i3S-Instituto de Investigação e Inovação em Saúde, Universidade do Porto, 4200-135 Porto, Portugal
4. IPATIMUP-Instituto de Patologia e Imunologia Molecular, Universidade do Porto, 4200-135 Porto, Portugal
5. INIAV, IP-National Institute for Agrarian and Veterinary Research, Vairão, 4485-655 Vila Do Conde, Portugal
* Correspondence: asazevedo@fe.up.pt; Tel.: +351-2250-8158; Fax: +351-225-081-449
† These authors contributed equally to this work.

Received: 19 June 2020; Accepted: 14 November 2020; Published: 17 November 2020

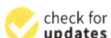

Abstract: Intraspecies diversity in biofilm communities is associated with enhanced survival and growth of the individual biofilm populations. Studies on the subject are scarce, namely, when more than three strains are present. Hence, in this study, the influence of intraspecies diversity in biofilm populations composed of up to six different *Escherichia coli* strains isolated from urine was evaluated in conditions mimicking the ones observed in urinary tract infections and catheter-associated urinary tract infections. In general, with the increasing number of strains in a biofilm, an increase in cell cultivability and a decrease in matrix production were observed. For instance, single-strain biofilms produced an average of 73.1 µg·cm^{-2} of extracellular polymeric substances (EPS), while six strains biofilms produced 19.9 µg·cm^{-2}. Hence, it appears that increased genotypic diversity in a biofilm leads *E. coli* to direct energy towards the production of its offspring, in detriment of the production of public goods (i.e., matrix components). Apart from ecological implications, these results can be explored as another strategy to reduce the biofilm burden, as a decrease in EPS matrix production may render these intraspecies biofilms more sensitive to antimicrobial agents.

Keywords: biofilms; *Escherichia coli*; intraspecies community; EPS matrix; peptide nucleic acid-fluorescence in situ hybridization; urinary tract infections; catheter-associated urinary tract infections; confocal laser scanning microscopy

1. Introduction

Microorganisms live in a wide variety of environments usually enclosed in communities attached to a surface. This type of community behavior can evolve towards complex multicellular structures, termed biofilms [1–3]. These are aggregates of microbial cells embedded in a matrix of extracellular polymeric substances (EPS) that provide several survival advantages, namely, nutrient capture, enzyme retention and resistance/tolerance to antimicrobial agents [4]. Within these structures, bacteria are highly sociable, communicating with each other by secreting important molecules (e.g., cell-signaling molecules, toxins and matrix components), leading to complex interactions during biofilm development [5,6]. This social environment may involve cooperation, competition, or even both.

Microbial competition can manifest as a response to space and nutrient limitation [7,8]. During microbial competition, microorganisms can inhibit the growth of and even kill neighboring cells by secreting broad-spectrum antibiotics [9] or secreting virulent proteins and toxins [10]. However, cooperation is also very prevalent in biofilm communities [11]. For instance, microorganisms can interact to increase their resistance, increasing the tolerance of the whole consortium to antimicrobial agents [12,13], or to enhance the biofilm-forming potential of the consortium [14]. In addition, metabolic cooperation and cross-feeding have been proven to increase the overall fitness of biofilms [15,16].

Another interesting theory adapted to the microbial world and, in particular, to the biofilm field, is the "public goods" dilemma [17–19]. This theory is based on the observation that, when in society, some bacteria cooperate by secreting a product/resource that becomes available to neighboring bacteria and, hence, benefits the overall consortium. Other bacteria, named cheaters, exploit the "public goods" without contributing for its production, leaving the metabolic burden of synthesizing these molecules to the producing bacteria [20]. Hence, cheaters are likely to outcompete the "public goods" producers and decrease the overall fitness of the consortium [21].

While several examples of cooperation can be found in the biofilm literature for interspecies biofilms, there are far fewer studies with intraspecies biofilms [22–24]. Moreover, and to the authors' knowledge, the number of strains assessed in intraspecies biofilms has always been lower than three. This begs the question: is there a maximum number of strains after which a cooperative behavior in intraspecies biofilms is no longer observed? To answer this question, and as a case study, we formed intraspecies biofilms with up to six strains of *Escherichia coli* isolates from urine, and analyzed their biofilm-forming ability under conditions mimicking the urinary tract infections (UTIs) and catheter-associated urinary tract infections (CAUTIs); UTIs are the most common type of healthcare-associated infection reported. Approximately 75% of hospital-acquired UTIs are associated with CAUTIs [25].

To assess cooperative or competitive behavior, the phylogenetic relatedness between the six *E. coli* strains was investigated and correlated to their performance as biofilm producers. As the self-produced EPS matrix is the most recognizable "public good" under the microbial biofilm context [15], the EPS production was grouped according to the number of strains present in the biofilm, as an indicator of social behavior. Additionally, the spatial location of species within the biofilm architecture was determined by employing a multiplex peptide nucleic acid fluorescence in situ hybridization (PNA-FISH) and confocal laser scanning microscopy (CLSM) analysis.

2. Results and Discussion

2.1. Single- and Multi-Strain Biofilm Growth

This work started with the expectation that related strains would cooperate in a biofilm consortium. However, the stage of biofilm development when this behavior, if existent, would occur, was not easily predictable. Moreover, inter-experimental variability in biofilm formation could overshadow the expected changes in metabolism. To increase the chances of picking up this behavior, 63 biofilm growth experiments (Table S1) were conducted, generating an equal number of biofilm growth curves for cultivable cell counts (Figure S1) and total biomass (Figure S2). We then calculated and compared the areas below the curves of the biofilm growth from 0 to 48 h using the trapezium rule [26,27] for both cultivable cell numbers (Figure 1a) and total biomass (Figure 1b).

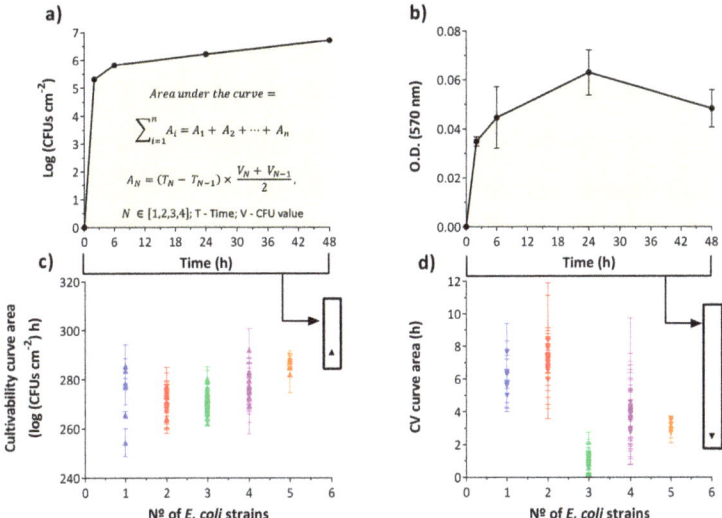

Figure 1. Biofilm formation profiles exhibited by the combination of *Escherichia coli* strains during 48 h, at 37 °C in AUM (artificial urine medium). Example of calculation of the area under the curve for cultivability (**a**) and total biomass (**b**). Cultivability areas showing a relationship between the number of cultivable cells and the number of strains within the biofilm (**c**). CV (crystal violet) areas show a trend of biomass reduction as the number of different strains within the biofilm increases (**d**). The results represent three independent experiments. Results are presented as the mean ± standard deviation. A—partial area; T—time; V—Log (CFUs·cm^{-2}) value or O.D.620 nm value.

For all consortia, from 2 h to 48 h, the cultivable cell counts significantly increased over time ($p < 0.05$). In particular, for single-strain biofilms, CFUs counts averaged from 3.6 log CFUs·cm^{-2} at 2 h to 6.5 log CFUs·cm^{-2} at 48 h ($p < 0.05$) (Figure S1a). However, for consortia of 1, 3 and 4 strains there was not a significant difference from 24 h to 48 h in terms of cultivability ($p > 0.05$), i.e., a stationary growth phase seemed to be reached. Concerning the 6 strains biofilm, CFUs counts averaged at 2 h, 5.3 log CFUs·cm^{-2}, significantly increased to 6.2 log CFUs·cm^{-2} at 24 h, and 6.7 log CFUs·cm^{-2} at 48 h, ($p < 0.05$) (Figure S1f).

When plotting the number of cultivable cells with the number of strains present in the biofilm (Figure 1c), an increase in the number of strains was accompanied with a slight increase in the number of cultivable cells. Nevertheless, there is no statistically significant difference between the cultivability of 1, 2 and 3 strains consortia ($p > 0.05$). Biofilms composed of 5 and 6 strains are statistically different from 1, 2 and 3 strains consortia ($p < 0.05$). While a slight increase in the number of cultivable cells might have been expected, since the number of cells in the initial suspension also increased with the number of strains, the total produced biomass decreased in general with an increase in the number of strains, particularly for biofilms composed of more than two strains (Figure 1d). In fact, the total biomass significantly decreased when comparing 1 and 2 strains consortia to the remaining biofilms ($p < 0.05$). This behavior is evident comparing the average optical density (O.D.$_{620\ nm}$) of 0.245 for single-strain and 0.048 for six-strains at 48 h ($p < 0.05$) (Figure S2). Still, an unexpected higher decrease was obtained for biofilms composed of three strains, not confirmed in later EPS quantification, which can evidence that loosely attached biofilm could have been dragged out during washing steps (i.e., EPS production still occurred but the physico-chemical forces of attachment to the surface was weaker).

For biofilms up to 5 strains, from 2 h to 48 h, the produced biomass significantly increased with time ($p < 0.05$) (Figure S2). However, when six strains were present, a significant increase in biomass production over time was not observed ($p > 0.05$) (Figure S2f). In addition, the biomass seemed to decrease for the 3 strains consortia during the incubation period ($p < 0.05$) (Figure S2c).

2.2. Biomass and Matrix Production as a Function of the Number of Strains in a Consortium

A cluster analysis (Figure 2) was conducted to provide a statistical basis on the observation that an increasing number of strains in a biofilm would affect its behavior, plotting the cultivable cell counts versus total biomass (Figure 2a) and versus EPS matrix (Figure 2b). Overall, a higher number of strains led to a lower amount of biomass production ($p < 0.05$). In particular, two strains biofilms were mainly clustered as low cell numbers and high biomass producers. Biofilms composed by three strains were clustered as very low biomass producers, contradicting the overall behavior. Biofilms composed by 4, 5 and 6 strains were clustered as high cell numbers and low biomass producers (Figure 2a).

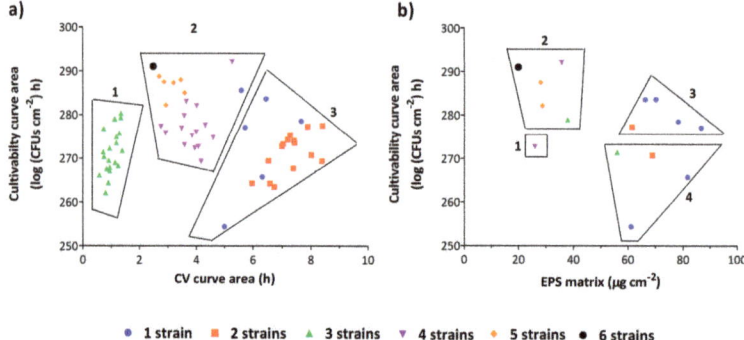

Figure 2. Cluster analysis for cultivability areas versus CV areas (**a**) and for cultivability areas versus EPS (extracellular polymeric substances) matrix (**b**) for 48 h-aged biofilms. Clusters are observable according to the number of strains in consortia. A trend for multi-strain biofilms to produce less EPS matrix is noticeable. The graph (**a**) is subdivided in three clusters: low cell numbers and biomass (1); high cell numbers and low biomass (2); low cell numbers and high biomass (3). The graph (**b**) is subdivided in four clusters: low cell numbers and EPS matrix (1); high cell numbers and low EPS matrix (2); high cell numbers and EPS matrix (3) and low cell numbers and high EPS matrix (4). The results represent three independent experiments. Results are presented as the mean.

To confirm these clusters, the EPS matrix was quantified for a subset of biofilms. Analyzing the clusters (Figure 2b), there is a tendency for multi-strain biofilms to produce less EPS matrix than single-strain biofilms. Biofilms composed by one and two strains were clustered as high EPS producers while biofilms with 4, 5 and 6 strains grouped as high cell numbers and low EPS producers. In fact, the produced EPS matrix decreased almost linearly with the increase in the number of strains in the consortia (Figure S3). Interestingly, for biofilms composed of three strains, the above-mentioned low biomass production was not confirmed by EPS matrix quantification by dry weight after lyophilization (Figure 2b).

Overall, this work shows that an increase in the number of *E. coli* strains in an intraspecies biofilm redirects the metabolism of the microorganisms towards offspring production at the expense of EPS matrix. However, more work is required in the future with other relevant bacterial species and other biofilm growth conditions (e.g., media culture, surfaces, hydrodynamic conditions) to investigate if the observed intraspecies phenomenon presented in this study is maintained.

2.3. How Long Does It Take for Microorganisms to Adapt Their Metabolism?

To better understand when the metabolism of the microorganisms is directed towards cell growth rather than EPS matrix production during biofilm growth, a cluster analysis for each of the time intervals of the experiment was performed (Figure 3). It is clear that, for 2 h-old biofilms, the trend for multi-strain biofilms to produce less biomass can already be observed (Figure 3a).

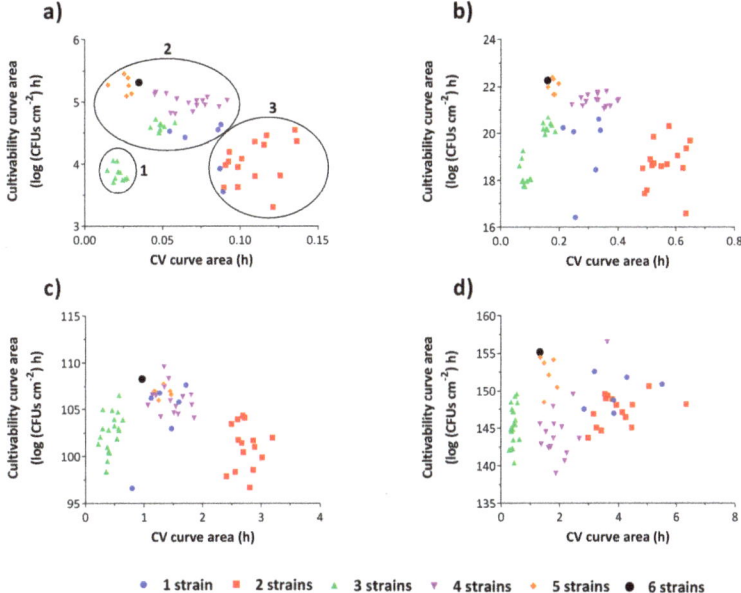

Figure 3. Cluster analysis for cultivability areas versus CV areas for each time point of the experiments: 0–2 h (**a**), 2–6 h (**b**), 6–24 h (**c**) and 24–48 h (**d**). The clustering phenomenon is more evident during the first hours of biofilm development, namely up to 24 h of growth. The graph (**a**) is subdivided in three clusters: low cell numbers and biomass (1); high cell numbers and low biomass (2); low cell numbers and high biomass (3). The results represent the mean of three independent experiments.

In fact, as the biofilm matures, the biofilm clustering according to the number of strains starts to be less evident (Figure 3c,d). After two hours of biofilm growth, two strains biofilms were clustered as low cell numbers and high biomass producers, while biofilms composed by 4, 5 and 6 strains and most of the biofilms composed by 1 strain were grouped as high cell numbers and low biomass producers. This behavior is maintained for the subsequent time points, with the exception of most of the biofilms composed by 4 strains which present low cell numbers after 48 h of growth. Interestingly, after 2 h, some of the three strains biofilms are grouped together with 4 strains biofilms. It is only afterwards that they develop the less expected behavior of very low biomass production. These results indicate that the differentiated behavior occurs predominantly within the first hours of biofilm development, which is expected. In fact, *E. coli* is known to rapidly direct its metabolism when adapting to diverse and sudden stress conditions [28,29]. In a study of Drazic et al. [30], major changes in the metabolic profile of *E. coli* occurred as early as after 5 min of hypochlorite-induced stress, in terms of relative concentrations of fatty acids, amino acids, acetic and formic acid, which were readily regenerated after 40 to 60 min.

2.4. Impact of Phylogenetic Closeness in Biomass Production for Two-Strain Biofilms

In theory, the microbial cooperation is promoted by high relatedness of microbial cells. To infer on this, seven housekeeping genes (*adk*, *fumC*, *gyrB*, *icd*, *mdh*, *purA* and *recA*) were sequenced in order to infer whether genetic similarity among the strains would impact the offspring and total biomass production of the overall consortia, according to the $\sum Cb_I$. According to this analysis, the percentage of different nucleotides among these isolates is below 1.8%. In a study of Lukjancenko et al. [31], the highest phylogenetic difference obtained, when comparing several *E. coli* strains using the same housekeeping genes, was around 2%, which seems to be in agreement with our findings.

Due to the lack of adequate methods to statistically assess the phylogenetic closeness impact of several strains in biofilm formation, only two-strain biofilms were analyzed. Urinary isolates (UI) 1, UI2 and UI6 present very low genetic variability between each other. UI4 and UI5 are also genetically similar. UI3 is the most genetically distant within these strains of *E. coli* (Figure 4a). The impact of the phylogeny was then assessed in terms of biofilm biomass (Figure 4b) and cell production (Figure 4c).

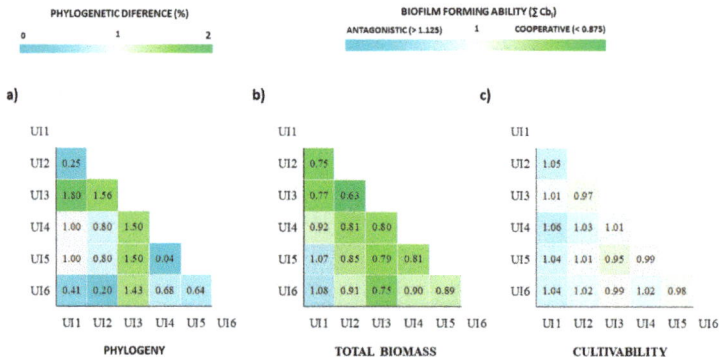

Figure 4. Heat maps showing the phylogenetic differences between the *E. coli* urinary isolates in percentage (**a**) and their biofilm-forming ability when combined with each other in pairs (**b**,**c**). Phylogenetic percentages were calculated using the different nucleotides in the 7 housekeeping genes between the six *E. coli* strains, based in the neighbor-joining method and pairwise distance. The biofilm-forming ability of the combined consortia was scored in terms of total produced biomass (**b**) and cultivability (**c**) according to the $\sum$ Combinatorial biofilm index ($\sum Cb_I$ scoring: cooperative (<0.875), neutral (0.875 < $\sum Cb_I$ < 1.125) and antagonistic (>1.125)] for 0–48 h period of biofilm formation. This analysis on total biomass suggests that both high and low phylogenetic distance between the strains can be accompanied with an increase in the produced biomass, namely, when UI3, the most distant, was paired with all the remaining, as well as when related strains (UI1 with UI2; UI4 with UI5) were combined. All the pairs in terms of cultivability were scored as neutral.

The biomass and cultivability of the biofilms were scored as cooperative, neutral or antagonistic according to the $\sum$ Combinatorial biofilm index ($\sum Cb_I$). Interestingly, in terms of total biomass, all the combinations of the UI3 (the most distant) with the remaining were scored as cooperative (0.63 < $\sum Cb_I$ < 0.80). Still, the combinations of related strains such as UI1 with UI2 as well as UI4 with UI5 were also scored as cooperative. This analysis suggests that both high and low phylogenetic distance between the strains can be accompanied with an increase in the produced biomass. A neutral score is obtained when analyzing the $\sum$ Cbi for all the consortia in terms of cultivability (Figure 4c). From this analysis, it appears that for two-strains biofilms, the phylogenetic relatedness is inversely proportional to the biomass production ability of the two-strain consortium. An open question remains on whether this behavior will still be observed when more than two-strain biofilms are analyzed in the future.

2.5. Spatial Organization of Biofilms Using PNA-FISH Combined with CLSM

It has been demonstrated that microorganisms locate and organize themselves within biofilms according to the nature of their microbial interactions. In general, microorganisms organize in three main forms: a segregation form associated with competition, a co-aggregation/intermixing structure related with cooperation and a layering arrangement found in cooperative or competitive behavior [32].

In the present study, to better understand the behavior between the strains, a multiplex PNA-FISH combined with CLSM was performed for the analysis of the spatial distribution of *E. coli* multi-strain biofilms. First, the hybridization of the PNA probes was previously optimized in terms of temperature and formamide concentration. Optimal conditions for multiplex FISH were obtained at 50 °C and 30% (*v/v*) formamide. PNA-UI126 was specific for UI2 and 6. However, probe PNA-UI5 exhibited a certain level of fluorescence for the remaining strains when alone. Nevertheless, this can be resolved by multiplex FISH analysis, making it possible to identify a consortium composed by three strains (Figure S4). The CLSM 3D images of the morphology of the biofilms, z planes and their cross-section are presented in Figure 5, Figure S5 and Figure S6 for 6 h, 24 h and 48 h of biofilm growth, respectively. Overall, the tested consortia showed, in general, a coaggregation structure. Concerning biofilms incubated for 6 h, aggregates could be found, such as the one at the center of Figure 5e, composed mainly by strains 3 and 5. In fact, the strains seem to be well mixed and aggregated to each other. Similar findings were obtained when *E. coli* is present alone in consortium with other species [33,34].

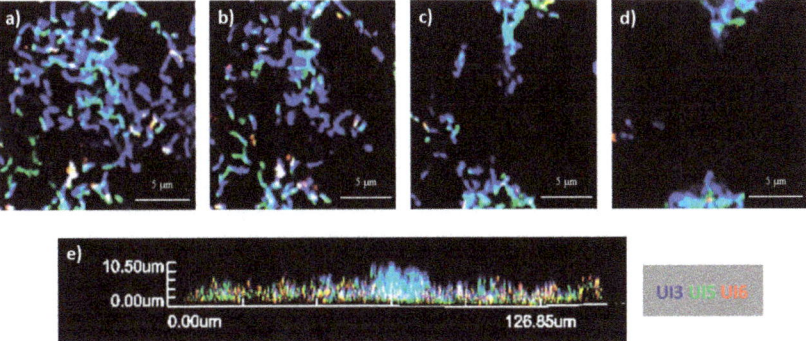

Figure 5. Three-dimensional organization of 6 h-aged biofilm formed in AUM and in polystyrene coupons by a consortium of three *E. coli* strains (UI3—blue, UI5—green and UI6—red). (**a**) Examples of CLSM (confocal laser scanning microscopy) images obtained of the layers within the biofilm at different heights (**a** = 0 μm; **b** = 0.7 μm; **c** = 2.1 μm; **d** = 3.5 μm). (**e**) Cross-section of the biofilm.

Intraspecies coaggregation is stated as important for the development of biofilms, enabling metabolic interactions, cell–cell communication and genetic exchange [35]. Therefore, we theorize that the strains can co-exist in the same space and are just enough far apart phylogenetically to cooperate when intraspecies diversity is increased in the surroundings. To understand this observed intraspecies phenomenon and to explain why an increase in diversity alters the EPS/cell numbers on these biofilms, we suggest that an intraspecies facultative cooperation strategy occurs, allowing them to save energy or to share resources. On the other hand, the proximity of the strains within the consortia may also facilitate the exchange of genes that confer advantages or the accumulation of mutations, helping them to adapt to the environmental conditions when the number of strains in a consortium is increased.

3. Materials and Methods

3.1. Bacterial Strains and Growth Conditions

In this study, six different *E. coli* strains were isolated from urine samples of patients using Cystine lactose electrolyte deficient agar (CLED) medium and MacConkey agar medium (Liofilchem, Roseto degli Abruzzi, Italy). Agar plates were incubated for 24 h at 37 °C. The identity of the six *E. coli* isolates was confirmed by sequencing the 16S ribosomal RNA (16S rRNA) gene, performed by StabVida, Lda (Caparica, Lisbon), and later confirmed using the Basic Local Alignment Search Tool (BLAST;

https://blast.ncbi.nlm.nih.gov). The *E. coli* strains were named urinary isolates (UI) followed by a number from 1 to 6 (e.g., UI1).

For each experiment, isolates were recovered from −80 °C glycerol stock cultures on Tryptic Soy Agar (TSA) (Merck, Darmstadt, Germany) and grown for 24 h at 37 °C.

3.2. Single- and Multi-Strain Biofilms Assays

For the preparation of each inoculum, isolated colonies for each strain were inoculated into artificial urine medium (AUM) [36] and incubated overnight (16–18 h), at 37 °C and 150 rpm. Subsequently, cell concentration was assessed by optical density at 620 nm (O.D.$_{620\,nm}$) and each inoculum was diluted in AUM in order to obtain a cell concentration of 10^6 CFUs·mL^{-1}.

In order to evaluate the biofilm-forming ability of each strain and in consortium, single- and multi-strain biofilms were grown as previously described [37]. Briefly, 200 µL of each inoculum prepared in AUM (10^6 CFUs·mL^{-1}) were added to each well of a 96-well tissue culture plate (Orange Scientific, Braine-l'Alleud, Belgium). Regarding multi-strain biofilms, an adequate volume of each strain culture was mixed, keeping a final volume of 200 µL with an initial concentration of 10^6 CFUs·mL^{-1} for each strain and added to each well. The plates were incubated at 37 °C, under static conditions, for 48 h. At predetermined time points (2, 6, 24 and 48 h), the biofilms were washed with 200 µL of 0.85 % (*w/v*) sterile saline solution to remove non-adherent and loosely attached cells. Then, biofilm formation was assessed by crystal violet (CV) staining (for total biomass quantification) and colony forming units (CFUs) counts (for cultivable cell counts). Quantification of extracellular polymeric matrix of single- and multi-strain biofilm was also performed for 48 h biofilms. These assays were performed with two or more independent experiments. Tested combinations are shown in Table S1 in Supplementary Information.

3.3. Biomass Quantification by Crystal Violet Staining

The produced biomass by single- and multi-strain biofilms in 96-well tissue culture plate was assessed by the CV staining [38]. The washed biofilms were fixed with 250 µL of 99% ethanol (*v/v*) for 15 min. Then, ethanol was removed, and the plates air-dried. Subsequently, biofilms were stained with 250 µL of CV (Merck, Germany) for 5 min. Microplates were rinsed with water, air-dried and the CV was resolubilized by adding 200 µL of 33 % (*v/v*) glacial acetic acid (Merck, Germany) to each well. Plates were stirred for 2 min and the content was transferred to new 96-well plates for O.D. (570 nm) measure using a microtiter plate reader (Spectra Max M2, Molecular Devices, Sunnyvale, CA, USA).

3.4. Cultivability Assessment

The number of cultivable biofilm cells was determined by CFUs counting as previously described by Azevedo, Almeida, Melo and Azevedo [37]. Briefly, after the washing step, 200 µL of 0.85 % (*w/v*) sterile saline solution were added into each well containing the biofilms. Biofilms were sonicated for 4 min (70 W, 35 kHz, Ultrasonic Bath T420, Elma, Singen, Germany) and 100 µL of the disrupted biofilms were serially diluted (1:10) in 0.85% (*w/v*) sterile saline solution and plated in triplicate in TSA plates (sonication conditions were previously optimized by Azevedo et al. [34]. The TSA plates were incubated at 37 °C for 14 h. The number of CFUs was expressed in logarithm per microtiter plate well's bottom and side area (log CFUs·cm^{-2}).

3.5. EPS Matrix Quantification by Dry Weight

EPS quantification was performed to a subset of biofilms (P1, P2, P3, P4, P5 and P6 (1 strain); P7 and P21 (2 strains); P22 and P41 (3 strains); P42 and P56 (4 strains); P57 and P62 (5 strains); P63 (6 strains)). For that, an extraction procedure was applied to separate the exopolymeric substances from the microbial cells [39,40]. The washed biofilms were sonicated in an ultrasonic bath for 4 min (70 W, 35 kHz, Ultrasonic Bath T420, Elma, Singen, Germany). The bacterial suspensions were transferred to universal tubes (50 mL) and sonicated (10 s, 25% amplitude). The bacterial suspensions were vortexed for 2 min and centrifuged for 10 min at 3000 rpm (at 4 °C). Then, the supernatants were filtered through a membrane (0.2 µm), using a syringe, to pre-weighed tubes. The tubes were frozen at −80 °C during 48 h for liquid extraction by lyophilization. After lyophilization, the tubes were weighed, and the total mass of the EPS matrix was determined.

3.6. Multilocus Sequence Typing for Phylogenetic Analysis

Multilocus Sequence Typing (MLST), as previously described by Liu et al. [41], was used to determine the diversity and phylogenetic relationships of the six *E. coli* strains. The sequencing of seven housekeeping genes, *adk* (Adenylate kinase), *fumC* (Fumarate hydratase), *gyrB* (DNA gyrase subunit B), *icd* (Isocitrate dehydrogenase), *mdh* (Malate dehydrogenase), *purA* (Adenylosuccinate synthetase) and *recA* (recA protein, repair and maintenance of DNA), was performed by StabVida, Lda (Caparica, Lisbon) following the protocols specified at the *E. coli* MLST website (http://mlst.warwick.ac.uk/mlst/dbs/Ecoli). For each obtained DNA sequence, the consensus sequence was generated after all gaps and single nucleotide changes were checked in the chromatograms for forward and reverse sequences using the Geneious 9.0.4 software (Biomatters Limited, New Zealand). Afterwards, sequences of all seven genes were concatenated for each isolate and aligned using Geneious 9.0.4 software. The phylogenetic analysis was inferred by the neighbor-joining algorithm using Geneious 9.0.4 software for the calculation of the pairwise distances in percentage [42].

3.7. Impact of the Phylogenetic Closeness in Biomass Production

In order to evaluate the phylogenetic impact in the biofilm development when the referred strains were combined, a scoring method was applied to the CV and CFUs areas (48 h growth) obtained for all the combinations. Therefore, the biofilm-forming ability and cultivability of the *E. coli* strains were scored according to the $\sum$ Combinatorial biofilm index ($\sum Cb_I$) adapted from Baptista et al. [43] presented in Equations (1) and (2):

$$Cb_{I(N)} = \frac{Curve\ Area_{(N)}}{Curve\ Area_{(Combined)}},\ N \in [1,2,3,4,5,6] \quad (1)$$

where Cb_I is the Cb index, which is calculated for each strain to be compared, dividing the curve area (total biomass or cultivability) of each strain for the curve area when those strains are combined. Then, the sum of the Cb_I for each strain in consortia gives the $\sum Cb_I$ as exemplified in Equation (2):

$$\sum_{i=1}^{n} Cb_{I(i)} = \left(Cb_{I(1)} + Cb_{I(2)} + \ldots + Cb_{I(n)}\right)/n \quad (2)$$

The obtained values for $\sum Cb_I$ are then scored according to the following criteria: <0.875—Cooperative; 0.875 to 1.125—Neutral; >1.125—Antagonistic. In addition, heat maps were constructed to better infer about the impact of the phylogenetic distance between the strains.

3.8. Optimization of the PNA-FISH Protocol

Two PNA-FISH probes were designed to target the *E. coli* strains (one probe for UI1, UI2 and UI6 strains; and another one for UI5 strain). Mismatches in the 16S rRNA sequences between the six *E. coli* strains were analyzed using Clustal Omega multiple sequence alignment tool (https://www.ebi.ac.uk/Tools/msa/clustalo/). Probes were selected according to their base pair (bp) length, mismatch localization, Guanine/Cytosine (GC) content, theoretical melting temperature point (T_m) and Gibbs free energy ($\Delta G < -13$) [27] (Table 1). The probes were attached to Alexa Fluor 488 (PNA-UI5) and Alexa Fluor 594 (PNA-UI126) signaling molecules via a double 8-amino-3, 6-dioxaoctanoic acid (AEEA) linker (Panagene, Daejeon, South Korea, HPLC purified > 90%). For UI3 and UI4 strains, 4′-6-Diamidino-2-phenylindole (DAPI; Merck, Germany) was used as a counterstain.

Table 1. Sequences of the PNA-FISH probes, their target positions in the 16S rRNA and theoretical values including bp (base pair), % GC, ΔG, and T_m.

PNA-Probes	Strains	Sequence	Position in 16S rRNA	bp	% GC	ΔG (kcal/mol)	T_m (°C)
PNA-UI126	UI1, 2 and 6	5'-GTGAGCCTTTACCC-3'	144 to 157	14	0.57	−16.43	73.30
PNA-UI5	UI5	5'-TCCATCGGGCAGT-3'	18 to 30	13	0.62	−15.88	75.96

_—mismatch position.

UI5 and UI2 strains were selected to optimize the hybridization conditions of the two PNA-FISH probes. A range of temperature and formamide concentrations were evaluated for a better microscopic signal using a LEICA DMLB2 epifluorescence microscope (Leica Microsystems Ltd.; Wetzlar, Germany) coupled with a Leica DFC300 FX camera (Leica Microsystems Ltd.; Wetzlar, Germany), with 100× oil immersion fluorescence objective. Images were acquired using Leica IM50 Image Manager, Image processing and Archiving software. The hybridization procedure in microscope slides was performed according to Almeida et al. [44]. Briefly, smears (30 µL) of each bacterial strain (OD_{620nm} = 0.1 ≈ 10^8 cells·mL^{-1}) in sterile distillate water were applied in microscope slides and immersed in 4% paraformaldehyde (30 µL) (Sigma-Aldrich, St. Louis, MO, USA) for 15 min. Then, 30 µL of 50% ethanol were added to the smears for 15 min and air-dried. Afterwards, the smears were covered with 20 µL of hybridization solution containing 10% dextran sulphate (Sigma-Aldrich, St. Louis, MO, USA), 10 mM NaCl (Sigma-Aldrich, St. Louis, MO, USA), 0.1% (wt/vol) sodium pyrophosphate (Sigma-Aldrich, St. Louis, MO, USA), 0.2% (wt/vol) polyvinylpyrrolidone (Sigma-Aldrich, St. Louis, MO, USA), 0.2% (wt/vol) Ficol (Sigma-Aldrich, St. Louis, MO, USA), 5 mM disodium EDTA (Sigma-Aldrich, St. Louis, MO, USA), 0.1% (vol/vol) Triton X-100 (Sigma-Aldrich, St. Louis, MO, USA), 50 mM Tris-HCl (Sigma-Aldrich, St. Louis, MO, USA), 30% or 50% (vol/vol) of formamide (Acros Organics, Belgium), and 200 nM of PNA probe. Smears with hybridization solution without PNA probe were performed as negative controls. Samples were covered with coverslips and placed in an incubator for a range of temperatures (48 °C to 54 °C) for 90 min. Then, the microscope slides were immersed in a pre-warmed washing solution containing 5 mM Tris base (Sigma-Aldrich, St. Louis, MO, USA), 15 mM NaCl (Sigma-Aldrich, St. Louis, MO, USA) and 1% (vol/vol) Triton X (pH = 10, Sigma-Aldrich, St. Louis, MO, USA), without their coverslips for 30 min at the same temperature of the hybridization step. The smears were covered with a drop of non-fluorescent immersion oil (Merck, Germany) and watched at the microscope. The microscope slides were stored for a maximum of 24 h in the dark at 4 °C before microscopy.

3.9. Study of the Spatial Organization in E. coli Multi-Strain Biofilms Using PNA-FISH Combined with Confocal Laser Scanning Microscopy Analysis

In order to assess the biofilm spatial organization and the strains distribution, the PNA-FISH and DAPI staining were performed directly in biofilms formed in polystyrene coupons as previously described [27,33]. Briefly, the biofilm formation was conducted as previously described. Then, 3 mL of the bacterial suspensions were added to each well of 12-well microtiter plates, with previously- placed sterilized polystyrene coupons (prepared according to Azevedo et al. [45]) at the bottom. The plates were then incubated for 6 h, 24 h and 48 h, under static conditions. After the incubation period, the coupons were carefully transferred and washed in another sterile 12-well microtiter plates with 3 mL of 0.85% (w/v) sterile saline solution and dried for 15 min at 60 °C. Afterwards, the biofilms in the coupons were placed carefully in a microscope slide, and the hybridization was performed as previously described for 90 min at 50 °C. When UI3 and UI4 were present, DAPI staining was performed. For this, a drop of DAPI solution (0.1 mg·mL^{-1}; Merck, Germany) was added to the coupons for 10 min in the dark at room temperature.

After the FISH procedure, the analysis of multi-strain biofilms structure and the location of the bacterial strains was made using a confocal laser scanning microscopy (Olympus BX61, Model FluoView 1000) and the multichannel simulated fluorescence projection of images and vertical cross-sections through the biofilm were generated by using the FluoView 1000 Software package (Olympus). During the analysis, a 60× water-immersion objective (60×/1.2 W) was used.

A laser excitation line 405 nm and emission filters BA 430-470 (blue channel) were used for DAPI observation; PNA-UI5 probe coupled to Alexa Fluor 488 was observed using a laser excitation line 488 nm and emission filters BA 505-540 (green channel); and for observation of PNA-UI126 probe coupled to Alexa Fluor 594, a laser excitation line 559 nm and emission filters BA 575-675 (red channel) was used.

3.10. Statistical Analysis

The results were compared using one-way analysis of variance (ANOVA) by applying the Tukey multiple-comparisons post-hoc test, using the Statistical Package for the Social Sciences (SPSS) Statistics 25 (IBM, Armonk, NY, USA). All tests were performed with a confidence level of 95%. The results were also compared by model-based clustering, using R software. The standard methodology selects the number of clusters according to the Bayesian information criterion (BIC) [46,47].

4. Conclusions

In conclusion, these results may represent another way to fight biofilm-related infections. We show that even in fully functional microorganisms, cells are induced to produce less EPS matrix when other strains are present. Nonetheless, most clinical biofilms are thought to be caused by a single strain. Hence, introducing multiple avirulent strains of the infecting microorganism at the site of infection, we might be inducing an EPS matrix-deficient biofilm which is, in theory, more susceptible to antibiotics/antimicrobial treatment. Moreover, as most of the antibiotics are most active in dividing cells [48], promoting cellular growth while increasing diversity, we might also increase susceptibility to antibiotics. For such strategy to work broadly, this approach must be applicable to intraspecies biofilms of other species and to pre-formed biofilms. Future lines of work will also include testing of these multi-strain biofilms in the presence of currently used antibiotics.

Supplementary Materials: The following are available online at http://www.mdpi.com/2079-6382/9/11/818/s1, Figure S1: Number of cultivable cells in single-strain biofilms and in multi-strain biofilms combining two, three, four, five and six *E. coli* strains, during 48 h. Standard deviations of three independent replicates are displayed. Figure S2. O.D. values for total biomass quantification (CV method) for single-strain biofilms and for multi-strain biofilms combining two, three, four, five and six *E. coli* strains, during 48 h. Standard deviations of three independent replicates are displayed; Figure S3. Mean EPS matrix concentration ± standard deviation of biofilms formed by consortia of 1 up to 6 different *E. coli* strains after 48 h of incubation at 37 °C in AUM. The produced EPS matrix decreases linearly with the addition of strains in consortia, adjusted with an R-squared of 0.94. Figure S4. Multiplex FISH using both PNA-UI5 and PNA-UI126 probes using UI5 and UI2, respectively, at 50 °C hybridization temperature and 30% formamide concentration. a–Green filter; b–Red filter; c–Filters overlapping. A magnification of 1500× was used. Figure S5. Three-dimensional organization of 24 h aged biofilm formed in AUM and in polystyrene coupons by a consortium of three *E. coli* strains (UI3-blue, UI5-green and UI6-red). (a) Examples of CLSM images obtained of the layers within the biofilm at different heights (a = 0 µm; c = 2 µm; d = 3 µm). (e) Cross section of the biofilm. Figure S6. Tri-dimensional organization of 48 h aged biofilm formed in AUM and in polystyrene coupons by a consortium of three *E. coli* strains (UI3-blue, UI5-green and UI6-red). (a) Examples of CLSM images obtained of the layers within the biofilm at different heights (a = 0 µm; b = 2 µm; c = 4 µm; d = 6 µm). (e) Cross section of the biofilm. Table S1: Number of possible combinations (P) of the six different *E. coli* strains used for biofilms formation assays.

Author Contributions: Conceptualization, A.S.A., C.A. and N.F.A.; Methodology, G.P.G. and J.B.; Formal Analysis, A.S.A., G.P.G., J.B. and J.P.; Investigation, A.S.A., G.P.G. and J.B.; Writing–Original Draft Preparation, A.S.A., G.P.G. and J.B.; Writing, A.S.A., C.A., F.J.M. and N.F.A.; Supervision, F.J.M. and N.F.A.; Project Administration, A.S.A. and N.F.A.; Funding Acquisition, A.S.A. and N.F.A. All authors have read and agreed to the published version of the manuscript.

Funding: This work was financially supported by Base Funding—UIDB/00511/2020 of the Laboratory for Process Engineering, Environment, Biotechnology and Energy—LEPABE—funded by national funds through the FCT/MCTES (PIDDAC); Project POCI-01-0145-FEDER-030431 (CLASInVivo) and project

POCI-01-0145-FEDER-029841 (POLY-PREVENTT), funded by FEDER funds through COMPETE2020—Programa Operacional Competitividade e Internacionalização (POCI) and by national funds (PIDDAC) through FCT/MCTES; Strategic funding of UIDB/04469/2020 of the Centre of Biological Engineering–CEB–funded by national funds through the FCT; Project BeMundus Brazil Europe/Erasmus Mundus scholarship granted by BM13DF0014.

Conflicts of Interest: The authors report no conflict of interest.

References

1. Costerton, J.W.; Cheng, K.-J.; Geesey, G.G.; Ladd, T.I.; Curtis, N.J.; Mrinal, D.; Marrie, T.J. Bacterial Biofilms in Nature and Disease. *Annu. Rev. Microbiol.* **1987**, *41*, 435–464. [CrossRef]
2. Donlan, R. Biofilms: Microbial Life on Surfaces. *Emerg. Infect. Dis.* **2002**, *8*, 881–890. [CrossRef]
3. Hall-Stoodley, L.; Costerton, J.W.; Stoodley, P. Bacterial Biofilms: From the Natural Environment to Infectious Diseases. *Nat. Rev. Genet.* **2004**, *2*, 95–108. [CrossRef]
4. Flemming, H.C.; Wingender, J. The Biofilm Matrix. *Nat. Rev. Microbiol.* **2010**, *8*, 623–633. [CrossRef]
5. Czárán, T.; Hoekstra, R.F. Microbial Communication, Cooperation and Cheating: Quorum Sensing Drives the Evolution of Cooperation in Bacteria. *PLoS ONE* **2009**, *4*, e6655. [CrossRef]
6. Azevedo, A.S.; Almeida, C.; Melo, L.F.; Azevedo, N.F. Impact of Polymicrobial Biofilms in Catheter-Associated Urinary Tract Infections. *Crit. Rev. Microbiol.* **2016**, *43*, 423–439. [CrossRef]
7. Hibbing, M.E.; Fuqua, C.; Parsek, M.R.; Peterson, S.B. Bacterial Competition: Surviving and Thriving in the Microbial Jungle. *Nat. Rev. Genet.* **2010**, *8*, 15–25. [CrossRef]
8. Rendueles, O.; Ghigo, J.-M. Mechanisms of Competition in Biofilm Communities. *Microbiol. Spectr.* **2015**, *3*, 3. [CrossRef]
9. Gao, C.; Zhang, M.; Wu, Y.; Huang, Q.; Cai, P. Divergent Influence to a Pathogen Invader by Resident Bacteria with Different Social Interactions. *Microbiol. Ecol.* **2018**, *77*, 76–86. [CrossRef]
10. Nadell, C.D.; Drescher, C.D.N.K.; Foster, K.R. Spatial Structure, Cooperation and Competition in Biofilms. *Nat. Rev. Genet.* **2016**, *14*, 589–600. [CrossRef]
11. López, D.; Vlamakis, H.; Kolter, R. Biofilms. *Cold Spring Harb. Perspect. Biol.* **2010**, *2*, a000398. [CrossRef]
12. Olsen, I. Biofilm-Specific Antibiotic Tolerance and Resistance. *Eur. J. Clin. Microbiol. Infect. Dis.* **2015**, *34*, 877–886. [CrossRef]
13. Lee, K.W.K.; Periasamy, S.; Mukherjee, M.; Xie, C.; Kjelleberg, S.; A Rice, S. Biofilm Development and Enhanced Stress Resistance of a Model, Mixed-Species Community Biofilm. *ISME J.* **2014**, *8*, 894–907. [CrossRef]
14. Kjaergaard, K.; Schembri, M.A.; Ramos, C.; Molin, S.; Klemm, P. Antigen 43 Facilitates Formation of Multispecies Biofilms. *Environ. Microbiol.* **2000**, *2*, 695–702. [CrossRef]
15. Flemming, H.-C.; Wingender, H.-C.F.J.; Szewzyk, U.; Steinberg, P.; Rice, S.A.; Kjelleberg, S.A.R.S. Biofilms: An Emergent form of Bacterial Life. *Nat. Rev. Genet.* **2016**, *14*, 563–575. [CrossRef]
16. Sztajer, H.; Szafranski, S.P.; Tomasch, J.; Reck, M.; Nimtz, M.; Rohde, M.; Wagner-Döbler, I. Cross-Feeding and Interkingdom Communication in Dual-Species Biofilms of Streptococcus Mutans and Candida Albicans. *ISME J.* **2014**, *8*, 2256–2271. [CrossRef]
17. West, S.A.; Griffin, A.S.; Gardner, A.; Diggle, S.P. Social Evolution Theory for Microorganisms. *Nat. Rev. Genet.* **2006**, *4*, 597–607. [CrossRef]
18. Xavier, J.B. Social Interaction in Synthetic and Natural Microbial Communities. *Mol. Syst. Biol.* **2011**, *7*, 483. [CrossRef]
19. West, S.A.; Diggle, S.P.; Buckling, A.; Gardner, A.; Griffins, A.S. The Social Lives of Microbes. *Annu. Rev. Ecol. Evol. Syst.* **2007**, *38*, 53–77. [CrossRef]
20. Jiricny, N.; Diggle, S.P.; A West, S.; Evans, B.A.; Ballantyne, G.; Ross-Gillespie, A.; Griffin, A.S. Fitness Correlates with the Extent of Cheating in a Bacterium. *J. Evol. Biol.* **2010**, *23*, 738–747. [CrossRef]
21. Nadell, C.D.; Xavier, J.B.; Foster, K.R. The Sociobiology of Biofilms. *FEMS Microbiol. Rev.* **2009**, *33*, 206–224. [CrossRef]
22. Stefanic, P.; Decorosi, F.; Viti, C.; Petito, J.; Cohan, F.M.; Mandic-Mulec, I. The Quorum Sensing Diversity within and between Ecotypes of Bacillus Subtilis. *Environ. Microbiol.* **2012**, *14*, 1378–1389. [CrossRef]

23. Lee, K.W.K.; Yam, J.K.H.; Mukherjee, M.; Periasamy, S.; Steinberg, P.D.; Kjelleberg, S.; Rice, S.A. Interspecific Diversity Reduces and Functionally Substitutes for Intraspecific Variation in Biofilm Communities. *ISME J.* **2016**, *10*, 846–857. [CrossRef]
24. Oluyombo, O.; Penfold, C.N.; Diggle, S.P. Competition in Biofilms between Cystic Fibrosis Isolates of Pseudomonas aeruginosa Is Shaped by R-Pyocins. *mBio* **2019**, *10*, e01828-18. [CrossRef]
25. CDCP, Centers for Disease Control and Prevention. Catheter-Associated Urinary Tract Infections (CAUTI). 2019. Available online: https://www.cdc.gov/hai/ca_uti/uti.html (accessed on 12 November 2019).
26. Azevedo, N.F.; Almeida, C.; Fernandes, I.; Cerqueira, L.; Dias, S.; Keevil, C.W.; Vieira, M.J. Survival of Gastric and Enterohepatic Helicobacter spp. in Water: Implications for Transmission. *Appl. Environ. Microbiol.* **2008**, *74*, 1805–1811. [CrossRef]
27. Almeida, C.; Azevedo, N.F.; Santos, S.R.B.; Keevil, C.W.; Vieira, M.J. Discriminating Multi-Species Populations in Biofilms with Peptide Nucleic Acid Fluorescence in Situ Hybridization (PNA FISH). *PLoS ONE* **2011**, *6*, e14786. [CrossRef]
28. Van Elsas, J.D.; Semenov, A.V.; Costa, R.; Trevors, J.T. Survival of Escherichia Coli in the Environment: Fundamental and Public Health Aspects. *ISME J.* **2011**, *5*, 367. [CrossRef]
29. López-Maury, L.; Marguerat, S.; Bähler, J. Tuning Gene Expression to Changing Environments: From Rapid Responses to Evolutionary Adaptation. *Nat. Rev. Genet.* **2008**, *9*, 583–593. [CrossRef]
30. Drazic, A.; Kutzner, E.; Winter, J.; Eisenreich, W. Metabolic Response of Escherichia Coli Upon Treatment with Hypochlorite at Sub-Lethal Concentrations. *PLoS ONE* **2015**, *10*, e0125823. [CrossRef]
31. Lukjancenko, O.; Wassenaar, T.M.; Ussery, D.W. Comparison of 61 Sequenced Escherichia Coli Genomes. *Microbiol. Ecol.* **2010**, *60*, 708–720. [CrossRef]
32. Liu, W.; Røder, H.L.; Madsen, J.S.; Bjarnsholt, T.; Sørensen, S.J.; Burmølle, M. Interspecific Bacterial Interactions Are Reflected in Multispecies Biofilm Spatial Organization. *Front. Microbiol.* **2016**, *7*, 1366. [CrossRef]
33. Azevedo, A.S.; Almeida, C.; Pereira, B.; Madureira, P.; Wengel, J.; Azevedo, N.F. Detection and Discrimination of Biofilm Populations Using Locked Nucleic Acid/2′-O-Methyl-Rna Fluorescence in Situ Hybridization (LNA/2′OMe-FISH). *Biochem. Eng. J.* **2015**, *104*, 64–73. [CrossRef]
34. Azevedo, A.S.; Almeida, C.; Pereira, B.; Melo, L.F.; Azevedo, N.F. Impact ofDelftia Tsuruhatensis and Achromobacter Xylosoxidans on Escherichia Colidual-Species Biofilms Treated with Antibiotic Agents. *Biofouling* **2016**, *32*, 227–241. [CrossRef]
35. Ledder, R.G.; Timperley, A.S.; Friswell, M.K.; Macfarlane, S.; McBain, A.J. Coaggregation between and among Human Intestinal and Oral Bacteria. *FEMS Microbiol. Ecol.* **2008**, *66*, 630–636. [CrossRef]
36. Brooks, T.; Keevil, C. A Simple Artificial Urine for the Growth of Urinary Pathogens. *Lett. Appl. Microbiol.* **1997**, *24*, 203–206. [CrossRef]
37. Azevedo, A.S.; Almeida, C.; Melo, L.F.; Azevedo, N.F. Interaction between Atypical Microorganisms and E. Coli in Catheter-Associated Urinary Tract Biofilms. *Biofouling* **2014**, *30*, 893–902. [CrossRef]
38. Stepanović, S.; Vuković, D.; Dakić, I.; Savić, B.; Švabić-Vlahović, M. A Modified Microtiter-Plate Test for Quantification of Staphylococcal Biofilm Formation. *J. Microbiol. Methods* **2000**, *40*, 175–179. [CrossRef]
39. Azeredo, J.; Lazarova, V.; Oliveira, R. Methods to Extract the Exopolymeric Matrix from Biofilms: A Comparative Study. *Water Sci. Technol.* **1999**, *39*, 243–250. [CrossRef]
40. Azeredo, J.; Henriques, M.; Sillankorva, S.; Oliveira, R. Extraction of Exopolymers from Biofilms: The Protective Effect of Glutaraldehyde. *Water Sci. Technol.* **2003**, *47*, 175–179. [CrossRef]
41. Liu, X.; Thungrat, K.; Boothe, D.M. Multilocus Sequence Typing and Virulence Profiles in Uropathogenic Escherichia Coli Isolated from Cats in the United States. *PLoS ONE* **2015**, *10*, e0143335. [CrossRef]
42. Kearse, M.; Moir, R.; Wilson, A.; Stones-Havas, S.; Cheung, M.; Sturrock, S.; Buxton, S.; Cooper, A.; Markowitz, S.; Duran, C.; et al. Geneious Basic: An Integrated and Extendable Desktop Software Platform for the Organization and Analysis of Sequence Data. *Bioinformatics* **2012**, *28*, 1647–1649. [CrossRef] [PubMed]
43. Baptista, J.; Simões, M.; Borges, A. Effect of Plant-Based Catecholic Molecules on the Prevention and Eradication of Pre-Established Escherichia Coli Biofilms: A Structure Activity Relationship Study. *Int. Biodeterior. Biodegrad.* **2018**, *141*, 101–113. [CrossRef]
44. Almeida, C.; Azevedo, N.F.; Fernandes, R.M.; Keevil, C.W.; Vieira, M.J. Fluorescence In Situ Hybridization Method Using a Peptide Nucleic Acid Probe for Identification of Salmonella spp. in a Broad Spectrum of Samples. *Appl. Environ. Microbiol.* **2010**, *76*, 4476–4485. [CrossRef] [PubMed]

45. Azevedo, N.F.; Pacheco, A.; Keevil, C.W.; Vieira, M.J. Adhesion of Water Stressed Helicobacter Pylori to Abiotic Surfaces. *J. Appl. Microbiol.* **2006**, *101*, 718–724. [CrossRef]
46. McLachlan, G. 9 The Classification and Mixture Maximum Likelihood Approaches to Cluster Analysis. *Handb. Stat.* **1982**, *2*, 199–208. [CrossRef]
47. Baudry, J.-P.; Raftery, A.E.; Celeux, G.; Lo, K.; Gottardo, R. Combining Mixture Components for Clustering. *J. Comput. Graph. Stat.* **2010**, *19*, 332–353. [CrossRef]
48. Kohanski, M.A.; Dwyer, D.J.; Collins, J.J. How Antibiotics Kill Bacteria: From Targets to Networks. *Nat. Rev. Genet.* **2010**, *8*, 423–435. [CrossRef]

Publisher's Note: MDPI stays neutral with regard to jurisdictional claims in published maps and institutional affiliations.

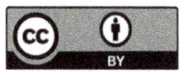

© 2020 by the authors. Licensee MDPI, Basel, Switzerland. This article is an open access article distributed under the terms and conditions of the Creative Commons Attribution (CC BY) license (http://creativecommons.org/licenses/by/4.0/).

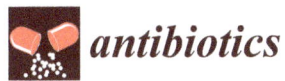

Article

Pitfalls Associated with Discriminating Mixed-Species Biofilms by Flow Cytometry

Tânia Grainha, Andreia P. Magalhães, Luís D. R. Melo * and Maria O. Pereira *

Centre of Biological Engineering, LIBRO—Laboratório de Investigação em Biofilmes Rosário Oliveira, University of Minho, Campus de Gualtar, 4710-057 Braga, Portugal; taniagrainha@ceb.uminho.pt (T.G.); amagalhaes@ceb.uminho.pt (A.P.M.)
* Correspondence: lmelo@deb.uminho.pt (L.D.R.M.); mopereira@deb.uminho.pt (M.O.P.); Tel.: +351-253-601-989 (L.D.R.M.); +351-253-604-402 (M.O.P.)

Received: 10 September 2020; Accepted: 21 October 2020; Published: 27 October 2020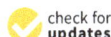

Abstract: Since biofilms are ubiquitous in different settings and act as sources of disease for humans, reliable methods to characterize and quantify these microbial communities are required. Numerous techniques have been employed, but most of them are unidirectional, labor intensive and time consuming. Although flow cytometry (FCM) can be a reliable choice to quickly provide a multiparametric analysis, there are still few applications on biofilms, and even less on the study of inter-kingdom communities. This work aimed to give insights into the application of FCM in order to more comprehensively analyze mixed-species biofilms, formed by different *Pseudomonas aeruginosa* and *Candida albicans* strains, before and after exposure to antimicrobials. For comparison purposes, biofilm culturability was also assessed determining colony-forming units. The results showed that some aspects, namely the microbial strain used, the morphological state of the cells and the biofilm matrix, make the accurate analysis of FCM data difficult. These aspects were even more challenging when double-species biofilms were being inspected, as they could engender data misinterpretations. The outcomes draw our attention towards the need to always take into consideration the characteristics of the biofilm samples to be analyzed through FCM, and undoubtedly link to the need for optimization of the processes tailored for each particular case study.

Keywords: *Pseudomonas aeruginosa*; *Candida albicans*; mixed-species biofilm analysis; flow cytometry

1. Introduction

The ability of microorganisms to form a biofilm is an important feature in clinical, industrial and environmental settings [1]. Biofilms are well-structured microbial communities adhered to biotic or abiotic surfaces enclosed within a self-produced extracellular polymeric matrix. The matrix is the major structural component of the biofilm [2] and is denominated as an extracellular polymeric substance (EPS). The EPS is composed of polysaccharides, proteins, nucleic acids, lipids and other biopolymers such as humic substances [3]. Most natural biofilms are polymicrobial and all members of the community contribute with their own EPS components, resulting in a more complex matrix [4].

The biofilms associated with numerous infectious diseases (e.g., infections of oral cavity, otitis, cystic fibrosis) are described as being of a polymicrobial nature with bacteria coexisting with pathogenic yeasts or filamentous fungi [5]. *Pseudomonas aeruginosa* is a ubiquitous bacterium and an opportunistic pathogen frequently isolated from healthy humans as part of the human microbiota and can coexist in mixed infections with the polymorphic fungus *Candida albicans* [6,7]. *C. albicans* is a commensal yeast able to initiate invasive growth and develop health problems in compromised individuals [8,9]. Notably, *C. albicans* is one of the few fungal species causing disease in humans [10]. *P. aeruginosa* and *C. albicans* represent an example of co-infection and are commonly related with chronic and healthcare-associated infections [11–13]. From a clinical point of view, it is crucial to entirely characterize the biofilm populations (single- and mixed-species) and understand the mechanisms underlying the changes that occur during co-infection as result of the established interactions. The monitoring of polymicrobial communities is routinely performed by culture-dependent approaches that require appropriate selective media and optimal growth conditions and is hindered by the presence of cells in a viable but poorly culturable state or underestimated by the presence of cellular aggregates [14,15]. Under these circumstances, standard microbiology methods are often unsuitable to diagnose polymicrobial biofilm infections. Molecular methodologies, such as quantitative real-time PCR (qPCR) [16,17] or fluorescence in situ hybridization using peptide nucleic acids (PNA FISH) [18–20], have helped in the characterization of members of microbial communities, affording a specific and sensitive quantification of specific species in biofilm samples that are unable to be detected by culturable methods. Nevertheless, these approaches cannot distinguish cellular subpopulations. Thus, flow cytometry (FCM) could present an accurate alternative to the analysis of biofilm cells, since it enables detailed investigation of cellular subpopulations due to its ability to perform multiparametric single-cell analysis [21]. The analysis of biofilm communities by this technique is particularly useful, since it allows a quick achievement of cell counts and provides an overview about the type of cells present in the samples, namely their size and complexity. In addition, this method allows for the discrimination between live and dead cells, also providing information about damaged cells [22]. Based on this, the goal of this study was to explore FCM analysis to characterize and discriminate mixed-species biofilm samples before and after being challenged by antimicrobial treatments.

Accordingly, the aspects that can influence FCM analysis as well as tips to circumvent them are presented through this work.

2. Results

2.1. Planktonic versus Biofilm Cells

Before biofilm analysis by FCM, an optimization of the process is desirable to adjust all sample analysis parameters. Firstly, as bacteria might be in the FCM detection limit, owing to its small size, a preliminary optimization was performed in order to guarantee the accurate detection of *P. aeruginosa* and thus the reliability of the results. Due to the complexity and heterogeneity of biofilms, optimizations using planktonic cells were performed. Since *P. aeruginosa* and *C. albicans* have distinct sizes and the flow cytometer allows for separation by size and complexity, it was assumed that their distinction on mixed communities should be well achieved using the same dyes. As can be observed in the dot plot (Figure 1), it was possible to define gates for each single-species planktonic culture tested.

Before examining the mixed-species biofilms, single-species biofilms of both species were also analyzed. The results obtained for these biological samples showed that cells from *C. albicans* biofilm populations are very different on cell size and complexity from the planktonic cells, leading to gating adjustments (Figure 1). In addition to the typical fungal cell gate previously defined for the planktonic cultures, several fluorescently labeled events up to the demarcated bacterial region were detected (Figure 2). To check whether this feature was particular for the *C. albicans* SC5314 strain, two more strains of each studied species (*P. aeruginosa* and *C. albicans*) were analyzed both on planktonic and biofilm states. Although this effect was not observed for *P. aeruginosa* PAO1, two more *P. aeruginosa* strains were also analyzed to strengthen the absence of that behavior. While this effect was not observed for any of the *P. aeruginosa* strains (Supplementary Figure S1), it was consistent on all *C. albicans* strains tested (Supplementary Figure S2).

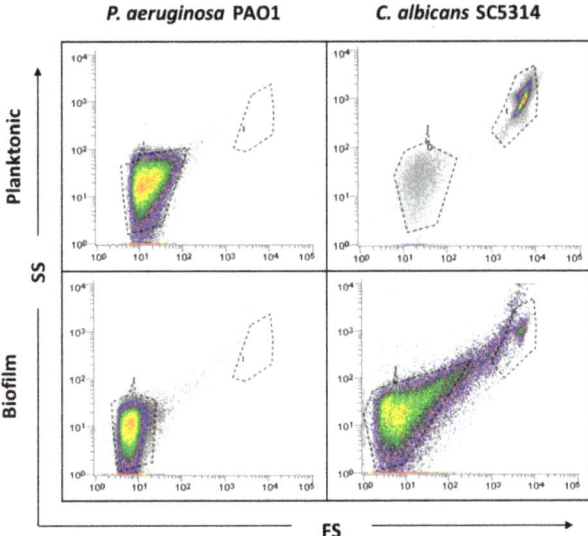

Figure 1. Representative dot plots obtained for planktonic cells and single biofilms of *P. aeruginosa* PAO1 and *C. albicans* SC5314 by flow cytometry (FCM).

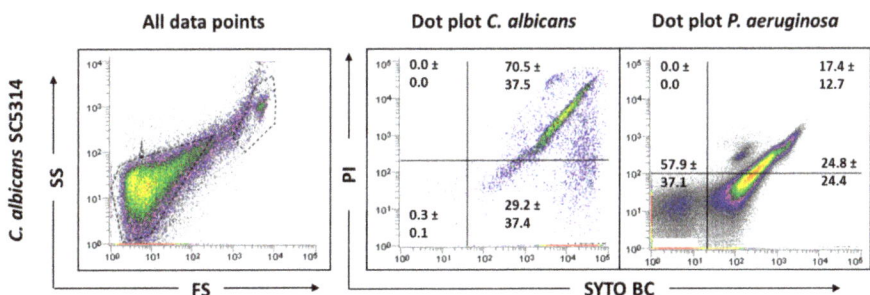

Figure 2. Representative dot plots obtained for *C. albicans* SC5314 biofilm by FCM. In 'all data points', the dot plots SS (Side Scatter) × FS (Forward Scatter) are represented, as acquired in the logarithm. Dot plots of *P. aeruginosa* and *C. albicans* represent the areas delineated to represent bacteria and fungi, respectively.

2.2. Effect of Hyphae and Biofilm Matrix on Flow Cytometry Analysis

In an attempt to understand the factors generating the differences observed in the *C. albicans* biofilm populations in comparison with planktonic cultures, two possibilities were inspected, the impact of hyphal growth and the effect of the biofilm matrix. Since *C. albicans* biofilm cells present different phases of growth, it is expected that cells with distinct hyphal lengths are also present. Additionally, the biofilms were grown in Roswell Park Memorial Institute (RPMI) 1640, a medium that favors hyphal growth; therefore, more elongated hyphae could appear in these samples compared with planktonic cultures [23]. Based on this knowledge, the possibility of hyphal growth introducing some heterogeneity in the population, with a consequent interference in the results, was raised. To evaluate this hypothesis, planktonic cultures of *C. albicans* SC5314 grown in Sabouraud Dextrose Broth (SDB) and in RPMI supplemented with serum 2% (*v/v*), to induce hyphal cell growth, were analyzed. It was noticed that the fungal population which had hyphae induction became more heterogenous (Supplementary Figure S3), thus allowing us to verify that the presence of hyphae could account for the observed differences. However, a closer inspection of the results for *C. albicans* 547096, a strain that does not have the ability to form hyphae in both planktonic and biofilm conditions, allowed us to notice a change between both modes of growth (Supplementary Figure S2). Despite it being clear that hyphal growth has some influence on the results, this did not entirely explain what happened in biofilm samples.

To deeply understand what influenced the results obtained in the biofilm samples, the possible interference of the biofilm matrix was also evaluated. The EPS matrix is composed of large amounts of eDNA [3,24] that can be bounded by the used fluorochromes, but, due to its small size, is only detected by the cytometer when it is attached to other matrix components. Therefore, efforts were done to extract the biofilm matrix, then the biofilm cells with and without the matrix were analyzed on the cytometer. The FCM of the biofilm matrix samples revealed a similar pattern to that obtained previously for *C. albicans* biofilms (Figure 3). Although this alteration between planktonic and biofilm samples was not previously clearly detected for *P. aeruginosa* strains, the analyses of the biofilm matrix samples allowed us to notice that the EPS matrix also play a role in the bacterial biofilm cell counts (Figure 3).

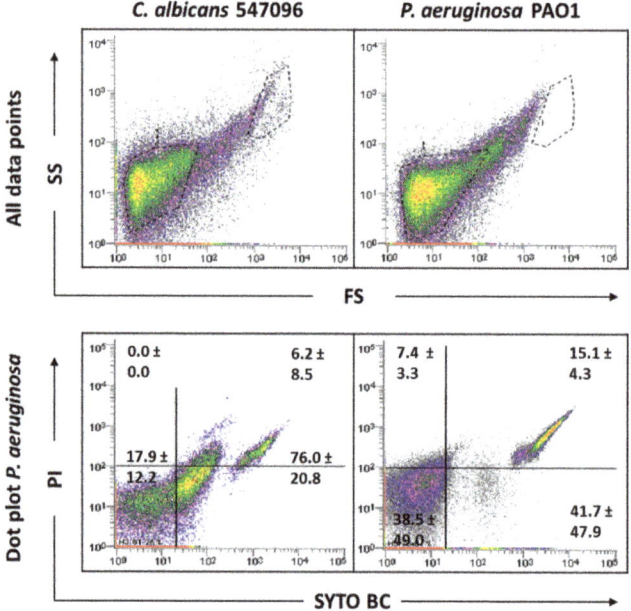

Figure 3. Representative dot plots obtained for biofilm matrix of *C. albicans* 547096 and *P. aeruginosa* PAO1 by FCM. In 'all data points', the dot plots SS (Side Scatter) × FS (Forward Scatter) are represented, as acquired in the logarithm. The dot plot of *P. aeruginosa* represents the areas delineated to represent bacteria.

The results indicate that both hyphal growth and the biofilm matrix account for altering the typical gate observed in *C. albicans* planktonic cultures. However, the presence of the EPS matrix has been shown to have greater impact on the FCM analysis. Although the *P. aeruginosa* gate does not differ between planktonic and biofilm, it was also evident that the matrix influences FCM analysis.

Overall, the data clearly highlighted that biofilm matrix extraction, before FCM analysis, is a requirement for this kind of methodology. Otherwise, it will not be possible to accurately analyze biofilm populations, due to the risk of populations not being properly differentiated, and consequently causing cell counts to be severely influenced by positively marked matrix events.

2.3. Influence of Sonication on Biofilm Cell Viability

As this study has mixed-species biofilms as the main focus, a sonication procedure was used based on a previous optimized protocol. The sonication time was evaluated to ensure that this procedure did not result in cell lysis (Supplementary information Figure S4). The results indicated that the matrix extraction with 30 s of sonication at 30% amplitude was not harmful to any of the strains tested ($p < 0.05$). However, these sonication conditions were not effective in removing the entire matrix of *C. albicans* SC5314 and 324LA/94 strains (Supplementary Figure S5). As can be observed in Figure 4, although some matrix has been removed from *C. albicans* 324LA/94 samples, the cellular suspensions still present some matrix traces, which are being gated where *P. aeruginosa* is usually gated, making the study of mixed-species biofilms containing this *C. albicans* strain unfeasible.

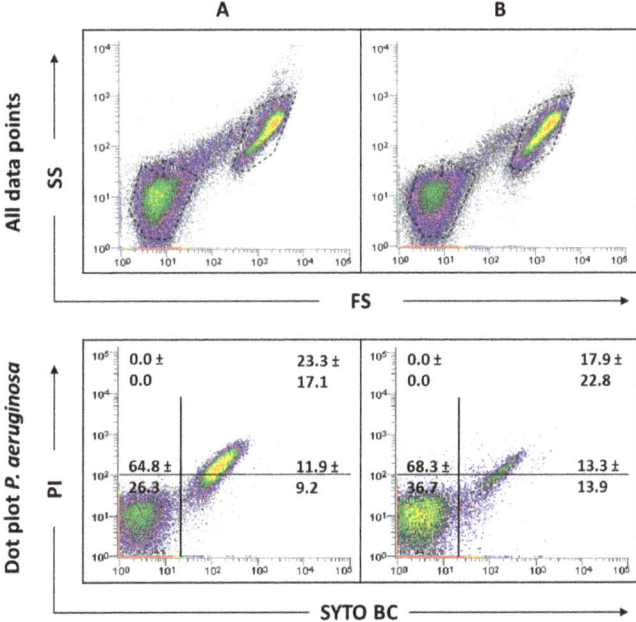

Figure 4. Representative dot plots obtained by FCM for *C. albicans* 324LA/94 biofilms before (**A**) and after (**B**) extraction of biofilm matrix.

2.4. Analysis of Mixed-Species Biofilms

To focus and frame the study, the number of strains used in the mixed biofilm formation were narrowed to one strain for each organism. In the case of *P. aeruginosa*, as no differences were observed between the strains tested in the FCM data analysis, the PAO1 strain was selected, because it is one of the most commonly used strains for biofilm research. Regarding *C. albicans*, to minimize the effects of the biofilm matrix and to eliminate hyphae influence, 547096 was the strain selected. The sonication parameters were tested in these mixed-species biofilms, and the results show that the matrix was effectively extracted (Figure 5).

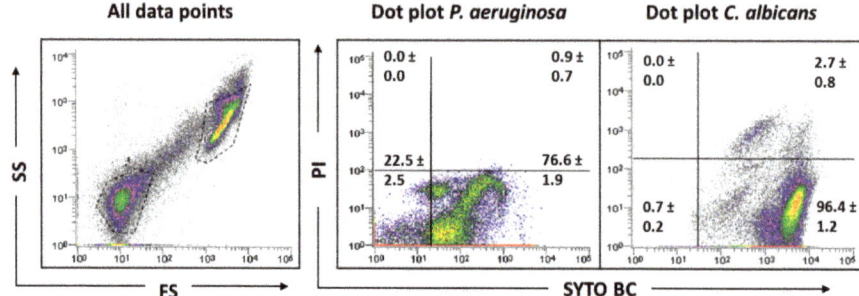

Figure 5. Representative dot plots obtained for *P. aeruginosa* PAO1 and *C. albicans* 547096 mixed-species biofilms by FCM. In 'all data points', the dot plots SS (Side Scatter) × FS (Forward Scatter) are represented, as acquired in the logarithm. Dot plots of *P. aeruginosa* and *C. albicans* represent the areas delineated to represent bacteria and fungi, respectively.

Indeed, the results showed a clear and distinct separation between bacterial and fungi populations, making the evaluation of this consortium by FCM possible. Since the *C. albicans* matrix, which was gated where *P. aeruginosa* is usually gated, does not appear because it was removed, bacterial cells will be more feasible counted.

2.5. Antimicrobial Effect on Mixed-Species Biofilms

Pre-established polymicrobial biofilms were treated with ciprofloxacin or linalool and their antimicrobial effect was evaluated by FCM (Figure 6) and colony-forming units (CFU) were counted (Table 1).

Table 1. FCM counting and colony-forming units (CFU) enumeration of pre-established mixed biofilms treated with two different concentrations of ciprofloxacin and linalool. Both 24 and 48 h-old untreated biofilms are included for comparison purposes. $\log_{10}$ values represent means ± standard deviations (sd).

Condition	*P. aeruginosa*		*C. albicans*	
	FCM Counts/mL	CFU/mL	FCM Counts/mL	CFU/mL
24 h-old biofilm	5.69 ± 0.03	6.99 ± 0.45	6.11 ± 0,17	6.51 ± 0.55
48 h-old biofilm	7.37 ± 0.02	8.53 ± 0.48	6.87 ± 0.10	7.46 ± 0.69
Ciprofloxacin (0.25 mg/L)	5.36 ± 0.24[#]	6.08 ± 0.94[#]	6.44 ± 0.23	6.64 ± 0.82
Ciprofloxacin (8 mg/L)	4.85 ± 0.62[#]	4.99 ± 1.31[*,#]	6.43 ± 0.23	6.82 ± 0.44
Linalool (0.3% v/v)	6.26 ± 0.21	7.62 ± 0.70	6.07 ± 0.19	2.02 ± 1.91[*,#]
Linalool (1.2% v/v)	6.27 ± 0.07	7.38 ± 0.41	6.28 ± 0.03	0.00[*,#]

[*] Significantly different compared with 24 h-old biofilm control ($p < 0.05$). [#] Significantly different compared with 48 h-old untreated biofilm ($p < 0.05$).

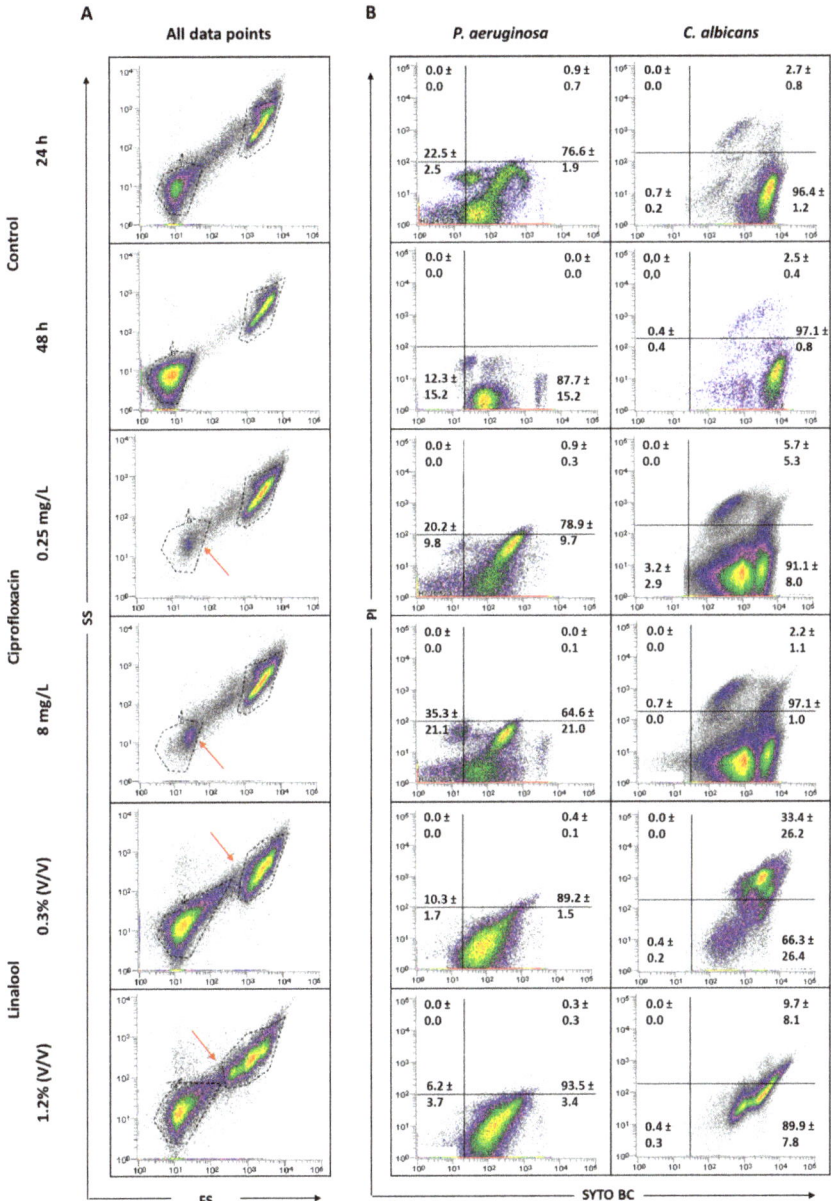

Figure 6. Representative all data points (**A**) and specific dot plots (**B**) obtained for *P. aeruginosa* PAO1 and *C. albicans* 547096 mixed-species biofilms by FCM. Dot plots of *P. aeruginosa* and *C. albicans* represent the areas delineated to represent bacteria and fungi, respectively. The arrows indicate alterations in the core of the population compared to the controls.

To understand the effect of the antimicrobials tested, it was considered important to verify the behavior of the total population in terms of size (FS) and complexity (SS). Figure 6 displays the graphs of all data points obtained for 24 and 48 h-old biofilms, and for the populations after antimicrobial treatments. The analysis of the dot plots indicated that there are no evident changes when comparing the 24 h-old biofilms of *P. aeruginosa* and *C. albicans* with the corresponding 48 h. The core of the fungal population presented a slight increase in the SYTO BC mean fluorescence intensity (MFI) from 2189 to 4208. Regarding the effect of the antimicrobials, the data revealed that, when using both ciprofloxacin concentrations, the core of the *P. aeruginosa* population is altered compared with the controls. In terms of viability, ciprofloxacin treatment does not appear to affect *P. aeruginosa* biofilm cells. In the case of *C. albicans*, no notable differences in terms of size and complexity were observed. Nevertheless, the yeast population seemed to be slightly destabilized, with the observation of two sub-populations, as well as a decrease in the SYTO BC uptake and an increase in the propidium iodide (PI) uptake compared with the 24 h-old biofilm control. These differences were more pronounced with the lowest concentration of ciprofloxacin ranging from 2182 to 1072 for SYTO BC MFI, and from 580 to 692 for PI MFI.

Using linalool, *P. aeruginosa* and *C. albicans* populations appeared altered, being more dispersed, suggesting a more heterogeneous population. With both linalool concentrations, *C. albicans* cells presented a reduced size and complexity (Figure 6). A population displacement along the PI axis was also observed, meaning that part of the cells is double stained. Furthermore, we observed a decrease in the SYTO BC uptake compared with the control, whereas SYTO BC MFI ranged from 2189 to 1604 and 1715 with the lowest and the highest concentration, respectively. Concerning *P. aeruginosa* populations, there was no effect observed in terms of viability and only a slight decrease in SYTO BC MFI was detected (from 117 in 24 h-old biofilm to 84 after biofilm treatment).

The cellular quantifications of the untreated and treated mixed biofilms are gathered in Table 1. Overall, FCM counts were somewhat lower than those detected by CFU, except when mixed biofilms were challenged with linalool, wherein *C. albicans* CFU counts were very low or even null. However, it must be taken into consideration that the standard deviation values associated with the CFU counts are higher than those observed for FCM, which might suggest more data variability between experiments.

Regarding the FCM results (Table 1) for *P. aeruginosa*, no significant differences were observed between ciprofloxacin-treated biofilms and the 24 h-old biofilm control. Furthermore, around 2 and 2.5-log reductions were achieved with the lowest and highest concentrations of ciprofloxacin, respectively, compared to the 48 h-old untreated biofilm. Taking into consideration CFU counts, the application of ciprofloxacin gave rise to some reductions in *P. aeruginosa* cells, notably when the higher concentration was used (about 2 and 3.5-log reductions compared with 24 and 48 h-old untreated biofilm, respectively). Ciprofloxacin treatment had no relevant effect on *C. albicans* as cell numbers remain unchanged for both concentrations, whatever the method used for biofilm cell counting.

The use of linalool had no relevant effect on *P. aeruginosa* viability and culturability compared with the 24 h-old biofilms. However, when compared with 48 h-old biofilms, although not statistically significant, about a 1-log reduction was observed when using either FCM or CFU. Concerning the fungus population in the mixed consortia, the use of FCM or CFU to count biofilm cells challenged by linalool gave rise to very distinct scenarios ($p < 0.05$). Indeed, through FCM, no significant alterations in the number of cells were noticeable in comparison with the respective controls. However, CFU counts revealed a clear negative effect of linalool in *C. albicans* culturability, achieving reductions of more than 4 or 5-log compared to the 24 or 48 h-old untreated biofilms, and even total eradication with the highest linalool concentration.

3. Discussion

The polymicrobial nature of most infections [5] leads to the growing need for the study of these complex communities. Currently, there are several techniques that can be employed to perform biofilm analysis that are often dependent on the investigation purpose. Although FCM has been essentially applied for studying planktonic cultures [25], there are some studies using biofilms [26–28]. Pan et al. (2014) compared three methods (FCM, CFU and a spectrophotometry method of optical density measurement) for the quantification of bacterial cells after exposure to nanoparticles and found that FCM measurement was the quickest and most accurate method for bacterial detection [29]. This methodology has also been successfully applied in the study of single-species biofilms and to investigate bacterial physiological responses [26,27]. FCM was also successfully applied in the study of cell viability in planktonic mixed cultures, using Gram-specific fluorescent staining [30].

Since the study of polymicrobial biofilm communities using FCM is less common, the rationale behind this study was to exploit and fruitfully apply this technique in the characterization and quantification of mixed-species biofilms while paying attention to the eventual hitches that this technique could engender and trying and to find solutions to surpass them.

Biofilms are complex microbial communities in which cells are embedded in an EPS matrix that cements cells together and provides heterogeneous microenvironments, leading to cells adopting different physiological states. Thus, biofilm cells differ phenotypically from their planktonic counterparts [31]. The results obtained in this study have shown that the analysis of biofilm cell viability using FCM is not straightforward, essentially due to the presence of cells with different morphologies and the biofilm matrix. *C. albicans* biofilms are typically formed by a mixture of vegetative cells, pseudohyphae and hyphae [32], with this mixture of morphologies having been detected by FCM. Due to the size and complexity of fungal cells, it was noticed that the counts made by FCM were influenced by the presence of hyphae, since they can be counted as more than a single event (Supplementary Figure S3).

The EPS matrix represents a significant part of the biofilms, playing an important role in their development and cohesion [33–35]. The matrix is suggested as the biofilms' house [36] because it protects biofilm cells from physical, chemical and biological adversities. The biofilm matrix contains several constituents, including eDNA [3,24], which, once attached to other matrix components, may be counted as positive events when passed in the flow cytometer, as highlighted by Figure 3. When the biofilm matrix was analyzed, several fluorescently labeled events, from the fungal cell gate previously defined up to the demarcated bacterial region, were detected. This squeezing of the events on the FS axis might be due to the heterogeneity of biofilm matrix components. These aspects may explain the impossibility of distinguishing the bacterial and fungal populations present in mixed cultures. Thus, matrix extraction is a crucial step before biofilm analysis by FCM. There are different methods that have been described for the extraction of EPS from single- and mixed-species biofilms, including centrifugation, filtration, heating, blending, sonication and treatments with agents or resins [37]. The EPS isolation method selected should be adapted accordingly to the type of biofilm under investigation. In the case of mixed-species biofilms, the selection and optimization of the extraction procedure was even more difficult. Moreover, it has to be taken into account that if the process becomes too complex or time consuming, the advantage of using FCM is lost. Sample sonication was the chosen methodology, but the matrix was not effectively extracted for the three *C. albicans* strains tested (Supplementary Figure S5) meaning that the success of the matrix extraction was strain dependent. These findings require longer sonication times and/or amplitudes to be tested in order to increase the amount of matrix extracted. Although it is known that sonication is an extraction method whose parameter optimization is microorganism dependent, in the case of mixed biofilms, there must be a commitment to reconcile the best possible parameters for all species present in the consortia. Thus, a reasonable time of sonication for both microbes present in the mixed cultures must be chosen, once the desirable target is achieved wherein the process does not affect the cellular viability of any of the tested species.

Based on previous studies, it can be assumed that, when using the same concentrations of antimicrobials agents, a greater antimicrobial effect occurs on planktonic cells, when comparing to the effect observed on biofilm cells, namely for ciprofloxacin [38] and linalool [39] towards *P. aeruginosa* and *C. albicans*, respectively. It is expected that, following an antimicrobial treatment, the composition and state of microbial populations might be altered [40]. Although, in some cases, there were no evident changes in the number of cells, it is important to emphasize some variations in SYTO BC and/or PI MFI, as well as variations in the core of the population (Figure 6). Ciprofloxacin is a broad-spectrum antibiotic of the fluoroquinolone class that acts on DNA gyrase (topoisomerase II) and topoisomerase IV, resulting in the inhibition of DNA replication, recombination and transcription, and thus causing bacterial death [41]. Ciprofloxacin affected the size and complexity of *P. aeruginosa* (Figure 6) and, regarding the results obtained by FCM, both concentrations of ciprofloxacin showed a bacteriostatic effect (Table 1) as the number of cells was lower after treatment compared with the 48 h-old untreated biofilm. Concerning CFU results, in addition to its bacteriostatic activity, a bactericidal activity was also observed to be more pronounced with the highest concentration of the antibiotic. These discrepancies between different methods are in accordance with the results observed by other authors [42]. Though ciprofloxacin is a bactericidal antibiotic according to classical testing, which uses planktonic cells, it is well known that cells from biofilm are more tolerant to the actions of antibiotics and harder to eradicate. Biofilm cells usually require higher doses to be eradicated by an antimicrobial [43]. The bacteriostatic effect observed here is due to the fact that cells were grown embedded in a biofilm. Both bacteriostatic and bactericidal effects of ciprofloxacin were previously reported in *Escherichia coli* [42]. Taking the 24 h-old biofilms as the reference, the application of ciprofloxacin did not alter the number of *C. albicans* cells; however, when the comparison is made with the 48 h-old untreated biofilm, a decrease in the number of cells was observed. These results indicate that ciprofloxacin might also have a fungistatic effect. Moreover, it was observed that the *C. albicans* population was divided into two sub-populations, shifted to the left with a reduced uptake of SYTO BC (Figure 6), meaning that a diminished metabolism of viable cells after ciprofloxacin treatment may have occurred. Indeed, a decrease in staining intensity was previously associated as an indicative characteristic of decreased metabolic state [26,44]. Although fluoroquinolones have no intrinsic antifungal growth-inhibitory activity, topoisomerase I and II are found in pathogenic fungi [45–47], which suggests that ciprofloxacin might be a strong candidate to interact with antifungal agents [48–50]. Linalool is a terpene alcohol commonly found as a component of the essential oils of aromatic plants. This compound has been reported as having antifungal activity, specifically against *C. albicans* [51,52]. A more recent study showed that linalool suppressed the expression of several virulence-related genes [53]. The effect of linalool on *C. albicans* cells showed marked differences between FCM and CFU counts. Although *C. albicans* did not suffer reductions in terms of FCM counts, the number of CFU was diminished after linalool application, meaning that their growth ability was affected. Even though no reduction in the FCM counts was observed, a clear alteration in population diversity, as well as a shift in the fungus population along the PI axis, was observed (Figure 6), meaning that cells are double stained with SYTO BC and PI. This increase in the number of cells being double stained suggests that linalool damages the cell membrane, allowing PI to enter into the cells. Thus, it can be assumed that part of the cell is in an intermediate physiological state between life and cell death, which may explain the reduction in the ability of fungi to grow on solid media. A double-stained population is considered injured, as discussed by Léonard et al. [54]. Therefore, the discrepancy between CFU and FCM counts may be explained by the emergence of viable but non-culturable cells; nonetheless, an additional non-culture-based method would be valuable to unambiguously assure this hypothesis. Indeed, the exposure of cell populations to antimicrobial action can lead to the appearance of different cell subpopulations, particularly an increase in the number of viable but non-culturable cells [55,56]. The differences here observed reflect the problem associated with CFU counting, since it does not allow for the detection of viable but non-culturable cells. Differences between culturable and FCM counts were previously reported by other authors [26,44]. The abovementioned linalool membrane effect was also observed in other studies, where it was reported that this antimicrobial agent acts by causing the disruption of the membrane integrity and interrupting the cell cycle [51,57]. Concerning *P. aeruginosa*, the application of both linalool concentrations did not alter the number of cells when compared to the 24 h-old biofilm control, but caused a decrease when the 48 h-old untreated biofilms were used for comparison, meaning that that linalool might have bacteriostatic activity. Similar bacteriostatic effects of linalool were previously reported for other bacteria, namely

Enterobacter cloacae, *E. coli*, *Proteus mirabilis*, *Salmonella enteritidis*, *Salmonella typhimurium*, *Staphylococcus epidermidis* and *Listeria monocytogenes* [58].

In addition to the discrepancies between FCM and CFU counts already mentioned, others were also observed (Table 1). In most cases, the number of culturable cells was higher than the FCM counts. This fact can be explained by the presence of injured cells that can reverse their state on fresh culture media and thus recover their growth ability. Moreover, in general, CFU results have higher variability between experiments, which leads to less accurate results.

Overall, this study showed that FCM can be a reliable methodology for the study of mixed-species biofilms, allowing for the discrimination of the stakeholders. However, for each consortium, previous optimization procedures must be followed, namely biofilm matrix extraction methodologies. Moreover, it was demonstrated that, when FCM is applied to scrutinize the mode of action of antimicrobial treatments, new insights can be provided due to the multiparametric analysis this technique allows.

A great step forward in the present research would be the clinical implementation of this methodology. Once the protocol is well developed and it is routinely applied, it is expected that it would be applied to real biofilm communities in clinical settings using blood samples or other samples where microorganisms are founded. Although FCM has been employed much more in the field of hematology, it has already been studied in different contexts. Microbial detection by FCM has already been proven to be possible using blood samples, as demonstrated in a previous work [59]. Clinical microbiology has undergone important changes during the last few years. Indeed, in recent years, microbiological techniques used in laboratories have been increasingly complemented by cutting-edge technologies such as FCM. The use of these practices presents several advantages to others, such as culture-dependent methods or microscopic approaches, since it provides multiparametric single-cell analysis very rapidly.

4. Materials and Methods

4.1. Microorganisms and Culture Conditions

Three reference strains of *P. aeruginosa*, two non-mucoid strains (PAO1 and UCBPP-PA14 (PA14)) and a mucoid strain (ATCC 39324), were used throughout this work. In addition, two clinical isolates of *C. albicans* (324LA/94, an oral isolate obtained from the culture collection of Cardiff Dental School (Cardiff, UK) and 547096, a urinary isolate obtained from the culture collection of the Biofilm Group of the Centre of Biological Engineering (Braga, Portugal)), and a reference strain, SC5314, were tested.

Prior to each assay, *P. aeruginosa* and *C. albicans* strains were subcultured from the frozen stock preparations onto Tryptic Soy Agar (TSA) and Sabouraud Dextrose Agar (SDA) plates, respectively. TSA and SDA were prepared from Tryptic Soy Broth (TSB; Liofilchem S.r.l., Roseto, Italy) or SDB (Liofilchem) supplemented with 1.2% (*w/v*) agar (Liofilchem). The plates were then incubated aerobically at 37 °C for 18–24 h.

Pure liquid cultures (pre-inocula) of *P. aeruginosa* were grown overnight in TSB, whereas *C. albicans* was maintained in SDB. For biofilm assays, 0.22 µm of filter-sterilized RPMI 1640 medium (Gibco® by Life Technologies™, Grand Island, NY, USA) at pH 7.0 was used.

4.2. Biofilm Formation

Biofilm assays were performed as previously described [60], with some modifications. Briefly, the initial cell suspension (pre-inocula) was centrifuged (3000× *g*, 4 °C, 10 min) and the pellet resuspended in RPMI 1640 to achieve a concentration of ~1 × 10^7 CFU per mL. Bacterial concentration was estimated using an ELISA microtiter plate reader at an optical density of 640 nm (OD$_{640}$ nm) (Sunrise-Basic Tecan, Männedorf, Switzerland), while yeast cells were enumerated by microscopy using a Neubauer counting chamber. For mixed-species cultures, a combination of 50% of the suspended inoculum of each species was used. Cellular suspensions were further transferred to 24-well plates

(Orange Scientific, Braine-l'Alleud, Belgium). Plates were then incubated aerobically for 24 h on a horizontal shaker at 120 rpm and 37 °C.

4.3. Hyphal Induction

In order to promote hyphal growth of *C. albicans* cells, planktonic cultures of *C. albicans* S5314 were grown overnight in RPMI supplemented with 2% (*v/v*) fetal bovine serum (Biochrom AG, Berlin, Germany) at 120 rpm and 37 °C. Cells were then analyzed by FCM.

4.4. Biofilm Quantification

4.4.1. Determination of Culturable Cells

After biofilm formation, wells were washed twice with sterile water after discarding the planktonic fraction. Afterwards, 500 µL of phosphate-buffered saline (PBS; 10 mM potassium phosphate, 150 mM NaCl; pH 7.0) was added to each well and the biofilms were scraped. In order to ensure the reproducibility of the scraping method, the conditions were strictly followed in all experiments by using a pipette tip and scraping each well about 1 min. To remove any aggregates, biofilm suspensions were vigorously vortexed (V1-Plus Biosan, Riga, Latvia) for 30 s. The resulting biofilm suspensions were then serially diluted in sterile water and plated onto agar plates (TSA for *P. aeruginosa* and SDA for *C. albicans*) for single-species biofilms. For mixed-species biofilms, *Pseudomonas* Isolation Agar (PIA; Sigma-Aldrich, St. Louis, MO, USA) and SDA supplemented with 30 mg/L gentamycin (Sigma-Aldrich, St. Louis, MO, USA) (to suppress the growth of *P. aeruginosa*) were used for the specific isolation of *P. aeruginosa* and *C. albicans*, respectively. Agar plates were incubated aerobically at 37 °C for 24–48 h for culturable cell counting. Values of culturable sessile cells were expressed as $\log_{10}$ CFU per mL and represent the average of the triplicates for each strain. At least two independent experiments were carried out in duplicate.

4.4.2. Extraction of Biofilm Matrix

For the extraction of the biofilm matrix, a previously described protocol was followed [61]. In brief, after washing and scraping the biofilm, all suspensions were sonicated for 30 s at 30% amplitude in a sonicator (Cole-Parmer 750-Watt Ultrasonic Homogenizer, Vernon Hills, IL, USA). The cells were then separated from the matrix by centrifugation at 3000× *g* for 5 min at 4 °C. The supernatant was filtered with a membrane pore size of 0.2 µm. The pellet, which corresponds to the cells of a biofilm without matrix, was resuspended in 1 mL of PBS to be analyzed further.

4.4.3. Flow Cytometry Assay

Biofilm cell viability was also determined by FCM. In brief, pre-formed biofilms were washed twice, scraped in 1 mL of PBS, vortexed at maximum speed (30 s) and analyzed by cytometry. In addition, the biofilm cells (without the EPS matrix) and the EPS matrix itself (after matrix extraction procedure) were also analyzed. Lastly, 0.5–2 µM of SYTO BC (Invitrogen™, Carlsbad, CA, USA) and 15 µM of PI (Invitrogen™, Carlsbad, CA, USA) were added to the tested suspensions. Samples were incubated in the dark for 20 min, at room temperature, and were analyzed further in an EC800™ flow cytometer (SANYO, Osaka, Japan). SYTO BC fluorescence was detected on the FL1 channel (PMT = 5) while PI fluorescence was detected on the FL4 channel (PMT = 3). SYTO BC absorbs at 485–487 nm and emits at 500–504 nm while PI excitation occurs at 535 nm and emission at 617 nm.

For all detected parameters, amplification was carried out using logarithmic scales. The cellular concentration was determined by acquiring the counts by the equipment. Multi-parametric analyses were performed on the scattering signals (forward scatter, FSC and side scatter, SSC), as well as on the FL1 (green fluorescence) and FL4 (red fluorescence) channels. When appropriate, a slight adjustment of the gate was made to guarantee the inclusion of the total population in the FCM analysis. For all assays, at least two independent experiments were carried out in duplicate.

4.5. Influence of Sonication on Biofilm Cell Viability

The biofilm suspensions obtained were pooled and sonicated for 30 s at 30% amplitude in a sonicator. A non-sonicated sample was included as a control. After this, for each sample, the values of biofilm-culturable cells were determined by CFU counting. On these samples, total cell counting was performed in duplicate for both species.

4.6. Antimicrobial Effect on Mixed-Species Biofilms

The antimicrobial effects of the antibiotic ciprofloxacin (Sigma-Aldrich) and the naturally occurring terpene alcohol, linalool (Sigma-Aldrich), were evaluated in mixed-species biofilms of *P. aeruginosa* PAO1 and *C. albicans* 547096. For this, 24 h-old pre-established mixed biofilms were exposed to defined concentrations of each antimicrobial: 0.3 or 1.2% v/v for linalool and 0.25 or 8 mg/L for ciprofloxacin. The rationale behind the use of these concentrations was based on the assumption that the lower concentrations had already been reported as inhibitory for planktonic culture; then, these concentrations were gradually boosted until we found one that had an inhibitory effect on biofilm without causing total cell eradication. Briefly, after biofilm formation, 500 µL of cell suspension was replaced by the antimicrobial solutions prepared at 2 times the desired concentration. Plates were then incubated aerobically at 37 °C for another 24 h. The results were assessed for biofilm cell culturability through CFU enumeration using selective growth media, as previously described, and by FCM. Both 24 and 48 h-old untreated biofilms were used to infer whether the antimicrobial agents demonstrated a bacteriostatic/bactericidal or fungistatic/fungicidal activity. At least two independent experiments were carried out.

4.7. Statistical Analysis

Data were analyzed using the Prism software package (GraphPad Software version 6.01). One-way ANOVA tests were performed, and means were compared by applying Tukey's multiple comparison test. The statistical analyses performed were considered significant when $p < 0.05$.

5. Conclusions

Overall, the obtained data allow us to strengthen the belief that FCM is a versatile and accurate technique to analyze biofilms; however, it is crucial to take into account some technical aspects to avoid erroneous interpretations. FCM analysis is strain dependent and, as the biofilm matrix is variable for each of microorganism, either grown in isolation or in polymicrobial consortia, the method of extraction (regardless of the one chosen for this purpose) must be personalized for each case. The use of FCM to analyze mixed biofilms challenged by the application of an antimicrobial can provide important insights, explaining the alterations in the behavior of the microbial community and suggesting antimicrobial modes of action in biofilm populations. These outcomes strengthen FCM as a promising technique to study heterogeneous biofilms and evaluate the efficacy of therapeutic approaches.

Throughout this work, the pitfalls related to FCM analysis of inter-kingdom polymicrobial biofilms were fully addressed and efforts were made to circumvent them in order to reliably characterize complex biofilm communities, which are still poorly explored using this approach. This work highlights the fact that this technique can be fruitfully used in the understanding of antimicrobial studies as long as specific and tailored optimization is carried out.

Supplementary Materials: The following are available online at http://www.mdpi.com/2079-6382/9/11/741/s1. Figure S1: Representative dot plots obtained for planktonic and biofilm cells of *P. aeruginosa*, Figure S2: Representative dot plots obtained for planktonic and biofilm cells of *C. albicans*, Figure S3: Representative dot plots obtained by FCM of planktonic cells of *C. albicans* SC5314 (A) and hyphal growth induction (B), Figure S4: Effect of sonication process on biofilm cell viability. CFU enumeration of *C. albicans* (A) and *P. aeruginosa* (B) biofilms before and after 30 s of sonication at 30% amplitude, Figure S5: Representative dot plots obtained for *P. aeruginosa* and *C. albicans* biofilms (A) and biofilm cells after matrix extraction (B) by FCM.

Author Contributions: Conceptualization, T.G., A.P.M., L.D.R.M. and M.O.P.; methodology, T.G., A.P.M. and L.D.R.M.; validation, T.G., M.O.P. and L.D.R.M.; formal analysis, T.G., A.P.M. and L.D.R.M.; investigation, T.G., A.P.M. and L.D.R.M.; data curation, T.G.; writing—original draft preparation, T.G.; writing—review and editing, M.O.P., L.D.R.M.; supervision, M.O.P. All authors have read and agreed to the published version of the manuscript.

Funding: This work was supported by the Portuguese Foundation for Science and Technology (FCT) under the scope of the strategic funding of the UID/BIO/04469/2020 unit and BioTecNorte operation (NORTE-01-0145-FEDER-000004), which was funded by the European Regional Development Fund under the scope of Norte2020–Programa Operacional Regional do Norte. The authors also acknowledge COMPETE2020 and FCT under the project POCI-01-0145-FEDER-029841 and FCT for the PhD grant to Tânia Grainha (grant number SFRH/BD/136544/2018).

Conflicts of Interest: The authors declare no conflict of interest.

References

1. Nickzad, A.; Déziel, E. The involvement of rhamnolipids in microbial cell adhesion and biofilm development—An approach for control? *Lett. Appl. Microbiol.* **2014**, *58*, 447–453. [CrossRef] [PubMed]
2. Branda, S.S.; Vik, Å.; Friedman, L.; Kolter, R. Biofilms: The matrix revisited. *Trends Microbiol.* **2005**, *13*, 20–26. [CrossRef] [PubMed]
3. Wingender, J.; Neu, T.R.; Flemming, H.-C. What are Bacterial Extracellular Polymeric Substances? *Microb. Extracell. Polym. Subst.* **1999**, 1–19. [CrossRef]
4. Decho, A.W.; Visscher, P.T.; Reid, R.P. Production and cycling of natural microbial exopolymers (EPS) within a marine stromatolite. *Palaeogeogr. Palaeoclim. Palaeoecol.* **2005**, *219*, 71–86. [CrossRef]
5. Peters, B.M.; Jabra-Rizk, M.A.; O'May, G.A.; Costerton, J.W.; Shirtliff, M.E. Polymicrobial interactions: Impact on pathogenesis and human disease. *Clin. Microbiol. Rev.* **2012**, *25*, 193–213. [CrossRef] [PubMed]
6. Fourie, R.; Ells, R.; Swart, C.W.; Sebolai, O.M.; Albertyn, J.; Pohl, C.H. Candida albicans and Pseudomonas aeruginosa Interaction, with Focus on the Role of Eicosanoids. *Front. Physiol.* **2016**, *7*, 64. [CrossRef]
7. Peleg, A.Y.; Hogan, D.A.; Mylonakis, E. Medically important bacterial-fungal interactions. *Nat. Rev. Microbiol.* **2010**, *8*, 340–349. [CrossRef]
8. Mallick, E.M.; Bennett, R.J. Sensing of the microbial neighborhood by Candida albicans. *PLoS Pathog.* **2013**, *9*, e1003661. [CrossRef]
9. Hirota, K.; Yumoto, H.; Sapaar, B.; Matsuo, T.; Ichikawa, T.; Miyake, Y. Pathogenic factors in Candida biofilm-related infectious diseases. *J. Appl. Microbiol.* **2017**, *122*, 321–330. [CrossRef]
10. Nobile, C.J.; Johnson, A.D. Candida albicans Biofilms and Human Disease. *Annu. Rev. Microbiol.* **2015**, *69*, 71–92. [CrossRef]
11. Bianchi, S.M.; Prince, L.R.; McPhillips, K.; Allen, L.; Marriott, H.M.; Taylor, G.W.; Hellewell, P.G.; Sabroe, I.; Dockrell, D.H.; Henson, P.W.; et al. Impairment of apoptotic cell engulfment by pyocyanin, a toxic metabolite of Pseudomonas aeruginosa. *Am. J. Respir. Crit. Care Med.* **2008**, *177*, 35–43. [CrossRef] [PubMed]
12. McAlester, G.; O'Gara, F.; Morrissey, J.P. Signal-mediated interactions between Pseudomonas aeruginosa and Candida albicans. *J. Med. Microbiol.* **2008**, *57*, 563–569. [CrossRef]
13. Percival, S.L.; Suleman, L.; Vuotto, C.; Donelli, G. Healthcare-Associated infections, medical devices and biofilms: Risk, tolerance and control. *J. Med. Microbiol.* **2015**, *64*, 323–334. [CrossRef]
14. Fux, C.A.; Costerton, J.W.; Stewart, P.S.; Stoodley, P. Survival strategies of infectious biofilms. *Trends Microbiol.* **2005**, *13*, 34–40. [CrossRef] [PubMed]
15. Carvalhais, V.; Pérez-Cabezas, B.; Oliveira, C.; Vitorino, R.; Vilanova, M.; Cerca, N. Tetracycline and rifampicin induced a viable but nonculturable state in *Staphylococcus epidermidis* biofilms. *Future Microbiol.* **2018**, *13*, 27–36. [CrossRef] [PubMed]
16. Vuong, J.; Collard, J.-M.; Whaley, M.J.; Bassira, I.; Seidou, I.; Diarra, S.; Ouédraogo, R.T.; Kambiré, D.; Taylor, T.H.; Sacchi, C.; et al. Development of Real-Time PCR Methods for the Detection of Bacterial Meningitis Pathogens without DNA Extraction. *PLoS ONE* **2016**, *11*, e0147765. [CrossRef]
17. Zemanick, E.T.; Wagner, B.D.; Sagel, S.D.; Stevens, M.J.; Accurso, F.J.; Harris, J.K. Reliability of quantitative real-time PCR for bacterial detection in cystic fibrosis airway specimens. *PLoS ONE* **2010**, *5*, e15101. [CrossRef]

18. Rodrigues, M.E.; Lopes, S.P.; Pereira, C.R.; Azevedo, N.F.; Lourenço, A.; Henriques, M.; Pereira, M.O. Polymicrobial Ventilator-Associated Pneumonia: Fighting In Vitro Candida albicans-Pseudomonas aeruginosa Biofilms with Antifungal-Antibacterial Combination Therapy. *PLoS ONE* **2017**, *12*, e0170433. [CrossRef]
19. Machado, A.; Almeida, C.; Salgueiro, D.; Henriques, A.; Vaneechoutte, M.; Haesebrouck, F.; Vieira, M.J.; Rodrigues, L.; Azevedo, N.F.; Cerca, N. Fluorescence in situ Hybridization method using Peptide Nucleic Acid probes for rapid detection of Lactobacillus and Gardnerella spp. *BMC Microbiol.* **2013**, *13*, 82. [CrossRef]
20. Almeida, C.; Azevedo, N.F.; Bento, J.C.; Cerca, N.; Ramos, H.; Vieira, M.J.; Keevil, C.W. Rapid detection of urinary tract infections caused by Proteus spp. using PNA-FISH. *Eur. J. Clin. Microbiol. Infect. Dis.* **2013**, *32*, 781–786. [CrossRef]
21. Müller, S.; Nebe-von-Caron, G. Functional single-cell analyses: Flow cytometry and cell sorting of microbial populations and communities. *FEMS Microbiol. Rev.* **2010**, *34*, 554–587. [CrossRef]
22. Davey, H.M.; Kell, D.B. Flow cytometry and cell sorting of heterogeneous microbial populations: The importance of single-cell analyses. *Microbiol. Rev.* **1996**, *60*, 641–696. [CrossRef] [PubMed]
23. Kucharíková, S.; lè ne Tournu, H.; Lagrou, K.; Van Dijck, P.; Bujdá ková, H. Detailed comparison of Candida albicans and Candida glabrata biofilms under different conditions and their susceptibility to caspofungin and anidulafungin. *J. Med. Microbiol.* **2011**, *60*, 1261–1269. [CrossRef] [PubMed]
24. Cheng, M.; Cook, A.E.; Fukushima, T.; Bond, P.L. Evidence of compositional differences between the extracellular and intracellular DNA of a granular sludge biofilm. *Lett. Appl. Microbiol.* **2011**, *53*, 1–7. [CrossRef]
25. Martins, N.; Costa-Oliveira, S.; Melo, L.D.R.; Ferreira, I.C.F.R.; Azeredo, J.; Henriques, M.; Silva, S. Susceptibility testing of Candida albicans and Candida glabrata to *Glycyrrhiza glabra* L. *Ind. Crops Prod.* **2017**, *108*, 480–484. [CrossRef]
26. Cerca, F.; Trigo, G.; Correia, A.; Cerca, N.; Azeredo, J.; Vilanova, M. SYBR green as a fluorescent probe to evaluate the biofilm physiological state of *Staphylococcus epidermidis*, using flow cytometry. *Can. J. Microbiol.* **2011**, *57*, 850–856. [CrossRef] [PubMed]
27. Kerstens, M.; Boulet, G.; Van Kerckhoven, M.; Clais, S.; Lanckacker, E.; Delputte, P.; Maes, L.; Cos, P. A flow cytometric approach to quantify biofilms. *Folia Microbiol.* **2015**, *60*, 335–342. [CrossRef]
28. Oliveira, F.; Lima, C.A.; Brás, S.; França, Â.; Cerca, N. Evidence for inter- and intraspecies biofilm formation variability among a small group of coagulase-negative staphylococci. *FEMS Microbiol. Lett.* **2015**, *362*, fnv175. [CrossRef]
29. Pan, H.; Zhang, Y.; He, G.-X.; Katagori, N.; Chen, H. A comparison of conventional methods for the quantification of bacterial cells after exposure to metal oxide nanoparticles. *BMC Microbiol.* **2014**, *14*, 222. [CrossRef]
30. Rüger, M.; Bensch, G.; Tüngler, R.; Reichl, U. A flow cytometric method for viability assessment of *Staphylococcus aureus* and *Burkholderia cepacia* in mixed culture. *Cytom. Part A* **2012**, *81A*, 1055–1066. [CrossRef] [PubMed]
31. Cos, P.; Toté, K.; Horemans, T.; Maes, L. Biofilms: An extra hurdle for effective antimicrobial therapy. *Curr. Pharm. Des.* **2010**, *16*, 2279–2295. [CrossRef]
32. Ramage, G.; Saville, S.P.; Thomas, D.P.; Lopez-Ribot, J.L. Candida Biofilms: An Update. *Eukaryot. Cell* **2005**, *4*, 633–638. [CrossRef] [PubMed]
33. Vilain, S.; Pretorius, J.M.; Theron, J.; Brözel, V.S. DNA as an adhesin: Bacillus cereus requires extracellular DNA to form biofilms. *Appl. Environ. Microbiol.* **2009**, *75*, 2861–2868. [CrossRef] [PubMed]
34. Tsuneda, S.; Aikawa, H.; Hayashi, H.; Yuasa, A.; Hirata, A. Extracellular polymeric substances responsible for bacterial adhesion onto solid surface. *FEMS Microbiol. Lett.* **2003**, *223*, 287–292. [CrossRef]
35. Hancock, R.E.W. A brief on bacterial biofilms. *Nat. Genet.* **2001**, *29*, 360. [CrossRef] [PubMed]
36. Flemming, H.-C.; Wingender, J. The biofilm matrix. *Nat. Rev. Microbiol.* **2010**, *8*, 623. [CrossRef] [PubMed]
37. Nielsen, P.H.; Jahn, A. Extraction of EPS. In *Microbial Extracellular Polymeric Substances*; Springer: Berlin/Heidelberg, Germany, 1999; pp. 49–72.
38. Dosler, S.; Karaaslan, E. Inhibition and destruction of Pseudomonas aeruginosa biofilms by antibiotics and antimicrobial peptides. *Peptides* **2014**, *62*, 32–37. [CrossRef]
39. Serra, E.; Hidalgo-Bastida, L.A.; Verran, J.; Williams, D.; Malic, S. Antifungal activity of commercial essential oils and biocides against Candida albicans. *Pathogens* **2018**, *7*, 15. [CrossRef]

40. Martínez, J.L. Effect of antibiotics on bacterial populations: A multi-hierachical selection process. *F1000Research* **2017**, *6*, 51. [CrossRef]
41. Van Bambeke, F.; Michot, J.-M.; Van Eldere, J.; Tulkens, P.M. Quinolones in 2005: An update. *Clin. Microbiol. Infect.* **2005**, *11*, 256–280. [CrossRef]
42. Silva, F.; Lourenço, O.; Queiroz, J.A.; Domingues, F.C. Bacteriostatic versus bactericidal activity of ciprofloxacin in *Escherichia coli* assessed by flow cytometry using a novel far-red dye. *J. Antibiot.* **2011**, *64*, 321–325. [CrossRef] [PubMed]
43. Høiby, N.; Ciofu, O.; Johansen, H.K.; Song, Z.J.; Moser, C.; Jensen, P.Ø.; Molin, S.; Givskov, M.; Tolker-Nielsen, T.; Bjarnsholt, T. The Clinical Impact of Bacterial Biofilms. *Int. J. Oral Sci.* **2011**, *3*, 55–65. [CrossRef]
44. Oliveira, A.; Ribeiro, H.G.; Silva, A.C.; Silva, M.D.; Sousa, J.C.; Rodrigues, C.F.; Melo, L.D.R.; Henriques, A.F.; Sillankorva, S. Synergistic antimicrobial interaction between honey and phage against *Escherichia coli* biofilms. *Front. Microbiol.* **2017**, *8*, 2407. [CrossRef]
45. Fostel, J.M.; Montgomery, D.A.; Shen, L.L. Characterization of DNA topoisomerase I from Candida albicans as a target for drug discovery. *Antimicrob. Agents Chemother.* **1992**, *36*, 2131–2138. [CrossRef] [PubMed]
46. Shen, L.L.; Baranowski, J.; Fostel, J.; Montgomery, D.A.; Lartey, P.A. DNA topoisomerases from pathogenic fungi: Targets for the discovery of antifungal drugs. *Antimicrob. Agents Chemother.* **1992**, *36*, 2778–2784. [CrossRef] [PubMed]
47. Shen, L.L.; Fostel, J.M. DNA Topoisomerase Inhibitors as Antifungal Agents. In *Advances in Pharmacology*; Academic Press: New York, NY, USA, 1994; Volume 29, pp. 227–244.
48. Stergiopoulou, T.; Meletiadis, J.; Sein, T.; Papaioannidou, P.; Tsiouris, I.; Roilides, E.; Walsh, T.J. Isobolographic analysis of pharmacodynamic interactions between antifungal agents and ciprofloxacin against Candida albicans and Aspergillus fumigatus. *Antimicrob. Agents Chemother.* **2008**, *52*, 2196–2204. [CrossRef]
49. Brilhante, R.S.N.; Caetano, E.P.; Sidrim, J.J.C.; Cordeiro, R.A.; Camargo, Z.P.; Fechine, M.A.B.; Lima, R.A.C.; Castelo Branco, D.S.C.M.; Marques, F.J.F.; Mesquita, J.R.L.; et al. Ciprofloxacin shows synergism with classical antifungals against *Histoplasma capsulatum var. capsulatum* and *Coccidioides posadasii*. *Mycoses* **2013**, *56*, 397–401. [CrossRef]
50. Stergiopoulou, T.; Meletiadis, J.; Sein, T.; Papaioannidou, P.; Tsiouris, I.; Roilides, E.; Walsh, T.J. Comparative pharmacodynamic interaction analysis between ciprofloxacin, moxifloxacin and levofloxacin and antifungal agents against Candida albicans and Aspergillus fumigatus. *J. Antimicrob. Chemother.* **2009**, *63*, 343–348. [CrossRef]
51. Zore, G.B.; Thakre, A.D.; Jadhav, S.; Karuppayil, S.M. Terpenoids inhibit Candida albicans growth by affecting membrane integrity and arrest of cell cycle. *Phytomedicine* **2011**, *18*, 1181–1190. [CrossRef]
52. Alviano, W.S.; Mendonca-Filho, R.R.; Alviano, D.S.; Bizzo, H.R.; Souto-Padron, T.; Rodrigues, M.L.; Bolognese, A.M.; Alviano, C.S.; Souza, M.M.G.; Mendonça-Filho, R.R.; et al. Antimicrobial activity of Croton cajucara Benth linalool-rich essential oil on artificial biofilms and planktonic microorganisms. *Oral Microbiol. Immunol.* **2005**, *20*, 101–105. [CrossRef]
53. Hsu, C.-C.; Lai, W.-L.; Chuang, K.-C.; Lee, M.-H.; Tsai, Y.-C. The inhibitory activity of linalool against the filamentous growth and biofilm formation in Candida albicans. *Med. Mycol.* **2013**, *51*, 473–482. [CrossRef]
54. Léonard, L.; Chibane, L.B.; Bouhedda, B.O.; Degraeve, P.; Oulahal, N. Recent advances on multi-parameter flow cytometry to characterize antimicrobial treatments. *Front. Microbiol.* **2016**, *7*, 1225. [CrossRef] [PubMed]
55. Pasquaroli, S.; Zandri, G.; Vignaroli, C.; Vuotto, C.; Donelli, G.; Biavasco, F. Antibiotic pressure can induce the viable but non-culturable state in Staphylococcus aureus growing in biofilms. *J. Antimicrob. Chemother.* **2013**, *68*, 1812–1817. [CrossRef]
56. Li, L.; Mendis, N.; Trigui, H.; Oliver, J.D.; Faucher, S.P. The importance of the viable but non-culturable state in human bacterial pathogens. *Front. Microbiol.* **2014**, *5*, 258. [CrossRef] [PubMed]
57. Khan, A.; Ahmad, A.; Akhtar, F.; Yousuf, S.; Xess, I.; Khan, L.A.; Manzoor, N. Ocimum sanctum essential oil and its active principles exert their antifungal activity by disrupting ergosterol biosynthesis and membrane integrity. *Res. Microbiol.* **2010**, *161*, 816–823. [CrossRef] [PubMed]
58. Soković, M.; Glamočlija, J.; Marin, P.D.; Brkić, D.; Griensven, L.J.L.D. van Antibacterial Effects of the Essential Oils of Commonly Consumed Medicinal Herbs Using an In Vitro Model. *Molecules* **2010**, *15*, 7532–7546. [CrossRef] [PubMed]

59. Costa, S.P.; Dias, N.M.; Melo, L.D.R.; Azeredo, J.; Santos, S.B.; Carvalho, C.M. A novel flow cytometry assay based on bacteriophage-derived proteins for Staphylococcus detection in blood. *Sci. Rep.* **2020**, *10*, 1–13. [CrossRef]
60. Stepanović, S.; Vuković, D.; Dakić, I.; Savić, B.; Švabić-Vlahović, M. A modified microtiter-plate test for quantification of staphylococcal biofilm formation. *J. Microbiol. Methods* **2000**, *40*, 175–179. [CrossRef]
61. Silva, S.; Henriques, M.; Martins, A.; Oliveira, R.; Williams, D.; Azeredo, J. Biofilms of non-Candida albicans Candida species: Quantification, structure and matrix composition. *Med. Mycol.* **2009**, *47*, 681–689. [CrossRef]

Publisher's Note: MDPI stays neutral with regard to jurisdictional claims in published maps and institutional affiliations.

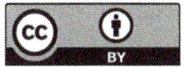

© 2020 by the authors. Licensee MDPI, Basel, Switzerland. This article is an open access article distributed under the terms and conditions of the Creative Commons Attribution (CC BY) license (http://creativecommons.org/licenses/by/4.0/).

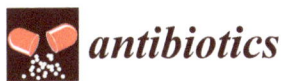

Article

Analysing the Initial Bacterial Adhesion to Evaluate the Performance of Antifouling Surfaces

Patrícia Alves [1], Joana Maria Moreira [1], João Mário Miranda [2,*] and Filipe José Mergulhão [1,*]

1. LEPABE—Laboratory for Process Engineering, Environment, Biotechnology and Energy, Faculty of Engineering, University of Porto, 4200-465 Porto, Portugal; up201510029@fe.up.pt (P.A.); joanarm@fe.up.pt (J.M.M.)
2. CEFT—Transport Phenomena Research Center, Faculty of Engineering, University of Porto, 4200-465 Porto, Portugal
* Correspondence: jmiranda@fe.up.pt (J.M.M.); filipem@fe.up.pt (F.J.M.); Tel.: +351-220414847 (J.M.M.); +351-225081668 (F.J.M)

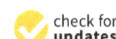

Received: 8 June 2020; Accepted: 15 July 2020; Published: 17 July 2020

Abstract: The aim of this work was to study the initial events of *Escherichia coli* adhesion to polydimethylsiloxane, which is critical for the development of antifouling surfaces. A parallel plate flow cell was used to perform the initial adhesion experiments under controlled hydrodynamic conditions (shear rates ranging between 8 and 100/s), mimicking biomedical scenarios. Initial adhesion studies capture more accurately the cell-surface interactions as in later stages, incoming cells may interact with the surface but also with already adhered cells. Adhesion rates were calculated and results shown that after some time (between 5 and 9 min), these rates decreased (by 55% on average), from the initial values for all tested conditions. The common explanation for this decrease is the occurrence of hydrodynamic blocking, where the area behind each adhered cell is screened from incoming cells. This was investigated using a pair correlation map from which two-dimensional histograms showing the density probability function were constructed. The results highlighted a lower density probability (below 4.0×10^{-4}) of the presence of cells around a given cell under different shear rates irrespectively of the radial direction. A shadowing area behind the already adhered cells was not observed, indicating that hydrodynamic blocking was not occurring and therefore it could not be the cause for the decreases in cell adhesion rates. Afterward, cell transport rates from the bulk solution to the surface were estimated using the Smoluchowski-Levich approximation and values in the range of 80–170 cells/cm^2.s were obtained. The drag forces that adhered cells have to withstand were also estimated and values in the range of 3–50×10^{-14} N were determined. Although mass transport increases with the flow rate, drag forces also increase and the relative importance of these factors may change in different conditions. This work demonstrates that adjustment of operational parameters in initial adhesion experiments may be required to avoid hydrodynamic blocking, in order to obtain reliable data about cell-surface interactions that can be used in the development of more efficient antifouling surfaces.

Keywords: bacterial adhesion; blocking effect; hydrodynamics; parallel plate flow cell

1. Introduction

Bacterial adhesion to a surface triggers a series of events that may lead to biofilm formation and fouling of that surface. Biofilms are bacterial cell communities that are embedded in a self-produced and highly hydrated matrix of extracellular polymeric substances (EPS). Living in biofilms is the most common state for bacteria in natural environments [1], and biofilms can be composed of single or multiple species that interact with each other [2]. Biofilms can cause deterioration of industrial equipment, food spoilage and disease [3,4], but they are also used in wastewater treatment systems and have been investigated for the production of valuable molecules, including recombinant proteins [5,6].

The first step in biofilm formation is the surface adsorption of molecules from the surrounding medium. This originates a conditioning film that can affect subsequent bacterial adhesion [7]. Initially, bacterial adhesion is reversible, but then the adhered organisms start to produce EPS and to anchor themselves irreversibly, leading to the development of the biofilm structure. Then, biofilms mature and release bacteria, often leading to serious bacterial transmission issues [1]. Microorganisms that adhere first have a pivotal role in linking the biofilm to the surface and their retention is crucial to maintain the biofilm on that surface when it is challenged by shear forces [8]. Thus, a better understanding of the initial adhesion process may provide clues to the development of antifouling surfaces.

One of the most promising strategies to prevent or delay biofilm formation on a given surface is to use a coating. In both medical and industrial settings, different types of antifouling coatings have been developed to prevent adhesion, which operate by contact killing or that release biocidal agents [9]. Release systems may promote the development of different types of resistance, and contact killing surfaces may originate a layer of dead cells and cellular debris that can serve as anchoring points for subsequent cell adhesion [7]. In that case, newly adhered cells can be protected from the biocidal agent by the layer formed by dead cells and debris. Anti-adhesion systems are, therefore, an attractive way of preventing or delaying biofilm formation [10]. The development of anti-adhesion coatings is an intense area of research, but these coatings have to be tested in environmental conditions that mimic their application scenario. Since medical and industrial biofilms often develop in areas where significant fluid motion exists, fluid displacement systems have been used to study these initial bacterial–surface interactions [11]. One of the most commonly used platforms for adhesion studies is the parallel plate flow cell (PPFC), which enables real-time monitoring of bacterial adhesion when the system is mounted on a microscope stage coupled to an image acquisition system [11].

A typical initial adhesion experiment performed in a PPFC with continuous monitoring of the number of adhered cells generates a pattern where a linear trajectory can be identified first, followed by a decrease in slope where adhesion seems to be leveling off [8]. It has been proposed that during the linear phase, cells arriving at the surface interact solely with the surface and that the rate at which organisms adhere in this phase is truly representative of the affinity of that organism to that surface [8]. It is also believed that at later stages, when the surface is partially covered, an arriving cell will interact with the surface but also with other adhered cells and that the observed adhesion rates level off due to hydrodynamic blocking [8]. As a consequence, these second adhesion rates would not be truly representative of the interaction between a single cell and the surface, as data would reflect contributions from different interactions that are hard to separate [8].

It has been demonstrated that hydrodynamic blocking can reduce the adhesion of cells by screening the surface behind already adhered cells [12]. If the surface is entirely free of cells, an incoming cell can freely attach as long as it can withstand the shear forces. However, when cells start to attach irreversibly, an incoming cell can no longer attach immediately behind an already adhered cell because that area is effectively screened. This creates a shadow where cell adhesion is prohibited (Figure 1). During colloidal particle deposition, it has been shown that the area blocked by one particle can represent 8 to 675 times the cross-sectional area of that particle [13,14]. In general, blocking is more likely to occur at high surface coverages, but local flow effects can introduce anisotropy in cell adhesion [12].

A detailed analysis of the hydrodynamic blocking has been presented in several works by Adamczyk and co-workers [15–17], but this approach is not straightforward to many researchers, and this may explain why a blocking analysis is absent from many studies dealing with adhesion under flow conditions. In a study by van Loenhout et al. [12], the hydrodynamic blocking effect on particle adsorption was assessed by performing experiments in laminar flow and Monte Carlo simulations to evaluate the effect of the hydrodynamic shadow on particle distribution. The spatial distribution and anisotropy were analysed through a two-dimensional (2D) map of a pair correlation function that was obtained from image analysis. This enabled the observation of the exclusion zone originating from the hydrodynamic blocking. The position of the adhered particles could be calculated and revealed the density of particles adhering around a given particle when compared to the overall density.

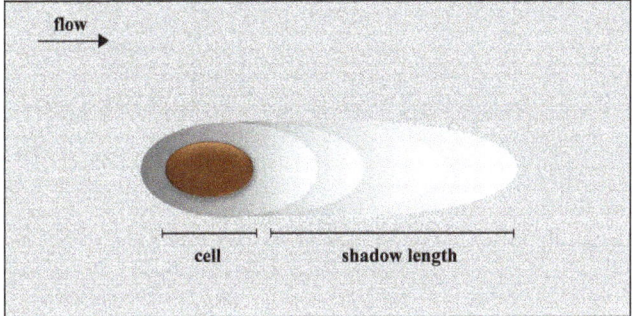

Figure 1. The hydrodynamic blocking effect. The area blocked by an adhered cell where further cell adhesion is prohibited is represented by the shadow.

The arrival of cells to the surface is dictated by mass transport, and in flow systems, this transport is achieved by convection and diffusion. Although solutions for the convective–diffusion equation can be obtained by complicated mathematical procedures, there are approximate solutions such as the Smoluchowski-Levich (SL) approximation that assumes that all microorganisms sufficiently close to a surface will adhere irreversibly [8]. On the other hand, adhered cells have to withstand hydrodynamic forces that may cause cell detachment, and therefore the adhesion rates observed in initial adhesion experiments are a balance between all these effects. It has also been shown that initial adhesion experiments can produce valuable data for the development of antifouling surfaces [10,18], and therefore the correct interpretation of that data is critical.

In this study, we have monitored in real-time the initial adhesion of *Escherichia coli* to a polydimethylsiloxane (PDMS) coating. *E. coli* was chosen as a model organism due to its relevance in both clinical and industrial settings, and PDMS is a very versatile polymer commonly used in both scenarios [19]. An interpretation of the events unfolding during initial adhesion is provided, showcasing the relative importance of cell transport to the surface, hydrodynamic blocking, and detachment forces.

2. Results and Discussion

Bacterial adhesion experiments were performed at different flow rates yielding a range of shear rates between 8 and 100/s, similar to relevant biomedical scenarios (Table S1) [20,21].

Figure 2 shows the number of cells adhered to the PDMS surface during the experimental time at different flow rates. In all tested conditions, an initial adhesion rate was determined by linear regression of the first experimental points (Figure 2, blue dashed line), and it was observed that after some time (between 5 and 9 min), the experimental points did not fit this initial regression. Thus, a second linear regression was made with the remaining points (Figure 2, red dashed line) so that a second adhesion rate could be determined. It was found that this second adhesion rate was lower (on average 55%) than the value determined with the first regression (in blue) (Figure 3a), but the most significant reduction was observed for the lower and higher flow rates (on average 76%; $p < 0.05$, Figure 3a). The flow rate of 2 mL/s presents the lowest reduction in the adhesion rate with a decrease of 20% (Figure 3a). Additionally, the adhesion rates were statistically different when comparing the results for the lower and the higher flow rates (1 and 2 mL/s with 8 and 10 mL/s, respectively) ($p < 0.05$).

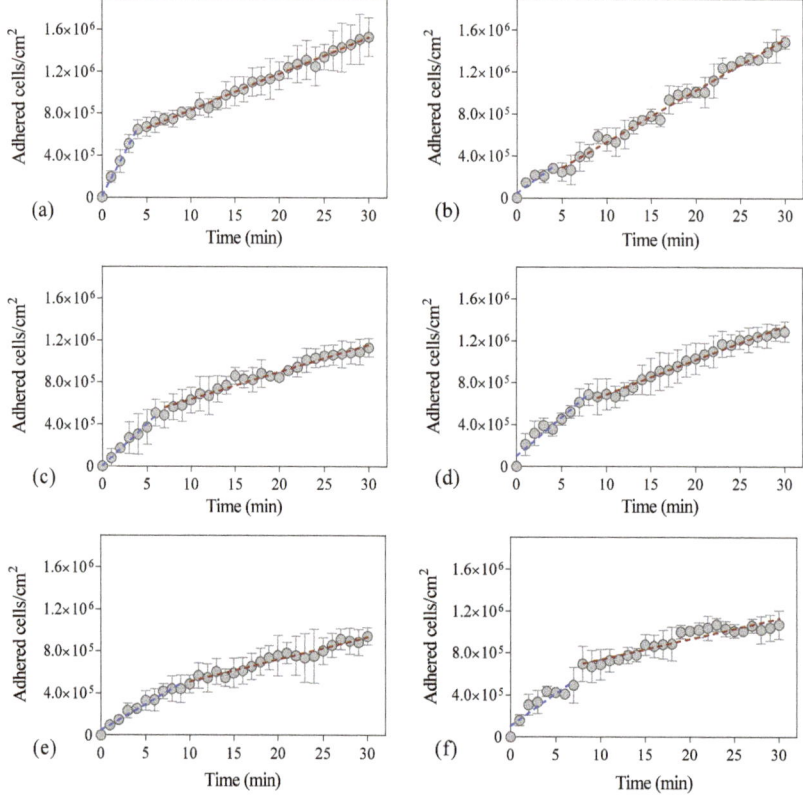

Figure 2. Number of *Escherichia coli* cells adhered to polydimethylsiloxane (PDMS) as a function of time. The dashed line indicates the best fit to a linear function for the initial adhesion rate (blue) and final adhesion rate (red) of the experiments. The adhesion assays were performed during 30 min at different flow rates: (**a**) 1 mL/s, (**b**) 2 mL/s, (**c**) 4 mL/s (**d**) 6 mL/s, (**e**) 8 mL/s, and (**f**) 10 mL/s corresponding to shear rates of 7.5/s, 15.0/s, 33.7/s, 51.6/s, 80.3/s, and 100.8/s, respectively, in a parallel plate flow cell (PPFC). Error bars indicate the standard deviation from three independent experiments.

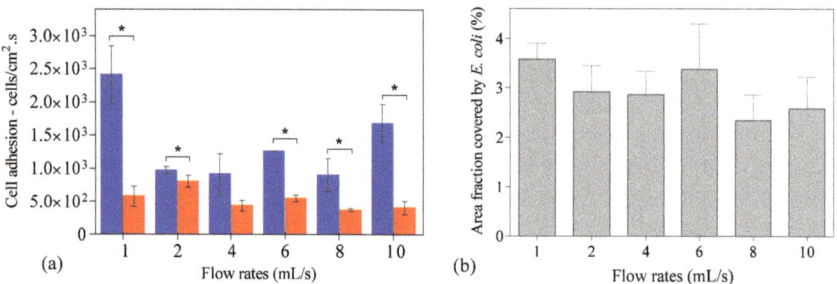

Figure 3. (**a**) Initial adhesion rates determined by linear regression of the first experimental points (blue bar) and for the remaining points (red bar) at different flow rates (1 to 10 mL/s). Statistical significance between the adhesion rates and the different flow rates was evaluated by one-way analysis of variance (one-way ANOVA, Tukey's post-hoc test) ($p < 0.05$); (**b**) Area fraction covered by *Escherichia coli* cells at the end of adhesion assay (30 min) on polydimethylsiloxane (PDMS) at different flow rates (1 to 10 mL/s).

It has been hypothesized that the main cause for this reduction in adhesion rate could be due to hydrodynamic blocking as arriving cells would interact with either already adhered cells or with the free surface [8]. Since the blocking effect is commonly evaluated as a function of the surface area coverage [12,22], this value was determined for the time where the slope decreased at each flow rate. Values between 0.8 to 1.8% were obtained, indicating low surface coverage at that time.

In order to assess if hydrodynamic blocking was occurring, we have performed an image analysis for each flow rate at the end of the adhesion assay (30 min), where surface coverage is at its highest value. It is precisely in those situations that blocking would be most likely to occur in our assays [12,22]. The image analysis revealed that the final surface coverage was similar for all tested flow rates (Figure 3b) and was below 4%.

Afterward, a pair correlation map was used to establish if significant areas were blocked by already adhered cells. Then, 2D histograms were created, showing the probability density function of the presence of cells around a given cell (Figure 4). The central cell was excluded from the calculations, which explains the low probability in the center of the image. Cells at a distance larger than 50 pixels (30.5 μm) were also excluded from the analysis as it has been shown that blocking is more effective at distances shorter than the cut-off value used in this work [23]. If hydrodynamic blocking was occurring, the pair correlation map should show a low probability of cell adhesion along the flow direction, as demonstrated in previous studies [12]. However, in our experiments, the pair correlation maps are symmetrical, as the density probability of the presence of a cell around a given cell was uniform (Figure 4) and had no directional bias. This demonstrates that hydrodynamic blocking was not occurring during our experiments, not at the end of the assay and surely not at the time point where the adhesion rates decreased.

In a previous study, it was shown that the size of the blocked area is a function of the dimensionless Péclet number [24]. In the present work, the Péclet number was below 0.4, which is much lower than the scenarios simulated in that study (2 to 100). Indeed, the size of the blocked area was shown to increase at higher shear rates and large particle sizes [12], and this may also explain why a shadow area was not observed in our work. Additionally, the low surface coverage may also have prevented the occurrence of blocking as it has been reported that even at surface coverages of about 10%, the blocking effect may not be significant [22].

Since hydrodynamic blocking was not occurring, other factors may explain the reduction in adhesion rates that we have observed (Figure 2). Higher flow velocities increase the number of contacts between planktonic cells and the surface, but the increased shear forces may also prevent adhesion or promote detachment [25,26]. In order to ascertain the effect of flow rate variation on the transport of cells from the bulk solution to the surface, the SL approximation was used [8]. Figure 5 shows that as the flow rate increases, mass transport is favored (values in the range of 80–170 cells/cm^2·s were obtained), and since the SL approximation considers that all cells in close proximity to the surface will adhere, higher adhesion rates are expected at higher flow rates. However, as the flow rate increases, the wall shear stress also increases, and therefore higher drag forces are expected (values in the range of 3–50×10^{-14} N were determined—Figure 5). It has been shown that sufficiently high shear stresses cause adhering bacteria to slide and roll over a surface, which may lead to detachment [27].

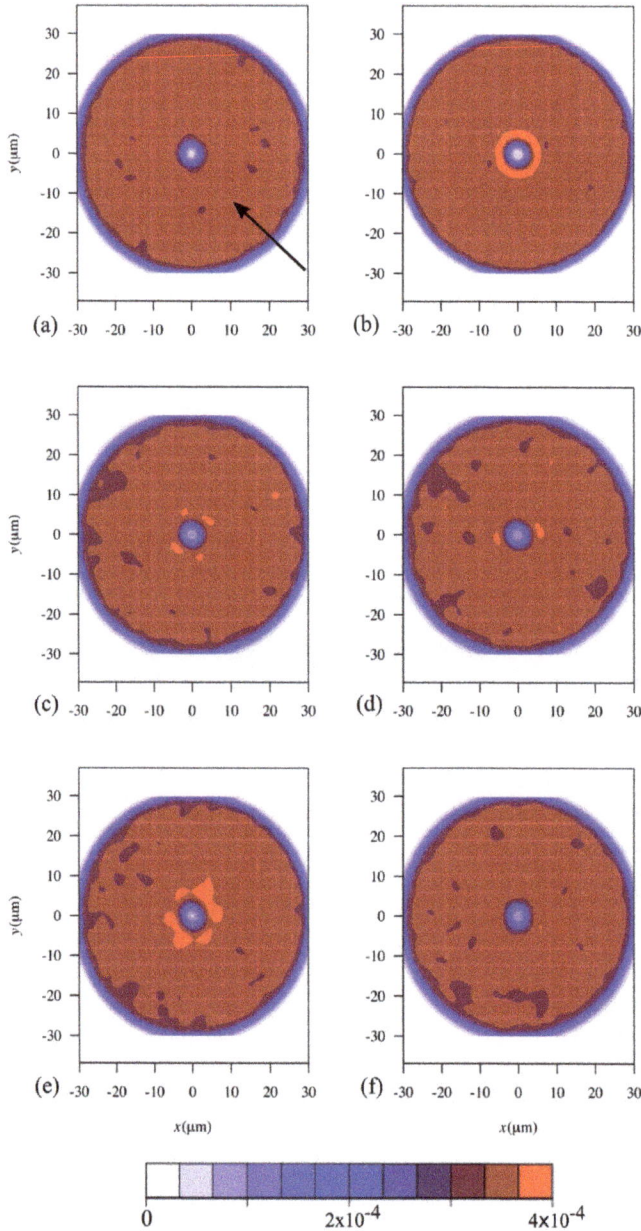

Figure 4. 2D histograms representing the probability density function of the presence of a cell around a given cell (reference cell is in the center). Results for different flow rates are shown: (**a**) 1 mL/s, (**b**) 2 mL/s, (**c**) 4 mL/s (**d**) 6 mL/s, (**e**) 8 mL/s, and (**f**) 10 mL/s corresponding to shear rates of 7.5/s, 15.0/s, 33.7/s, 51.6/s, 80.3/s, and 100.8/s, respectively, in a PPFC. The number of independent cells measured for each flow rate was (**a**) $1.53 \times 10^6 \pm 1.84 \times 10^5$ cells/cm^2; (**b**) $1.49 \times 10^6 \pm 6.14 \times 10^4$ cells/cm^2; (**c**) $1.13 \times 10^6 \pm 8.87 \times 10^4$ cells/cm^2; (**d**) $1.29 \times 10^6 \pm 9.84 \times 10^4$ cells/cm^2; (**e**) $9.41 \times 10^5 \pm 8.25 \times 10^4$ cells/cm^2 and (**f**) $1.07 \times 10^6 \pm 1.37 \times 10^5$ cells/cm^2. The direction of the flow in all histograms is depicted by an arrow located on panel (a).

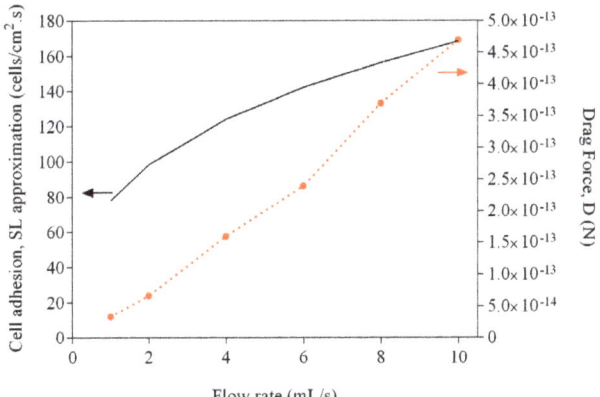

Figure 5. Variation of the drag force (D) and values obtained with the Smoluchowski-Levich (SL) approximation as a function of the flow rate (1 to 10 mL/s). The full line represents the predicted adhesion rate using the SL approximation and the dashed line represents the drag force.

It is known that the strength of adhesion can depend on the history of the contact between a bacterium and a surface and that factors like the residence time and the shear applied during adhesion are strong modulators [28,29]. Additionally, these forces are strongly depending on chemistry [30] and mechanical properties of the surface [31]. It is likely that for each experimental condition tested, the relative importance of mass transport and detachment changes, and this may induce variations in the observed cell adhesion. In any case, since blocking is not occurring, the experimental values obtained at this second stage are also a reflection of the interaction between single cells and the surface.

3. Materials and Methods

3.1. Bacteria and Culture Conditions

E. coli JM109(DE3) from Promega (USA) was selected for this study because it has been used in previous works from our group for the evaluation of initial adhesion in antifouling surfaces [10,18,32,33] and because it was shown to have similar biofilm formation behavior to different clinical isolates, including *E. coli* CECT 434 [21]. The inoculum was prepared as previously described [34]. Briefly, 500 µL of a glycerol stock (kept at −80 °C) was added to a total volume of 0.2 L of the inoculation medium composed by 5.5 g/L glucose (Chem-Lab nv, Zedelgem, Belgium), 2.5 g/L peptone (Oxoid, Basingstoke, Hampshire, England), 1.25 g/L yeast extract in phosphate buffer (1.88 g/L KH_2PO_4 and 2.60 g/L Na_2HPO_4; Chem-Lab nv, Zedelgem, Belgium) at pH 7.0. The culture was incubated overnight at 37 °C, with orbital agitation (160 rpm in a shaker: IKA KS 130 basic, Staufen, Germany). Subsequently, this culture was centrifuged (at 3202 *g* for 10 min at 25 °C) to harvest the cells, and these were washed twice with 0.05 M of citrate buffer (composed by citric acid, Scharlau, Barcelona, Spain; pH 5.0) to remove any traces of the culture medium [35]. Cells were again harvested by centrifugation and resuspended in citrate buffer by vortexing in order to reach an optical density of 0.1 ($OD_{610\,nm}$). A calibration curve was used to determine the cell density (7.6×10^7 cells/mL). This suspension was used to perform adhesion experiments.

3.2. Surface Preparation and Experimental Setup

Adhesion experiments were performed in a PPFC, as described by Moreira et al. [20]. The PPFC used in the present work has a rectangular cross-section of 0.8 × 1.6 cm and a length of 25.42 cm. Briefly, glass slides (7.6 × 2.6 × 0.1 cm, VWR, Carnaxide, Portugal) were washed with a 0.5% detergent solution (Sonasol Pril, Henkel Ibérica SA, Barcelona, Spain) for 30 min and then the detergent was rinsed with distilled water. Subsequently, the surfaces were immersed in 3% sodium hypochlorite for 30 min. Finally, the surfaces were rinsed with distilled water and prepared for coating. PDMS (Sylgard 184 Part A, Dow Corning; viscosity = 1.1 cm^2/s; specific density = 1.03, Midland, MI, USA) was prepared by performing the following steps: i) the curing agent (Sylgard 184 Part B, Dow Corning, Midland, MI, USA) was added to the PDMS at a 1:10 ratio; ii) the mixture was placed in the vacuum chamber in which the pump was turned on and off periodically thus changing the pressure and collapsing air bubbles that may have formed. Subsequently, the mixture was used to coat glass slides by spin-coating (Spin150 PolosTM, Caribbean, Netherlands) at 4000 rpm for 60 s in order to obtain a thickness of 10 µm. The PPFC was mounted in a microscope (Nikon Eclipse LV100, Tokyo, Japan).

3.3. Adhesion Experiments

The bacterial suspension was introduced in the flow cell for 30 min at flow rates of 1, 2, 4, 6, 8, and 10 mL/s. The flow rates were adjusted with a valve. Adhesion was followed by brightfield microscopy, and three trials were performed for each flow rate. Images were taken at 60 s intervals to enable a more accurate adhesion analysis. Obtained images were processed using ImageJ (version 1.38e) software [36] and for each flow rate tested, the number of adhered cells per unit area was determined as a function of time (Code 1—supplementary material). Initial adhesion rates were obtained by linear regression analysis of initial points. After some time, from 5 to 9 min, the adhesion rate decreased, and the remaining points were subjected to a second linear regression. The difference between the first and second slopes was analysed. Standard deviations on the triplicate sets were calculated for all analysed parameters. Graph production and statistical analysis were performed using GraphPad Prism 6.01 (La Jolla, USA). The differences between the slopes as well as the variation of the adhesion rates with the shear conditions were evaluated using one-way analysis of variance (one-way ANOVA, Tukey's post-hoc test). All statistical analysis used a 95% confidence limit, so that p values equal to or greater than 0.05 were not considered statistically significant.

The percentage area fraction covered by *E. coli* cells was determined for different flow rates (1 to 10 mL/s). For this, ImageJ macro scripts were created to convert the images to an 8-bit greyscale file format and thresholds were applied to determine the occupied area (Code 2—supplementary material).

3.4. Blocking Analysis

After each 30 min trial, 5 images were taken in different regions of the surface to obtain a large set of adhered cells. Using ImageJ, the images were inverted, and the maxima detected (Figure S1). Each maximum corresponds to a cell. The respective coordinates were obtained and a pair correlation map was constructed [12]. Results are presented in the form of a 2D density probability function. The probability density function can be used to calculate, by integration, the probability of a cell being found around another cell at a region defined by Δx and Δy, where x and y are the coordinates centered in the reference cell. The probability density function was calculated using an R language script (see R scripts—supplementary materials). To find the probability density function, a threshold R_{max} was defined. Pairs at a distance larger than R_{max} were not considered to construct the probability density function.

3.5. Mass Transfer and Drag Force

The theoretical mass transport was estimated though the SL equation (approximate solution) [8] for each flow rate:

$$SL = 0.538 \frac{D_\infty C_b}{R_b} \left(\frac{Pe\, h_0}{x} \right)^{1/3}, \qquad (1)$$

where D_∞ is the diffusion coefficient (approximately 4.0×10^{-13} m^2/s for *E. coli* [37]), C_b is the bacterial concentration (7.6×10^{13} cell/m^3), h_0 is the height of the rectangular channel (0.08 m) and x is the distance for which an average velocity variation below 15% was determined (m) as detailed in

Moreira, et al. [20]. R_b corresponds to the microbial radius (4.5×10^{-7} m) assuming that *E. coli* has a cylindrical shape estimated accordingly to the equation [15]:

$$R_b = \frac{1}{\ln\left(\frac{L}{b}\right) - 0.11}\left(\frac{L}{2}\right), \qquad (2)$$

where L and b are the length and the diameter of the *E. coli* used in this study, respectively.

The SL equation also includes the Péclet number (Pe) which represents the ratio between convective and diffusional mass transport, given for the parallel plate configuration as:

$$Pe = \frac{3 v_{av} R_b^3}{2\left(\frac{h_0}{2}\right)^2 D_\infty}, \qquad (3)$$

where v_{av} is the average flow velocity (m/s) determined in Moreira et al. [20].

It is assumed that gravity effects and hydrodynamic lift are negligible compared to the drag force [38], which was estimated by the following equation [38]:

$$D = 32.0 \tau_w R_b^2 + O(\text{Re}_c), \qquad (4)$$

where τ_w corresponds to the wall shear stress.

The flow within the near-wall region can be characterized using the local Reynolds number (Re_c), based on the shear rate, γ, [38], as follows:

$$\text{Re}_c = \rho \gamma R_b^2 / \mu, \qquad (5)$$

where ρ, is the density (993.37 kg/m^3), and μ is the dynamic viscosity of the fluid (0.000694 kg/m.s). The values for τ_w and γ were obtained by Computational Fluid Dynamics as described in [20] and are listed in Table S1 (Supplementary material).

Re_c is always lower than 1, as $R_b \ll h_0$, and so the inertial effects are negligible in the near-wall region and terms of higher order, $O(\text{Re}_c)$, in Equation (4) are negligible [38].

4. Conclusions

Bacterial adhesion studies are important not only because they provide an understanding of the early stages of biofilm formation but also because they may provide clues for the development of more efficient antifouling surfaces. These studies should be performed in conditions that mimic the real-life scenario not only regarding the surfaces and bacteria under evaluation but also in defined hydrodynamic conditions prevailing on that scenario. When real-time monitoring of initial adhesion is performed, a decrease in the initial adhesion rates is often observed along the experimental time. This decrease is often associated with hydrodynamic blocking, which can occur at significant surface coverage values. For low surface coverage situations, this decrease is most likely caused by cell detachment, which occurs when the force exerted on a single bacterium overcomes the adhesion force between the cell and that surface. Initial adhesion experiments should, therefore, be conducted so that low surface coverage values are obtained (by adapting the test conditions, namely the assay time), and the absence of blocking should be verified so that reliable results can be obtained. This enables the performance evaluation of different coatings so that more efficient antifouling surfaces can be developed.

Supplementary Materials: The following are available online at http://www.mdpi.com/2079-6382/9/7/421/s1, Figure S1: Steps of the method. From left to right: initial image, inverted image and maxima; R scripts—Relative positions script and Histogram script; Code 1—Cell adhesion analysis; Code 2—Surface coverage; Table S1: Shear rate and wall shear stress at the different flow rates tested (determined by Computational Fluid Dynamics) and examples of biomedical scenarios where these shear rates can be found.

Author Contributions: Conceptualization, P.A., J.M.M. (Joana Maria Moreira), J.M.M. (João Mário Miranda) and F.J.M.; methodology, P.A., J.M.M. (João Mário Miranda) and F.J.M.; investigation, P.A., J.M.M. (Joana Maria Moreira) and J.M.M. (João Mário Miranda); resources, J.M.M. (João Mário Miranda) and F.J.M.; data curation, P.A., J.M.M. (João Mário Miranda) and F.J.M.; writing—original draft preparation, P.A. and F.J.M.; supervision, J.M.M. (João Mário Miranda) and F.J.M.; funding acquisition, J.M.M. (João Mário Miranda), F.J.M. All authors have read and agreed to the published version of the manuscript.

Funding: This research was funded by Base Funding—UIDB/00511/2020 of the Laboratory for Process Engineering, Environment, Biotechnology and Energy—LEPABE and Base Funding—UIDB/00532/2020 of the Transport Phenomena Research Center—CEFT—funded by national funds through the FCT/MCTES (PIDDAC). P.A. acknowledges the receipt of a Ph.D. grant from the Portuguese Foundation from Science and Technology (FCT) (PD/BD/114317/2016). The authors would like to acknowledge the support from the EU COST Actions ENIUS (CA16217) and ENBA (CA15216).

Conflicts of Interest: The authors declare no conflict of interest.

References

1. Gusnaniar, N.; van der Mei, H.C.; Qu, W.; Nuryastuti, T.; Hooymans, J.M.M.; Sjollema, J.; Busscher, H.J. Physico-chemistry of bacterial transmission versus adhesion. *Adv. Colloid Interface Sci.* **2017**, *250*, 15–24. [CrossRef] [PubMed]
2. Costa, A.M.; Mergulhão, F.J.; Briandet, R.; Azevedo, N.F. It is all about location: How to pinpoint microorganisms and their functions in multispecies biofilms. *Future Microbiol.* **2017**, *12*, 987–999. [CrossRef] [PubMed]
3. Brooks, J.D.; Flint, S.H. Biofilms in the food industry: Problems and potential solutions. *Int. J. Food Sci. Technol.* **2008**, *43*, 2163–2176. [CrossRef]
4. Miquel, S.; Lagrafeuille, R.; Souweine, B.; Forestier, C. Anti-biofilm activity as a health issue. *Front. Microbiol.* **2016**, *7*, 592. [CrossRef] [PubMed]
5. Soares, A.; Azevedo, A.; Gomes, L.C.; Mergulhão, F.J. Recombinant protein expression in biofilms. *AIMS Microbiol.* **2019**, *5*, 232–250. [CrossRef]
6. Soares, A.; Gomes, L.C.; Mergulhão, F.J. Comparing the Recombinant Protein Production Potential of Planktonic and Biofilm Cells. *Microorganisms* **2018**, *6*, 48. [CrossRef]
7. Moreira, J.; Gomes, L.; Whitehead, K.; Lynch, S.; Tetlow, L.; Mergulhão, F. Effect of surface conditioning with cellular extracts on *Escherichia coli* adhesion and initial biofilm formation. *Food Bioprod. Process.* **2017**, *104*, 1–12. [CrossRef]
8. Busscher, H.J.; van der Mei, H.C. Microbial adhesion in flow displacement systems. *Clin. Microbiol. Rev.* **2006**, *19*, 127–141. [CrossRef] [PubMed]
9. Ramstedt, M.; Ribeiro, I.A.C.; Bujdakova, H.; Mergulhão, F.J.M.; Jordao, L.; Thomsen, P.; Alm, M.; Burmølle, M.; Vladkova, T.; Can, F.; et al. Evaluating efficacy of antimicrobial and antifouling materials for urinary tract medical devices: Challenges and recommendations. *Macromol. Biosci.* **2019**, *19*, e1800384. [CrossRef] [PubMed]
10. Lopez-Mila, B.; Alves, P.; Riedel, T.; Dittrich, B.; Mergulhão, F.; Rodriguez-Emmenegger, C. Effect of shear stress on the reduction of bacterial adhesion to antifouling polymers. *Bioinspir. Biomim.* **2018**, *13*, 065001. [CrossRef] [PubMed]
11. Azeredo, J.; Azevedo, N.F.; Briandet, R.; Cerca, N.; Coenye, T.; Costa, A.R.; Desvaux, M.; Di Bonaventura, G.; Hébraud, M.; Jaglic, Z. Critical review on biofilm methods. *Crit. Rev. Microbiol.* **2017**, *43*, 313–351. [CrossRef]
12. van Loenhout, M.T.; Kooij, E.S.; Wormeester, H.; Poelsema, B. Hydrodynamic flow induced anisotropy in colloid adsorption. *Colloids Surf. A Physicochem. Eng. Asp.* **2009**, *342*, 46–52. [CrossRef]
13. Meinders, J.; Noordmans, J.; Busscher, H. Simultaneous monitoring of the adsorption and desorption of colloidal particles during deposition in a parallel plate flow chamber. *J. Colloid Interface Sci.* **1992**, *152*, 265–280. [CrossRef]
14. Dabroś, T.; Van de Ven, T. Kinetics of coating by colloidal particles. *J. Colloid Interface Sci.* **1982**, *89*, 232–244. [CrossRef]
15. Adamczyk, Z. Modeling adsorption of colloids and proteins. *Curr. Opin. Colloid Interface Sci.* **2012**, *17*, 173–186. [CrossRef]
16. Adamczyk, Z.; Warszyński, P.; Szyk-Warszyńska, L.; Weroński, P. Role of convection in particle deposition at solid surfaces. *Colloids Surf. A Physicochem. Eng. Asp.* **2000**, *165*, 157–187. [CrossRef]

17. Adamczyk, Z. Particle adsorption and deposition: Role of electrostatic interactions. *Adv. Colloid Interface Sci.* **2003**, *100*, 267–347. [CrossRef]
18. Alves, P.; Gomes, L.C.; Vorobii, M.; Rodriguez-Emmenegger, C.; Mergulhão, F.J. The potential advantages of using a poly(HPMA) brush in urinary catheters: Effects on biofilm cells and architecture. *Colloids Surf. B Biointerfaces* **2020**, *191*, 110976. [CrossRef] [PubMed]
19. Carlsen, P.N. *Polydimethylsiloxane: Structure and Applications*; Nova Science Publishers, Inc.: New York, NY, USA, 2020.
20. Moreira, J.; Araújo, J.; Miranda, J.M.; Simões, M.; Melo, L.; Mergulhão, F. The effects of surface properties on *Escherichia coli* adhesion are modulated by shear stress. *Colloids Surf. B Biointerfaces* **2014**, *123*, 1–7. [CrossRef]
21. Gomes, L.; Moreira, J.; Teodósio, J.; Araújo, J.; Miranda, J.; Simões, M.; Melo, L.; Mergulhão, F. 96-well microtiter plates for biofouling simulation in biomedical settings. *Biofouling* **2014**, *30*, 535–546. [CrossRef]
22. Van der Mei, W.N.; Krom, B.; Sjollema, J. Analysis of the contribution of sedimentation to bacterial mass transport in a parallel plate flow chamber Part II: Use of fluorescence imaging. *Colloids Surf. B Biointerfaces* **2011**, *87*, 427–432. [CrossRef]
23. Sjollema, J.; Busscher, H. Deposition of polystyrene particles in a parallel plate flow cell. 2. Pair distribution functions between deposited particles. *Colloids Surf.* **1990**, *47*, 337–352. [CrossRef]
24. Dabros, T. Interparticle hydrodynamic interactions in deposition processes. *Colloids Surf.* **1989**, *39*, 127–141. [CrossRef]
25. Lecuyer, S.; Rusconi, R.; Shen, Y.; Forsyth, A.; Vlamakis, H.; Kolter, R.; Stone, H.A. Shear stress increases the residence time of adhesion of *Pseudomonas aeruginosa*. *Biophys. J.* **2011**, *100*, 341–350. [CrossRef]
26. Dickinson, R.B.; Cooper, S.L. Analysis of shear-dependent bacterial adhesion kinetics to biomaterial surfaces. *AIChE J.* **1995**, *41*, 2160–2174. [CrossRef]
27. Nejadnik, M.R.; van der Mei, H.C.; Busscher, H.J.; Norde, W. Determination of the shear force at the balance between bacterial attachment and detachment in weak-adherence systems, using a flow displacement chamber. *Appl. Environ. Microbiol.* **2008**, *74*, 916. [CrossRef]
28. Marshall, B.T.; Sarangapani, K.K.; Lou, J.; McEver, R.P.; Zhu, C. Force history dependence of receptor-ligand dissociation. *Biophys. J.* **2005**, *88*, 1458–1466. [CrossRef]
29. Xu, L.C.; Vadillo-Rodriguez, V.; Logan, B.E. Residence time, loading force, pH, and ionic strength affect adhesion forces between colloids and biopolymer-coated surfaces. *Langmuir* **2005**, *21*, 7491–7500. [CrossRef]
30. Garrett, T.R.; Bhakoo, M.; Zhang, Z. Bacterial adhesion and biofilms on surfaces. *Prog. Nat. Sci.* **2008**, *18*, 1049–1056. [CrossRef]
31. Lichter, J.A.; Thompson, M.T.; Delgadillo, M.; Nishikawa, T.; Rubner, M.F.; Van Vliet, K.J. Substrata mechanical stiffness can regulate adhesion of viable bacteria. *Biomacromolecules* **2008**, *9*, 1571–1578. [CrossRef]
32. Alves, P.; Gomes, L.C.; Rodríguez-Emmenegger, C.; Mergulhão, F.J. Efficacy of a poly(MeOEGMA) brush on the prevention of *Escherichia coli* biofilm formation and susceptibility. *Antibiotics* **2020**, *9*, 216. [CrossRef] [PubMed]
33. Alves, P.; Nir, S.; Reches, M.; Mergulhão, F. The effects of fluid composition and shear conditions on bacterial adhesion to an antifouling peptide-coated surface. *MRS Commun.* **2018**, *8*, 938–946. [CrossRef]
34. Teodósio, J.; Simões, M.; Melo, L.; Mergulhão, F. Flow cell hydrodynamics and their effects on *E. coli* biofilm formation under different nutrient conditions and turbulent flow. *Biofouling* **2011**, *27*, 1–11. [CrossRef] [PubMed]
35. Simões, M.; Simões, L.C.; Cleto, S.; Pereira, M.O.; Vieira, M.J. The effects of a biocide and a surfactant on the detachment of *Pseudomonas fluorescens* from glass surfaces. *Int. J. Food Microbiol.* **2008**, *121*, 335–341. [CrossRef]
36. Schneider, C.A.; Rasband, W.S.; Eliceiri, K.W. NIH Image to ImageJ: 25 years of image analysis. *Nat. Methods* **2012**, *9*, 671. [CrossRef]
37. Xia, Z.; Woo, L.; van de Ven, T.G. Microrheological aspects of adhesion of *Escherichia coli* on glass. *Biorheology* **1989**, *26*, 359–375. [CrossRef] [PubMed]
38. Boulbene, B.; Morchain, J.; Bonin, M.M.; Janel, S.; Lafont, F.; Schmitz, P. A combined computational fluid dynamics (CFD) and experimental approach to quantify the adhesion force of bacterial cells attached to a plane surface. *AIChE J.* **2012**, *58*, 3614–3624. [CrossRef]

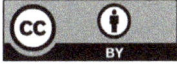

© 2020 by the authors. Licensee MDPI, Basel, Switzerland. This article is an open access article distributed under the terms and conditions of the Creative Commons Attribution (CC BY) license (http://creativecommons.org/licenses/by/4.0/).

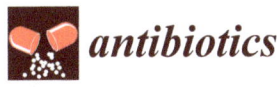 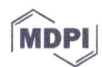

Article

Carbon Nanotube/Poly(dimethylsiloxane) Composite Materials to Reduce Bacterial Adhesion

Márcia R. Vagos [1], Marisa Gomes [1], Joana M. R. Moreira [1], Olívia S. G. P. Soares [2], Manuel F. R. Pereira [2,*] and Filipe J. Mergulhão [1,*]

1. LEPABE—Laboratory for Process Engineering, Environment, Biotechnology and Energy, Faculty of Engineering, University of Porto, Rua Roberto Frias, 4200-465 Porto, Portugal; marciavagos@gmail.com (M.R.V.); marisagomes@fe.up.pt (M.G.); joanarm@fe.up.pt (J.M.R.M.)
2. LCM—Laboratory of Catalysis and Materials, Associate Laboratory LSRE/LCM, Department of Chemical Engineering, Faculty of Engineering, University of Porto, Rua Roberto Frias s/n, 4200-465 Porto, Portugal; salome.soares@fe.up.pt
* Correspondence: fpereira@fe.up.pt (M.F.R.P.); filipem@fe.up.pt (F.J.M.); Tel.: +351-22-508-1468 (M.F.R.P.); +351-22-508-1556 (F.J.M.)

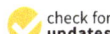

Received: 15 June 2020; Accepted: 17 July 2020; Published: 22 July 2020

Abstract: Different studies have shown that the incorporation of carbon nanotubes (CNTs) into poly(dimethylsiloxane) (PDMS) enables the production of composite materials with enhanced properties, which can find important applications in the biomedical field. In the present work, CNT/PDMS composite materials have been prepared to evaluate the effects of pristine and chemically functionalized CNT incorporation into PDMS on the composite's thermal, electrical, and surface properties on bacterial adhesion in dynamic conditions. Initial bacterial adhesion was studied using a parallel-plate flow chamber assay performed in conditions prevailing in urinary tract devices (catheters and stents) using *Escherichia coli* as a model organism and PDMS as a control due to its relevance in these applications. The results indicated that the introduction of the CNTs in the PDMS matrix yielded, in general, less bacterial adhesion than the PDMS alone and that the reduction could be dependent on the surface chemistry of CNTs, with less adhesion obtained on the composites with pristine rather than functionalized CNTs. It was also shown CNT pre-treatment and incorporation by different methods affected the electrical properties of the composites when compared to PDMS. Composites enabling a 60% reduction in cell adhesion were obtained by CNT treatment by ball-milling, whereas an increase in electrical conductivity of seven orders of magnitude was obtained after solvent-mediated incorporation. The results suggest even at low CNT loading values (1%), these treatments may be beneficial for the production of CNT composites with application in biomedical devices for the urinary tract and for other applications where electrical conductance is required.

Keywords: carbon nanotubes; poly(dimethylsiloxane); adhesion; *Escherichia coli*

1. Introduction

The recent advancements in carbon nanotube (CNT) science have opened up promising possibilities for the development of novel materials and devices in the biomedical field [1]. Their nano-dimensional structure allied to a unique set of properties, such as a large aspect ratio, high surface energy density, electrical and thermal conductivity, as well as superior mechanical strength, flexibility, and ability to blend with other materials to form nanocomposites, have prompted their integration in biomaterials with enhanced properties [2–4].

In the last decade, CNT-polymer nanocomposites have been extensively used in pharmaceutical and medical fields, often showing remarkable improvements in the mechanical, electrical, optical, thermal, and structural properties of the composite material in relation to the polymer alone [2]. Due to their vast potential in the biomedical nanotechnology field, CNTs have been used not only in the construction of biosensors for the detection of biomolecules and cells but also in the development of drug delivery systems [1,5,6].

Studies on the direct cell-CNT interactions have provided indications that nanotubes have the potential to strongly adhere to cell membranes, so there has been an interest in the use of CNTs as coatings for cell culture substrates or medical implants to increase cell attachment and growth [7–9]. Likewise, CNT incorporation into polymers has shown to enhance cell attachment and proliferation, with beneficial implications in cell culture substrates and tissue engineering scaffolds [10–17]. However, as far as implantable medical devices are concerned, microbial adhesion on the implant surface often results in severe infections and failure of the implant. Therefore, contrary to having surfaces with enhanced cell attachment capability, developing surfaces capable of reducing bacterial adhesion becomes a major concern. The antibiofouling properties of CNTs, which are mainly related to their resistance against protein adhesion and other fouling components, also make them an attractive nanomaterial for a wide range of applications [4]. Their antimicrobial activity mainly depends on their length, physical disposition (degree of entanglement), and number of layers [18]. Different studies have indeed reported the efficacy of multiwalled carbon nanotube (MWCNT)/polymer composites in the reduction of bacterial adhesion and biofilm formation [19–22]. Modification of the surface of CNTs has also proved to play an important role in their antifouling potential [10,23].

In the biomedical industry, poly(dimethylsiloxane) (PDMS) has been widely used in the fabrication of medical devices and implants [24]. Particularly in the fabrication of urinary tract devices, PDMS is often used due to its high biocompatibility, mechanical resistance, and good chemical stability [25,26]. Despite these excellent properties, as with any other silicone material, PDMS is prone to non-specific surface adsorption of proteins and bacteria, which can be a disadvantage in the biomedical field. Recently, different studies have reported the increase of the antifouling properties of PDMS by the incorporation of MWCNTs [27–30].

Regarding CNT/PDMS composites, several reports have been published on their mechanical, electrical, and thermal properties, showing that the CNT incorporation can be beneficial [3,31–38]. Another example of the application of these composites is in the fabrication of electrically conductive materials for implants with sensing capacity [39–43]. Therefore, a deeper investigation of the interactions between bacterial cells and CNT-polymer composites at the interface level could provide insights into the use of CNT-based coatings in medical implants. Testing of these new composites should be performed in hydrodynamic conditions that are relevant for their final application [44] as flow affects the transport of bacteria to the surface and also the forces that adhered cells have to withstand [45]. Additionally, it has been shown that initial adhesion can provide very useful information regarding the antifouling performance of a surface or a coating [46,47].

The present study aimed at evaluating the bacterial adhesion behavior onto CNT/PDMS composite coatings. In order to assess the influence of CNT surface chemistry and dispersion state on cell adhesion, pristine, functionalized, and ball-milled CNTs were used. The materials were characterized in terms of thermal stability, surface hydrophobicity and morphology, and direct current (DC) electrical conductivity. Bacterial adhesion assays were performed in a parallel-plate flow chamber (PPFC) system using *Escherichia coli* as model bacteria.

2. Results and Discussion

2.1. Materials Characterization

The values of Brunauer–Emmett–Teller surface area (S_{BET}) obtained for the pristine-CNT (p-CNT), functionalized-CNT (f-CNT), ball-milled p-CNT (p-BM) and ball-milled f-CNT (f-BM) samples were 289 $m^2\,g^{-1}$, 361 $m^2\,g^{-1}$, 375 $m^2\,g^{-1}$ and 348 $m^2\,g^{-1}$, respectively. These values indicate that the four samples of CNTs have different textural properties due to structural changes on f-CNT induced during the nitric acid treatment and also due to the milling process. It has been shown that acidic functionalization increases structural defects of the CNTs and opens their end caps [48,49], increasing the available area for adsorption [50]. The ball-milling treatment breaks the tubes, being responsible for the increase in the surface area observed for sample p-BM [51]. In the case of the sample f-BM, the surface area remains almost unchanged, probably due to the lower ball-milling treatment time applied to this sample and due to a higher agglomeration of the material (induced by the oxygen-containing surface groups and the ball-milling). The different textural properties of the two types of CNTs used may affect the bonding strength between the nanotubes and the PDMS chains.

Temperature programmed desorption (TPD) analysis was performed to assess the content of functional groups introduced on the surface of the CNTs by the acid treatment and compare it to p-CNT. In this analysis, the amount of CO and CO_2 released from the CNT sample reflects the type of oxygenated groups present at their surfaces, which in turn depends on the applied treatment. Results are shown in Figure 1, where it can be seen that f-CNT contained a large amount of oxygenated surface groups, which corroborates the acidic character of this sample when compared to p-CNT.

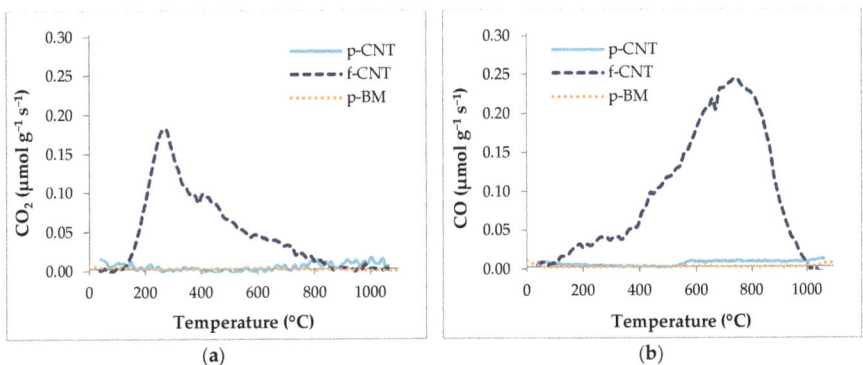

Figure 1. Temperature programmed desorption results of CO_2 spectra (**a**) and CO spectra (**b**) of carbon nanotube (CNT) samples: pristine-CNT (p-CNT), functionalized-CNT (f-CNT) and ball-milled p-CNT (p-BM).

In fact, the surface of CNTs after functionalization with HNO_3 contains a large amount of carboxylic acid groups (released as CO_2 below 400 °C), lactones (released as CO_2 around 650 °C) and some carboxylic anhydrides (released as CO and CO_2 at around 550 °C). Phenol groups (released as CO at around 700 °C) and carbonyl/quinone groups (released as CO at around 850 °C) are also present [52,53]. The ball-milling treatment does not change the chemical surface of the CNTs [51].

The results of the thermogravimetric analysis (TGA) are shown in Figure 2. In the TGA spectra, it can be seen that PDMS started to pyrolyze at 450 °C, with a rapid mass loss until 600 °C. The composite samples showed a very different thermal behavior, with a smooth decomposition resulting in a lower percentage of mass loss. The p-CNT/PDMS sample showed the highest stability, suggesting that the interfacial bonding with PDMS was stronger for this material. Furthermore, it seems that the texture of the CNTs is not a critical factor in the thermal stability of the composite (p-BM/PDMS curve). However, with f-BM/PDMS, there was a significant difference in the decomposition, showing a higher weight loss compared to the other composites. This seems to indicate that the surface chemistry of the CNTs plays a more important role in the filler-polymer interactions than their structure since the oxygen-containing groups of the functionalized CNTs introduce polar moieties in the matrix, which have low affinity for the PDMS chains due to sterical and electrostatic repulsions [54–57].

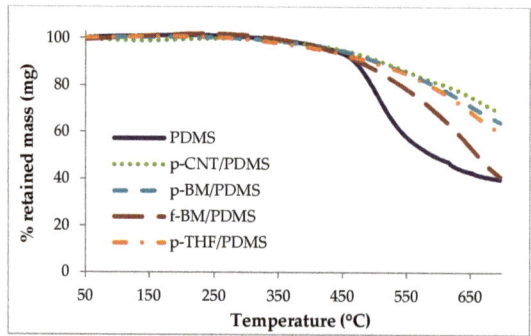

Figure 2. Thermogravimetric spectra of poly(dimethylsiloxane) (PDMS), p-CNT/PDMS, p-BM/PDMS, ball-milled f-CNT (f-BM)/PDMS and THF-treated p-CNT (p-THF)/PDMS composites.

Interestingly, the addition of tetrahydrophuran (THF) in the fabrication of the composites through the solution mixing method did not seem to have a negative impact on the polymer-CNT bondings, as can be seen from the TGA curve of THF-treated p-CNT (p-THF)/PDMS, which is very similar to that of p-BM/PDMS, suggesting that THF, even after being removed from the composite, served as an interfacial agent with PDMS. In general, from these results, it can be concluded that the interactions between the PDMS matrix and the CNTs are effective, resulting in an enhancement of the thermal stability of all the composites.

The results of the contact angle (CA) measurements are shown in Figure 3 and Table 1. All the surfaces produced were hydrophobic (negative ΔG_s^{TOT} value). In addition, in all the surfaces, the acid-base forces had a greater contribution to the overall surface energy than the Lifshitz–van der Waals' forces, showing the importance of the electron donor forces. The results showed that the p-CNT/PDMS and p-BM/PDMS surfaces were more hydrophobic than the f-CNT/PDMS and f-BM/PDMS surfaces, respectively ($p < 0.05$). Surprisingly, the p-THF/PDMS was found to be less hydrophobic than the THF-treated f-CNT (f-THF)/PDMS surface ($p < 0.05$), which was the most hydrophobic one. The surface with the least hydrophobic character was f-BM/PDMS, and all the other surfaces were more hydrophobic than PDMS ($p < 0.05$).

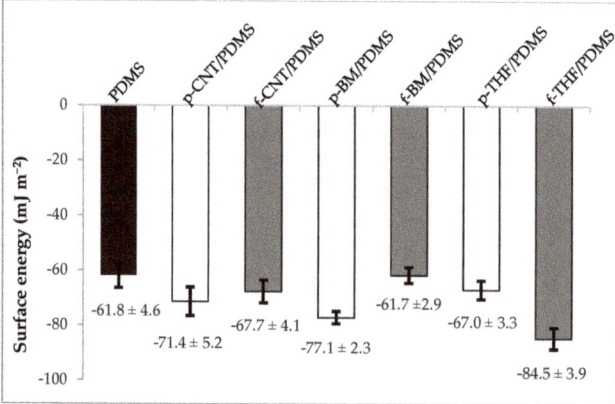

Figure 3. Surface free energy and adhesion energy of PDMS (black bar), p-CNT/PDMS, p-BM/PDMS and p-THF/PDMS composites (white bars); and f-CNT/PDMS, f-BM/PDMS and THF-treated f-CNT (f-THF)/PDMS composites (gray bars).

Table 1. Contact angle results and the calculated values of the surface energy of the samples.

Sample	θ_w	θ_{br}	θ_{form}	γ_s^-	ΔG_s^{LW}	ΔG_s^{AB}	ΔG_s^{TOT}
PDMS	113.6° ± 0.6	87.6° ± 1.8	111.2° ± 0.6	4.5 ± 0.9	−2.9 ± 0.5	−58.9 ± 4.3	−61.8 ± 4.4
p-CNT/PDMS	117.0° ± 0.7	80.4° ± 0.7	110.4° ± 0.8	2.5 ± 0.4	−1.2 ± 0.1	−70.2 ± 2.9	−71.4 ± 2.9
f-CNT/PDMS	116.6° ± 0.6	76.6° ± 1.5	111.1° ± 0.5	3.0 ± 0.6	−0.6 ± 0.2	−67.0 ± 3.7	−67.7 ± 3.7
p-BM/PDMS	121.5° ± 0.3	88.8° ± 0.9	115.7° ± 0.4	1.9 ± 0.3	−3.2 ± 0.3	−73.8 ± 2.2	−77.1 ± 2.2
f-BM/PDMS	113.6° ± 0.4	71.3° ± 1.4	109.1° ± 0.6	4.0 ± 0.7	−0.1 ± 0.1	−61.5 ± 3.3	−61.7 ± 3.3
p-THF/PDMS	116.6° ± 0.3	80.5° ± 1.7	112.0° ± 0.5	3.2 ± 0.7	−1.2 ± 0.3	−65.7 ± 3.8	−67.0 ± 3.8
f-THF/PDMS	125.6° ± 0.4	92.3° ± 1.5	118.6° ± 0.9	1.2 ± 0.4	−4.3 ± 0.5	−80.1 ± 3.7	−84.5 ± 3.8

θ_w, θ_{br} and θ_{form}: the average of measured contact angles with water, α-bromonaphthalene and formamide, respectively; γ_s^-: electron donor parameter; ΔG_s^{LW} and ΔG_s^{AB}: Lifshitz–van der Waals and acid-base free energies of the surface, respectively; ΔG_s^{TOT}: free energy of interaction between two entities of the surfaces immersed in water. Values of γ_s^-, ΔG_s^{LW}, ΔG_s^{AB} and ΔG_s^{TOT} are in mJ m^{-2}.

These results are in agreement with a previous study carried out by Beigbeder and its co-workers, where MWCNTs/PDMS composites showed a higher hydrophobicity when compared with unfilled PMDS [30]. It should be noted that these two groups of surfaces with opposing tendencies were also prepared using two different methods—bulk mixing and solution mixing. The surfaces produced by the bulk mixing process were more hydrophobic with p-CNT then with f-CNT, which can be explained because p-CNT is very hydrophobic, thus raising the overall hydrophobicity of the composite, whereas f-CNT has an acidic character due to the oxygenated surface groups, therefore yielding less hydrophobic composites [58]. However, the p-THF/PDMS and f-THF/PDMS composites showed an opposite tendency. It has been shown that THF can easily disperse CNTs [59], with reportedly improved results for functionalized CNTs [35]. However, in the present work, no comparative assessment was made on the dispersion of the two composites, so this aspect requires further analysis.

In order to assess the effect of the ball-milling procedure, Scanning Electron Microscopy (SEM) analysis of the surface of the p-CNT/PDMS, f-CNT/PDMS, p-BM/PDMS, and f-BM/PDMS composite samples was performed (Figure 4). The images show some sections of the composite surfaces where the CNTs were more densely packed. It can be seen in these regions that the CNTs formed small elevations and were closer to the surface. The p-CNT, f-CNT, p-BM, and f-BM samples all presented a similar morphological aspect; however, a decrease in the length of the MWCNTs is noticed as a result of the ball-milling treatment. It has been previously shown that ball-milling cuts the tubes (decreasing their lengths) and promotes their disentanglement [51].

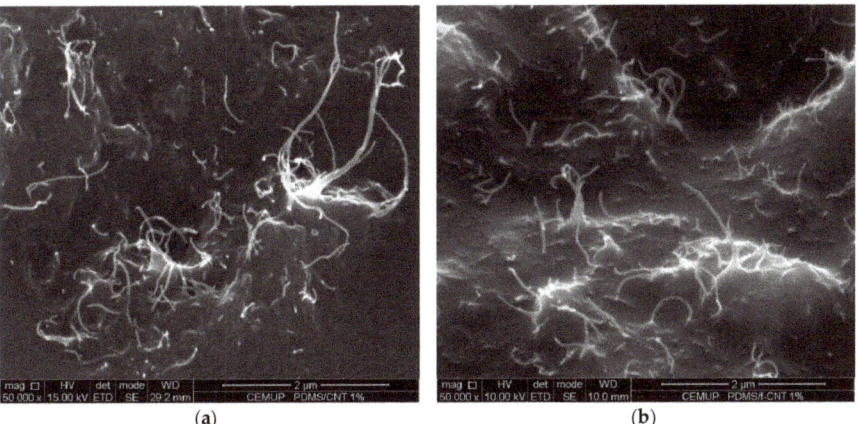

Figure 4. *Cont.*

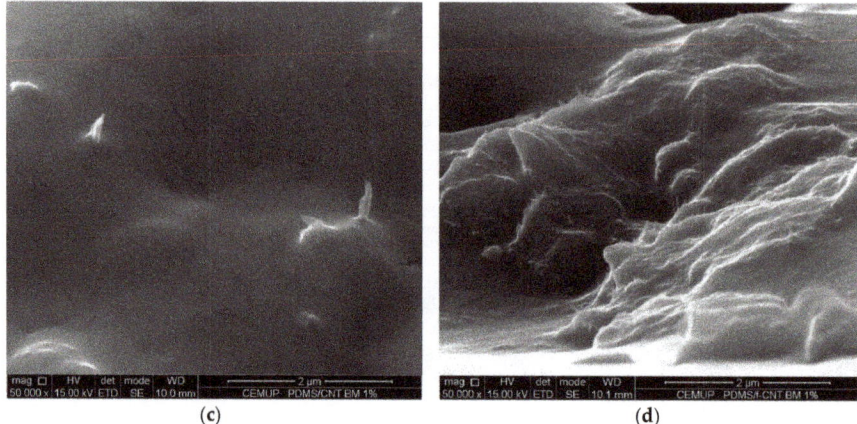

Figure 4. Scanning electron microscopy images of samples' surfaces (magnification 50,000×); (**a**) p-CNT/PDMS; (**b**) f-CNT/PDMS; (**c**) p-BM/PDMS; and (**d**) f-BM/PDMS.

Electrical measurements were performed to evaluate the influence of the different MWCNT surface treatments in the overall electrical response of the composites (Table 2). Despite the excellent electrical properties of CNTs, and their role in the enhancement of the final conductivity of a polymer composite [60,61], the present results revealed that the composites produced by the bulk mixing process (p-CNT/PDMS, f-CNT/PDMS, p-BM/PDMS, and f-BM/PDMS) did not exhibit any increase in electrical conductivity, as can be seen from the very low conductance values, which were all of the same order of magnitude as that of PDMS. This fact indicates that the CNTs were not well-enough dispersed in these samples to establish a percolative path for the current to flow with the CNT concentrations used.

Table 2. Direct current mean conductance of the different composite coatings measured in a specified voltage interval (−100–100 Volt, for the glass, PDMS, p-CNT/PDMS, f-CNT/PDMS, p-BM/PDMS, and f-BM/PDMS samples, and −10–10 Volt for the p-THF/PDMS and f-THF/PDMS samples).

Sample	Conductance (S)
PDMS	$1.9 \cdot 10^{-12} \pm 9.9 \cdot 10^{-14}$
p-CNT/PDMS	$1.9 \cdot 10^{-12} \pm 5.8 \cdot 10^{-14}$
f-CNT/PDMS	$1.3 \cdot 10^{-12} \pm 5.0 \cdot 10^{-14}$
p-BM/PDMS	$1.3 \cdot 10^{-12} \pm 5.8 \cdot 10^{-14}$
f-BM/PDMS	$1.4 \cdot 10^{-12} \pm 6.0 \cdot 10^{-14}$
p-THF/PDMS	$1.5 \cdot 10^{-5} \pm 4.2 \cdot 10^{-7}$
f-THF/PDMS	$6.9 \cdot 10^{-7} \pm 2.0 \cdot 10^{-8}$

However, the f-THF and p-THF samples showed a significant increase in electric conductance by five to seven orders of magnitude, respectively, which indicates that even at CNT concentrations as low as 1%, there is an enhancement in conduction driven by their better dispersion in PDMS, which made possible the formation of effective conduction paths along the nanotubes. In fact, the use of an adequate solvent to wet CNTs has already proven its worth in the improvement of the electrical properties of the CNT/PDMS composites [62]. Note that the top micrometer PDMS layer covering the CNTs, which was thicker in the case of the coatings fabricated by bulk mixing, may have acted as an insulating layer, hampering the measurements of current flowing through them, which could also explain why conductance values of different orders of magnitude were obtained.

A tendency for higher values of conductance of the composites prepared with non-functionalized CNTs (p-CNT/PDMS and p-THF/PDMS), compared with the functionalized ones, was observed. These results are supported by previous studies that have shown an electrical conductivity of p-CNT/polymer composites several orders higher than that of carboxylic f-CNT/polymer composites [63,64]. In the case of the samples treated with THF, this increase is even more significant. In fact, values obtained with p-THF/PDMS were nearly two orders of magnitude larger than those obtained with f-THF/PDMS. According to Carabineiro, et al. [65], as π orbitals are responsible for CNTs conductance [66], the lower conductivity obtained for the composites with f-CNT can be explained by the defects caused on the π orbitals during the functionalization process.

2.2. E. coli Adhesion Assays

The results of the bacterial adhesion assays with *E. coli* are presented in Figure 5. The bars correspond to the cell density after a 30 min adhesion assay. Results show that p-CNT/PDMS, p-BM/PDMS, f-BM/PDMS, and p-THF/PDMS surfaces yielded lower *E. coli* adhesion than with PDMS ($p < 0.0001$), while f-CNT/PDMS and f-THF/PDMS surfaces had no effect on cell adhesion ($p > 0.05$). All the composite coatings had the same or lower adhesion than the PDMS control. The coatings that had the lowest cell density after 30 min were those with non-functionalized CNTs (p-samples), while those with functionalized CNTs (f-samples) always presented a higher adhesion ($p < 0.0001$), clearly showing an effect of CNT chemistry on cell adhesion behavior.

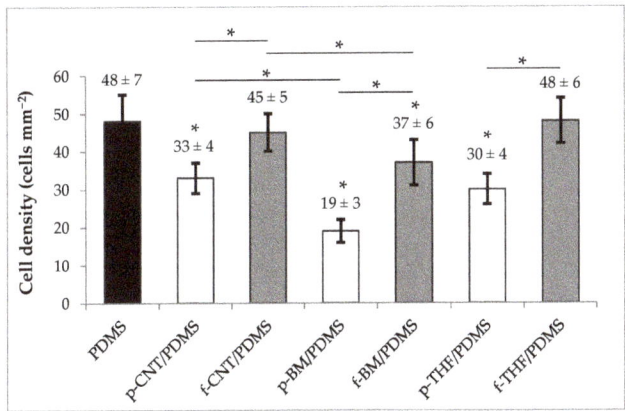

Figure 5. Bar chart of the average cell densities of PDMS (black bar), p-CNT/PDMS, p-BM/PDMS, and p-THF/PDMS (white bars); and f-CNT/PDMS, f-BM/PDMS, and f-THF/PDMS (gray bars) coatings, obtained with three independent tests. Error bars correspond to standard deviation. * indicates $p < 0.0001$, and consequently statistically different from the control.

From the results, it was also observed that there was a reduction in cell adhesion from p-CNT/PDMS to p-BM/PDMS, as well as from f-CNT/PDMS to f-BM/PDMS ($p < 0.0001$). Since the only difference between them was the milling of the CNTs, this was probably driven by a better degree of dispersion in PDMS achieved for the ball-milled nanotubes, which therefore influenced the distribution of the nanotubes near the interface and possibly the surface roughness of the coatings. On the other hand, using THF to disperse the CNTs also seemed to influence cell adhesion, with an intensification of the response obtained for p-CNT/PDMS and f-CNT/PDMS. This may also suggest that the CNTs in the p-THF/PDMS and f-THF/PDMS surfaces were able to interact more efficiently with the cells, possibly due to their availability at the surface.

Comparing these results with those obtained for the surface energy, it can be noted that for p-CNT/PDMS, f-CNT/PDMS, p-BM/PDMS and f-BM/PMDS surfaces there seemed to be a correlation with the hydrophobic character, where a lower hydrophobicity seemed to favor cell adhesion. These results are in agreement with our previous work, whose findings revealed that even at lower loading values (0.1 wt %), functionalized CNTs could increase cell adhesion by 40% when compared to the PDMS surface with p-CNTs [67]. However, in the p-THF/PDMS and f-THF/PDMS surfaces, an opposite relationship was observed. In fact, other studies have been supporting the theory that hydrophobic surfaces promote cell adhesion [68,69], showing that this relation between hydrophobicity and cell adhesion is not so stringent [70,71]. The fact that these coatings were produced using a different method, which possibly resulted in better dispersion of the CNTs, may have had an influence on their distribution at the surface and thus on the measured surface energy. However, the adhesion values obtained followed the same trend as the remaining groups of surfaces, which suggests that other types of forces and interactions may be driving bacterial adhesion in these composites. It should be noted that in previous works from our group, we have shown that a significant reduction in initial bacterial adhesion may indicate an antifouling behavior in longer biofilm formation assays performed in the hydrodynamic conditions of urinary catheters and stents [46,47].

Although the p-BM/PDMS was the most promising surface, with a reduction in cell adhesion of approximately 60%, p-THF/PDMS composites also showed very encouraging results. Along with the reduction in cell adhesion of about 40%, these surfaces have shown a great improvement in electrical conduction (by seven orders of magnitude when compared to PDMS), which poses advantages in biomedical applications where sensing capabilities are required and similar values of shear stress are applied [72–74].

3. Materials and Methods

3.1. CNT Modification

The original CNT sample was commercially available pristine MWCNTs (Nanocyl^{TM} NC3100, Sambreville, Belgium) produced by catalytic chemical vapor deposition with an average length and diameter of 1.5 µm and 9.5 nm, respectively. p-CNTs were first functionalized by a well-established oxidation treatment with nitric acid (HNO_3) [49] to produce f-CNTs with oxygenated moieties. Briefly, a sample of p-CNT was oxidized in reflux with HNO_3 in a Pyrex round-bottom flask containing 300 mL of HNO_3 7 M and 3 g of p-CNT, connected to a condenser and the liquid phase was heated at 130 °C with a heating mantle for 180 min. After this process, the f-CNTs were washed with distilled water to neutral pH and dried at 110 °C overnight.

Additionally, both p-CNT and f-CNT samples were mechanically treated by ball-milling (Retsch MM200, Haan, Germany) at 15 vibrations s^{-1} for 180 and 90 min to produce the p-BM and f-BM samples, respectively.

3.2. CNT/PDMS Composite Fabrication

The composite materials were fabricated using two different processes—bulk mixing and solution mixing. The first method—bulk mixing—consisted of the direct incorporation of the CNT samples into the PDMS matrix (Sylgard 184 Part A, Dow Corning, Midland, MI, USA; viscosity = 1.1 cm^2 s^{-1}; specific density = 1.03) at 1 wt % CNT loading. Firstly, the CNT samples were dispersed in the PDMS matrix by shear mixing with a magnetic bar at 500 rpm for 30 min, allowing for a rough dispersion of the aggregates. The ball-milling technique enables a better dispersion of the CNT when compared with p-CNT and f-CNT. The CNT/PDMS mixture was then subjected to a sonication procedure (Hielscher UP400S, Teltow, Germany, at 200 Watt and 12 kHz) for at least 60 min until the CNTs were all macroscopically dispersed. However, even after sonication, there were some clusters of CNTs suspended in the composite. After that, a 30 min ultrasound bath (Selecta Ultrasons, Barcelona, Spain) step was added to eliminate the bubbles. The curing agent (Sylgard 184 Part B, Dow Corning) was then added to the base polymer in an A:B proportion of 10:1 and carefully stirred to homogenize the two components without re-introducing bubbles. The composite materials were then deposited as thin layers on top of glass slides by spin coating (Spin150 Polos^{TM}, Caribbean, the Netherlands) for 1 min at 6000 rpm for the p-CNT/PDMS and f-CNT/PDMS composites, and at 2000 rpm for the p-BM/PDMS and f-BM/PDMS composites. The former required a higher spin speed since the mixture was more viscous due to the higher degree of aggregation of the CNTs.

The second method used to fabricate the composite materials—solution mixing—consisted of first dispersing the CNTs in THF for about 16 h (resulting in the p-THF and f-THF samples) and then mixing this CNT suspension with the PDMS for additional 6 h at the same 1 wt % CNT loading. Again, the curing agent was added in a 10:1 proportion. The resulting mixture was deposited on the glass slides by manually spreading in such a way to form a uniform layer, and the films were cured in the same conditions as the other materials. The six different materials produced are summarized in Table 3.

Table 3. Description of the materials prepared through the bulk mixing and solution mixing processes.

Material	CNT Treatment	Method
p-CNT/PDMS	none	bulk mixing
f-CNT/PDMS	oxidation with nitric acid	bulk mixing
p-BM/PDMS	ball-milling	bulk mixing
f-BM/PDMS	oxidation with nitric acid; ball-milling	bulk mixing
p-THF/PDMS	none	solution mixing
f-THF/PDMS	oxidation with nitric acid	solution mixing

3.3. Characterization

The four samples of CNTs—p-CNT, f-CNT, p-BM and f-BM—were characterized by N_2 adsorption isotherms determined at −196 °C with a Quantachrome NOVA 4200e apparatus (Quantachrome Instruments, Boynton Beach, USA). Their textural properties were compared by measuring the (S_{BET}) of the various materials. The p-CNT and f-CNT were further characterized by TPD to compare their surface chemistry. The samples were heated from room temperature to 1100 °C at a heating rate of 5 °C min^{-1} with a total flow rate of the helium carrier gas of 25 cm^3 min^{-1} in an AMI-300 (Altamira Instruments, Pittsburgh, USA) apparatus. About 0.09 g of each sample was analyzed by tracking the m/z signals of 18 (H_2O), 28 (CO), and 44 (CO_2) with a Dycor Dymaxion mass spectrometer (Ametek Process Instruments, Pittsburgh, USA). The signals were then processed and analyzed to obtain the total amount of CO and CO_2 released from the samples. To assess the effect of the incorporation of the CNTs on the thermal stability of the composites, PDMS, p-CNT, p-BM, f-BM and p-THF/composite samples were analyzed by TGA (Netzsch STA 409 PC/PG, Selb, Germany). Samples were heated up to 700 °C at a heating rate of 10 °C min^{-1}, under nitrogen flow, and the weight loss monitored to compare the on-set temperature of decomposition among the tested samples.

To obtain an estimative of the surface hydrophobicity of the various composite materials, static CA measurements were performed (Dataphysics Contact Angle System OCA) using the sessile drop technique. Calculations of the surface tension and surface free energy of the solid surfaces (s) were based on the thermodynamic theory [75] by using the Young–Good–Girifalco–Fowkes Equation (1) [76,77], where γ_s^{LW} and γ_s^{AB} are the Lifshitz–van der Waals and the Lewis acid-base components of the samples' surface tension, respectively, and γ_s^+ and γ_s^- are the electron acceptor and electron donor parameters, respectively. γ_s^{LW} and γ_s^{AB} were obtained by measuring the contact angle (θ) of three different liquids (l) with known surface tension components—water, α-bromonaphthalene, and formamide—followed by the simultaneous resolution of three equations of the type of the Equation (1) where the subscript **s** refers to the surface and the subscript **l** refers to the liquid. The global surface energy (γ_s^{TOT}) was then determined by the sum of these two components using Equation (2):

$$(1 + cos\theta)\gamma_l^{TOT} = 2\left(\sqrt{\gamma_s^{LW}\gamma_l^{LW}} + \sqrt{\gamma_s^+\gamma_l^-} + \sqrt{\gamma_s^-\gamma_l^+} \right), \quad (1)$$

$$\gamma_s^{TOT} = \gamma_s^{LW} + \gamma_s^{AB} = \gamma_s^{LW} + 2\sqrt{\gamma_s^+\gamma_s^-}, \quad (2)$$

From Equations (1) and (2), the hydrophobicity of the surfaces was determined as a measure of the free energy of interaction between two entities of that surfaces immersed in water (w)—ΔG_s^{TOT}. According to the thermodynamic theory, a surface is hydrophobic if the interaction between the two entities is stronger than the interaction of each entity with water ($\Delta G_s^{TOT} < 0$ mJ m^{-2}) and hydrophilic otherwise ($\Delta G_s^{TOT} > 0$ mJ m^{-2}). ΔG_s^{TOT} was calculated according to Equations (3)–(5), where the surface tension components of the interacting entities are considered:

$$\Delta G_s^{TOT} = -2\gamma_s^{TOT} = \Delta G_s^{LW} + \Delta G_s^{AB}, \tag{3}$$

$$\Delta G_s^{LW} = -2\left(\sqrt{\gamma_s^{LW}} - \sqrt{\gamma_w^{LW}}\right)^2, \tag{4}$$

$$\Delta G_s^{AB} = -4\left(\sqrt{\gamma_s^+\gamma_s^-} + \sqrt{\gamma_w^+\gamma_w^-} - \sqrt{\gamma_s^+\gamma_w^-} - \sqrt{\gamma_w^+\gamma_s^-}\right), \tag{5}$$

ΔG_s^{LW} and ΔG_s^{AB} represent the Lifshitz–van der Waals and the acid-base free energies of cohesion of the surface, respectively [75].

The surface of the various samples was further characterized by SEM. Images of the cross-sections of the coatings were also obtained. SEM analyses were performed using a High-resolution Environmental Scanning Electron Microscope with X-Ray Microanalysis and Electron Backscattered Diffraction analysis—Quanta 400 FEG ESEM (Hillsboro, OR, USA).

Additionally, to assess the effect of the introduction of CNTs in the PDMS matrix on the conductivity properties of the composites, DC electrical conductivity tests were performed. A DC-voltage (V) signal in the range −100–+100 Volt or −10–+10 Volt was applied on each sample produced by the bulk mixing and solution mixing procedure, respectively. The corresponding current (I) was measured at 21 points in 10 runs using two copper contacts that were placed on top of the coating with a separation of 2 cm and then connected to a power source (Keithley Programmable Single Channel DC Power Supplier, Cleveland, OH, USA). The current-voltage curves were obtained and an average value of conductance (I/V) was calculated from a linear fit of the curves.

3.4. Cell Cultivation and Harvesting

E. coli JM109(DE3) from Promega (Madison, WI, USA) was selected for this study because it has been used in previous works from our group for the evaluation of initial adhesion in antifouling surfaces [67] and because it has was shown to have similar biofilm formation behavior to different clinical isolates, including *E. coli* CECT434 [78]. A starter cell culture was obtained using the same procedure as described in Moreira, et al. [79]. In brief, the cells were collected from a cryo-preserved batch (1 mL aliquots in glycerol stock kept at a constant −80 °C) and thawed at room temperature. Then, 200 mL of culture medium, prepared as previously described [80], were inoculated with 500 μL of cell suspension and incubated overnight at 37 °C with a constant orbital agitation of 120 rpm. A volume of 60 mL of the cultured bacteria was centrifuged (Eppendorf Centrifuge 5810R, Hamburg, Germany) at 3202× *g* for 10 min, resuspended in citrate buffer at pH 5 and centrifuged again in the same conditions. The final cell suspension was then diluted in citrate buffer until an optical density (OD$_{600\,nm}$) of 0.1, corresponding to a cell density of 7.6×10^7 cells mL^{-1}.

3.5. E. coli Adhesion Assays

The bacterial adhesion assays on the coated slides were performed in a PPFC coupled to a system containing a reactor connected to a centrifugal pump and tubing system, which was fed with a steady flow of the *E. coli* suspension. A flow rate of 2 mL s^{-1} was used, which yields a shear rate of 15 s^{-1} and a shear stress of 0.01 Pa [68]. This shear rate is typical for urinary catheters [81] and stents [82], where *E. coli* is one of the most relevant microbial colonizers [45]. The equipment was also coupled to a water bath to keep a constant temperature of 37 °C. For each sample, the medium with *E. coli* was allowed to flow for 30 min, after which the coatings were removed and stained with

4′-6-diamidino-2-phenylindole for later visualization under fluorescence microscopy (Nikon Eclipse LV100 series, magnification 100×, Nikon Corporation, Tokyo, Japan) and total cell counts. The final cell density of each sample was taken into account in the evaluation of bacterial cell adhesion.

3.6. Statistical Analysis

Differences between the final cell densities on each surface were tested using a one-way analysis of variance followed by Tukey's test for pairwise comparisons. Three independent assays were conducted for each surface. Results were considered statistically different when a confidence level >95% was reached ($p < 0.05$). The standard deviation between the three values obtained from the independent experiments is represented by error bars.

4. Conclusions

MWCNT/PDMS composite materials with 1 wt % of MWCNTs loading were produced using two different procedures, bulk mixing (p-CNT/PDMS, f-CNT/PDMS, p-BM/PDMS, and f-BM/PDMS) and solution mixing (p-THF/PDMS and f-THF/PDMS). The materials were characterized in terms of surface energy, thermal stability, electrical conductivity and surface topology. Adhesion assays with *E. coli* were performed in an attempt to establish a relationship between the materials' properties and the tendency for cell adhesion. The results showed that p-CNT were successfully functionalized through oxidation treatment, and p-CNT/PDMS and f-CNT/PDMS had different textural properties, which were reflected in the enhancement of thermal stability of the composites. The conductivity measurements showed a considerable improvement in DC electrical conductivity in the p-THF/PDMS and f-THF/PDMS composites, with possible applications in biosensing devices.

The *E. coli* adhesion assays resulted in reduced adhesion on the composite materials, with the lowest adhesion obtained on the p-BM/PDMS sample, and the highest obtained on the f-THF/PDMS sample. The CA measurements suggested that for the composites produced by bulk mixing (p-CNT/PDMS, f-CNT/PDMS, p-BM/PDMS, and f-BM/PDMS) the adhesion was favored by lower hydrophobicity, while for the p-THF/PDMS and f-THF/PDMS composites the opposite was observed. The p-THF/PDMS sample seemed to be the best compromise between cell adhesion and electrical conductivity.

Author Contributions: Conceptualization, J.M.R.M., O.S.G.P.S., M.F.R.P., and F.J.M.; methodology, M.R.V., J.M.R.M., and O.S.G.P.S.; investigation, M.R.V. and M.G.; resources, M.F.R.P. and F.J.M.; data curation, M.R.V., J.M.R.M., M.G., and O.S.G.P.S.; writing—original draft preparation, M.R.V., J.M.R.M., and M.G.; supervision, O.S.G.P.S., M.F.R.P., and F.J.M.; funding acquisition, M.F.R.P. and F.J.M. All authors have read and agreed to the published version of the manuscript.

Funding: This work was financially supported by Base Funding—UIDB/50020/2020 of the Associate Laboratory LSRE-LCM and by Base Funding—UIDB/00511/2020 of the Laboratory for Process Engineering, Environment, Biotechnology and Energy—LEPABE—funded by national funds through the FCT/MCTES (PIDDAC). OSGPS acknowledges FCT funding under the Scientific Employment Stimulus—Institutional Call CEECINST/00049/2018.

Conflicts of Interest: The authors declare no conflict of interest.

References

1. Saliev, T. The Advances in Biomedical Applications of Carbon Nanotubes. *C J. Carbon Res.* **2019**, *5*, 29. [CrossRef]
2. Špitalský, Z.; Tasis, D.; Papagelis, K.; Galiotis, C. Carbon nanotube–Polymer composites: Chemistry, processing, mechanical and electrical properties. *Prog. Polym. Sci.* **2010**, *35*, 357–401. [CrossRef]
3. Chua, T.P.; Mariatti, M.; Aziz, A.; Rashid, A.A. Effects of surface-functionalized multi-walled carbon nanotubes on the properties of poly(dimethyl siloxane) nanocomposites. *Compos. Sci. Technol.* **2010**, *70*, 671–677. [CrossRef]
4. Upadhyayula, V.K.K.; Gadhamshetty, V. Appreciating the role of carbon nanotube composites in preventing biofouling and promoting biofilms on material surfaces in environmental engineering: A review. *Biotechnol. Adv.* **2010**, *28*, 802–816. [CrossRef] [PubMed]

5. Eatemadi, A.; Daraee, H.; Karimkhanloo, H.; Kouhi, M.; Zarghami, N.; Akbarzadeh, A.; Abasi, M.; Hanifehpour, Y.; Joo, S.W. Carbon nanotubes: Properties, synthesis, purification, and medical applications. *Nanoscale Res. Lett.* **2014**, *9*, 1–13. [CrossRef] [PubMed]
6. He, H.; Pham-Huy, L.A.; Dramou, P.; Xiao, D.; Zuo, P.; Pham-Huy, C. Carbon Nanotubes: Applications in Pharmacy and Medicine. *BioMed Res. Int.* **2013**, *2013*, 578290–578302. [CrossRef] [PubMed]
7. Li, X.; Liu, X.; Huang, J.; Fan, Y.; Cui, F.-Z. Biomedical investigation of CNT based coatings. *Surf. Coat. Technol.* **2011**, *206*, 759–766. [CrossRef]
8. Matsuoka, M.; Akasaka, T.; Totsuka, Y.; Watari, F. Strong adhesion of Saos-2 cells to multi-walled carbon nanotubes. *Mater. Sci. Eng. B* **2010**, *173*, 182–186. [CrossRef]
9. Matsuoka, M.; Akasaka, T.; Totsuka, Y.; Watari, F. Carbon nanotube-coated silicone as a flexible and electrically conductive biomedical material. *Mater. Sci. Eng. C* **2012**, *32*, 574–580. [CrossRef]
10. Venkatesan, J.; Jayakumar, R.; Mohandas, A.; Bhatnagar, I.; Kim, S.-K. Antimicrobial Activity of Chitosan-Carbon Nanotube Hydrogels. *Materials* **2014**, *7*, 3946–3955. [CrossRef]
11. Newman, P.; Minett, A.; Ellis-Behnke, R.; Zreiqat, H. Carbon nanotubes: Their potential and pitfalls for bone tissue regeneration and engineering. *Nanomed. Nanotechnol. Boil. Med.* **2013**, *9*, 1139–1158. [CrossRef] [PubMed]
12. Fabbro, A.; Prato, M.; Ballerini, L. Carbon nanotubes in neuroregeneration and repair. *Adv. Drug Deliv. Rev.* **2013**, *65*, 2034–2044. [CrossRef]
13. Hirata, E.; Akasaka, T.; Uo, M.; Takita, H.; Watari, F.; Yokoyama, A. Carbon nanotube-coating accelerated cell adhesion and proliferation on poly (L-lactide). *Appl. Surf. Sci.* **2012**, *262*, 24–27. [CrossRef]
14. Harrison, B.S.; Atala, A. Carbon nanotube applications for tissue engineering. *Biomaterials* **2007**, *28*, 344–353. [CrossRef] [PubMed]
15. Abarrategi, A.; Gutierrez, M.C.; Moreno-Vicente, C.; Hortiguela, M.J.; Ramos, V.; López-Lacomba, J.L.; Ferrer, M.L.; Del Monte, F. Multiwall carbon nanotube scaffolds for tissue engineering purposes. *Biomaterials* **2008**, *29*, 94–102. [CrossRef]
16. Zanello, L.P.; Zhao, B.; Hu, H.; Haddon, R. Bone Cell Proliferation on Carbon Nanotubes. *Nano Lett.* **2006**, *6*, 562–567. [CrossRef]
17. Lobo, A.O.; Antunes, E.F.; Machado, A.H.A.; Pacheco-Soares, C.; Trava-Airoldi, V.J.; Corat, E.J. Cell viability and adhesion on as grown multi-wall carbon nanotube films. *Mater. Sci. Eng. C* **2008**, *28*, 264–269. [CrossRef]
18. Teixeira-Santos, R.; Gomes, M.; Mergulhão, F. Carbon Nanotube-Based Antimicrobial and Antifouling Surfaces. In *Engineered Antimicrobial Surfaces*; Springer Singapore: Singapore, 2020; pp. 65–93. [CrossRef]
19. Kim, K.-I.; Kim, D.-A.; Patel, K.D.; Shin, U.S.; Kim, H.-W.; Lee, J.-H.; Lee, H.-H. Carbon nanotube incorporation in PMMA to prevent microbial adhesion. *Sci. Rep.* **2019**, *9*, 4921. [CrossRef]
20. Lin, C.-W.; Aguilar, S.; Rao, E.; Mak, W.H.; Huang, X.; He, N.; Chen, D.; Jun, D.; Curson, P.A.; McVerry, B.T.; et al. Direct grafting of tetraaniline via perfluorophenylazide photochemistry to create antifouling, low bio-adhesion surfaces. *Chem. Sci.* **2019**, *10*, 4445–4457. [CrossRef]
21. Jing, H.; Sahle-Demessie, E.; Sorial, G.A. Inhibition of biofilm growth on polymer-MWCNTs composites and metal surfaces. *Sci. Total. Environ.* **2018**, *633*, 167–178. [CrossRef]
22. Zhang, Q.; Arribas, P.; Remillard, E.M.; García-Payo, M.C.; Khayet, M.; Vecitis, C.D. Interlaced CNT Electrodes for Bacterial Fouling Reduction of Microfiltration Membranes. *Environ Sci Technol* **2017**, *51*, 9176–9183. [CrossRef] [PubMed]
23. Zhang, Q.; Nghiem, J.; Silverberg, G.J.; Vecitis, C.D. Semiquantitative Performance and Mechanism Evaluation of Carbon Nanomaterials as Cathode Coatings for Microbial Fouling Reduction. *Appl. Environ. Microbiol.* **2015**, *81*, 4744–4755. [CrossRef]
24. Gomes, M.; Gomes, L.C.; Teixeira-Santos, R.; Mergulhão, F.J. PDMS in Urinary Tract Devices: Applications, Problems and Potential Solutions. In *Polydimethylsiloxane: Structure and Applications*, 1st ed.; Carlsen, P.N., Ed.; Nova Science Publishers: Hauppauge, NY, USA, 2020; pp. 95–144.
25. Shen, Q.; Shan, Y.; Lü, Y.; Xue, P.; Liu, Y.; Liu, X. Enhanced Antibacterial Activity of Poly (dimethylsiloxane) Membranes by Incorporating SiO(2) Microspheres Generated Silver Nanoparticles. *Nanomaterials* **2019**, *9*, 705. [CrossRef] [PubMed]
26. Keskin, D.; Mokabbar, T.; Pei, Y.; Van Rijn, P. The Relationship between Bulk Silicone and Benzophenone-Initiated Hydrogel Coating Properties. *Polymers* **2018**, *10*, 534. [CrossRef] [PubMed]

27. Ji, Y.; Sun, Y.; Lang, Y.; Wang, L.; Liu, B.; Zhang, Z. Effect of CNT/PDMS Nanocomposites on the Dynamics of Pioneer Bacterial Communities in the Natural Biofilms of Seawater. *Materials* **2018**, *11*, 902. [CrossRef]
28. Sun, Y.; Zhang, Z. Anti-biofouling property studies on carboxyl-modified multi-walled carbon nanotubes filled PDMS nanocomposites. *World J. Microbiol. Biotechnol.* **2016**, *32*, 148. [CrossRef]
29. Martinelli, E.; Suffredini, M.; Galli, G.; Glisenti, A.; Pettitt, M.E.; Callow, M.E.; Callow, J.A.; Williams, D.; Lyall, G. Amphiphilic block copolymer/poly(dimethylsiloxane) (PDMS) blends and nanocomposites for improved fouling-release. *Biofouling* **2011**, *27*, 529–541. [CrossRef]
30. Beigbeder, A.; Degée, P.; Conlan, S.L.; Mutton, R.J.; Clare, A.S.; Pettitt, M.E.; Callow, M.E.; Callow, J.A.; Dubois, P. Preparation and characterisation of silicone-based coatings filled with carbon nanotubes and natural sepiolite and their application as marine fouling-release coatings. *Biofouling* **2008**, *24*, 291–302. [CrossRef]
31. Paul, J.; Sindhu, S.; Nurmawati, M.H.; Valiyaveettil, S. Mechanics of prestressed polydimethylsiloxane-carbon nanotube composite. *Appl. Phys. Lett.* **2006**, *89*, 184101–184103. [CrossRef]
32. Park, I.-S.; Kim, K.J.; Nam, J.-D.; Lee, J.; Yim, W. Mechanical, dielectric, and magnetic properties of the silicone elastomer with multi-walled carbon nanotubes as a nanofiller. *Polym. Eng. Sci.* **2007**, *47*, 1396–1405. [CrossRef]
33. Hu, C.H.; Liu, C.H.; Chen, L.Z.; Fan, S.S. Semiconductor behaviors of low loading multiwall carbon nanotube/poly(dimethylsiloxane) composites. *Appl. Phys. Lett.* **2009**, *95*, 103103. [CrossRef]
34. Khosla, A.; Gray, B. Preparation, characterization and micromolding of multi-walled carbon nanotube polydimethylsiloxane conducting nanocomposite polymer. *Mater. Lett.* **2009**, *63*, 1203–1206. [CrossRef]
35. Hong, J.; Lee, J.; Hong, C.K.; Shim, S.E. Effect of dispersion state of carbon nanotube on the thermal conductivity of poly(dimethyl siloxane) composites. *Curr. Appl. Phys.* **2010**, *10*, 359–363. [CrossRef]
36. Kim, T.-H.; Kim, H.-S. Effect of acid-treated carbon nanotube and amine-terminated polydimethylsiloxane on the rheological properties of polydimethylsiloxane/carbon nanotube composite system. *Korea Aust. Rheol. J.* **2010**, *22*, 205–210.
37. Lee, J.-B.; Khang, D.-Y. Electrical and mechanical characterization of stretchable multi-walled carbon nanotubes/polydimethylsiloxane elastomeric composite conductors. *Compos. Sci. Technol.* **2012**, *72*, 1257–1263. [CrossRef]
38. Kim, T.A.; Kim, H.S.; Lee, S.S.; Park, M. Single-walled carbon nanotube/silicone rubber composites for compliant electrodes. *Carbon* **2012**, *50*, 444–449. [CrossRef]
39. Sepúlveda, A.; Fachin, F.; De Villoria, R.G.; Wardle, B.; Viana, J.C.; Pontes, A.; Rocha, L. Nanocomposite Flexible Pressure Sensor for Biomedical Applications. *Procedia Eng.* **2011**, *25*, 140–143. [CrossRef]
40. Sinha, N.; Yeow, J.T.W. Carbon Nanotubes for Biomedical Applications. *IEEE Trans. NanoBioscience* **2005**, *4*, 180–195. [CrossRef]
41. So, H.-M.; Sim, J.W.; Kwon, J.; Yun, J.; Baik, S.; Chang, W.S. Carbon nanotube based pressure sensor for flexible electronics. *Mater. Res. Bull.* **2013**, *48*, 5036–5039. [CrossRef]
42. Ivanov, I.N.; Goehegan, D.B. Carbon Nanotube Temperature and Pressure Sensors. U.S. Patent 8,568,027 B2, 3 March 2011.
43. Xu, J.; Su, W.; Li, Z.; Liu, W.; Liu, S.; Ding, X. A modularized and flexible sensor based on MWCNT/PDMS composite film for on-site electrochemical analysis. *J. Electroanal. Chem.* **2017**, *806*, 68–74. [CrossRef]
44. Alves, P.; Nir, S.; Reches, M.; Mergulhão, F.J. The effects of fluid composition and shear conditions on bacterial adhesion to an antifouling peptide-coated surface. *MRS Commun.* **2018**, *8*, 938–946. [CrossRef]
45. Ramstedt, M.; Ribeiro, I.A.C.; Bujdakova, H.; Mergulhão, F.J.M.; Jordao, L.; Thomsen, P.; Alm, M.; Burmølle, M.; Vladkova, T.; Can, F.; et al. Evaluating Efficacy of Antimicrobial and Antifouling Materials for Urinary Tract Medical Devices: Challenges and Recommendations. *Macromol. Biosci.* **2019**, *19*, e1800384. [CrossRef] [PubMed]
46. Lopez-Mila, B.; Alves, P.; Riedel, T.; Dittrich, B.; Mergulhão, F.J.; Rodriguez-Emmenegger, C. Effect of shear stress on the reduction of bacterial adhesion to antifouling polymers. *Bioinspiration Biomim.* **2018**, *13*, 065001. [CrossRef]
47. Alves, P.; Gomes, L.C.; Vorobii, M.; Rodriguez-Emmenegger, C.; Mergulhão, F.J. The potential advantages of using a poly(HPMA) brush in urinary catheters: Effects on biofilm cells and architecture. *Colloids Surf. B Biointerfaces* **2020**, *191*, 110976. [CrossRef]

48. Soares, O.S.G.; Órfão, J.; Pereira, M.F.R. Pd–Cu and Pt–Cu Catalysts Supported on Carbon Nanotubes for Nitrate Reduction in Water. *Ind. Eng. Chem. Res.* **2010**, *49*, 7183–7192. [CrossRef]
49. Rocha, R.P.; Silva, A.M.; Romero, S.M.; Pereira, M.F.R.; Figueiredo, J.L. The role of O- and S-containing surface groups on carbon nanotubes for the elimination of organic pollutants by catalytic wet air oxidation. *Appl. Catal. B Environ.* **2014**, *147*, 314–321. [CrossRef]
50. Atieh, M.A.; Bakather, O.Y.; Al-Tawbini, B.; Bukhari, A.A.; Abuilaiwi, F.; Fettouhi, M. Effect of Carboxylic Functional Group Functionalized on Carbon Nanotubes Surface on the Removal of Lead from Water. *Bioinorg. Chem. Appl.* **2011**, *2010*, 603978–603987. [CrossRef]
51. Soares, O.S.G.; Gonçalves, A.; Jaén, J.J.D.; Órfão, J.; Pereira, M.F.R. Modification of carbon nanotubes by ball-milling to be used as ozonation catalysts. *Catal. Today* **2015**, *249*, 199–203. [CrossRef]
52. Figueiredo, J.L.; Pereira, M.F.R.; Freitas, M.M.A.; Órfão, J.J.M. Modification of the surface chemistry of activated carbons. *Carbon* **1999**, *37*, 1379–1389. [CrossRef]
53. Gonçalves, A.; Figueiredo, J.L.; Órfão, J.; Pereira, M.F.R. Influence of the surface chemistry of multi-walled carbon nanotubes on their activity as ozonation catalysts. *Carbon* **2010**, *48*, 4369–4381. [CrossRef]
54. Huang, Y.Y.; Terentjev, E. Dispersion of Carbon Nanotubes: Mixing, Sonication, Stabilization, and Composite Properties. *Polymers* **2012**, *4*, 275–295. [CrossRef]
55. Wang, P.; Geng, S.; Ding, T. Effects of carboxyl radical on electrical resistance of multi-walled carbon nanotube filled silicone rubber composite under pressure. *Compos. Sci. Technol.* **2010**, *70*, 1571–1573. [CrossRef]
56. Hwang, S.-H.; Park, Y.-B.; Yoon, K.H.; Bang, D.S. Smart Materials and Structures Based on Carbon Nanotube Composites. In *Carbon Nanotubes—Synthesis, Characterization, Applications*; Yellampalli, S., Ed.; IntechOpen: London, UK, 2011; pp. 371–396. [CrossRef]
57. Camponeschi, E.L. Dispersion and Alignment of Carbon Nanotubes in Polymer Based Composites. Ph.D. Thesis, Georgia Institute of Technology, Atlanta, GA, USA, 2007.
58. Silva, T.L.S.; Morales-Torres, S.; Figueiredo, J.L.; Silva, A.M. Multi-walled carbon nanotube/PVDF blended membranes with sponge- and finger-like pores for direct contact membrane distillation. *Desalination* **2015**, *357*, 233–245. [CrossRef]
59. Wang, D.; Lu, S.; Jiang, S.P. Tetrahydrofuran-functionalized multi-walled carbon nanotubes as effective support for Pt and PtSn electrocatalysts of fuel cells. *Electrochim. Acta* **2010**, *55*, 2964–2971. [CrossRef]
60. Sekitani, T.; Nakajima, H.; Maeda, H.; Fukushima, T.; Aida, T.; Hata, K.; Someya, T. Stretchable active-matrix organic light-emitting diode display using printable elastic conductors. *Nat. Mater.* **2009**, *8*, 494–499. [CrossRef]
61. Shin, M.K.; Oh, J.; Lima, M.; Kozlov, M.; Kim, S.J.; Baughman, R.H. Elastomeric Conductive Composites Based on Carbon Nanotube Forests. *Adv. Mater.* **2010**, *22*, 2663–2667. [CrossRef]
62. Hong, J.S.; Lee, J.H.; Nam, Y.W. Dispersion of solvent-wet carbon nanotubes for electrical CNT/polydimethylsiloxane composite. *Carbon* **2013**, *61*, 577–584. [CrossRef]
63. Li, Q.; Xue, Q.; Hao, L.; Gao, X.; Zheng, Q. Large dielectric constant of the chemically functionalized carbon nanotube/polymer composites. *Compos. Sci. Technol.* **2008**, *68*, 2290–2296. [CrossRef]
64. Yu, A.; Itkis, M.E.; Bekyarova, E.; Haddon, R.C. Effect of single-walled carbon nanotube purity on the thermal conductivity of carbon nanotube-based composites. *Appl. Phys. Lett.* **2006**, *89*, 133102. [CrossRef]
65. Carabineiro, S.A.C.; Pereira, M.F.R.; Nunes-Pereira, J.; Silva, J.; Caparrós, C.; Sencadas, V.; Lanceros-Méndez, S. The effect of nanotube surface oxidation on the electrical properties of multiwall carbon nanotube/poly(vinylidene fluoride) composites. *J. Mater. Sci.* **2012**, *47*, 8103–8111. [CrossRef]
66. Charlier, J.-C.; Blase, X.; Roche, S. Electronic and transport properties of nanotubes. *Rev. Mod. Phys.* **2007**, *79*, 677–732. [CrossRef]
67. Vagos, M.R.; Moreira, J.M.; Soares, O.S.G.; Pereira, M.F.; Mergulhão, F.J. Incorporation of carbon nanotubes in polydimethylsiloxane to control *Escherichia coli* adhesion. *Polym. Compos.* **2018**, *40*, E1697–E1704. [CrossRef]
68. Moreira, J.; Araújo, J.; Miranda, J.; Simões, M.; Melo, L.; Mergulhão, F. The effects of surface properties on *Escherichia coli* adhesion are modulated by shear stress. *Colloids Surf. B Biointerfaces* **2014**, *123*, 1–7. [CrossRef] [PubMed]
69. Krishnan, S.; Weinman, C.J.; Ober, C.K. Advances in polymers for anti-biofouling surfaces. *J. Mater. Chem.* **2008**, *18*, 3405–3413. [CrossRef]

70. Oliveira, K.; Oliveira, T.; Teixeira, P.; Azeredo, J.; Henriques, M.; Oliveira, R. Comparison of the Adhesion Ability of Different *Salmonella* Enteritidis Serotypes to Materials Used in Kitchens. *J. Food Prot.* **2006**, *69*, 2352–2356. [CrossRef] [PubMed]
71. Moreira, J.M.R.; Simões, M.; Melo, L.; Mergulhão, F.J. *Escherichia coli* adhesion to surfaces–a thermodynamic assessment. *Colloid Polym. Sci.* **2014**, *293*, 177–185. [CrossRef]
72. Huiszoon, R.C.; Subramanian, S.; Rajasekaran, P.R.; Beardslee, L.A.; Bentley, W.E.; Ghodssi, R. Flexible Platform for In Situ Impedimetric Detection and Bioelectric Effect Treatment of *Escherichia coli* Biofilms. *IEEE Trans. Biomed. Eng.* **2019**, *66*, 1337–1345. [CrossRef]
73. Liang, T.; Qu, Q.; Chang, Y.; Gopinath, S.C.B.; Liu, X.T. Diagnosing ovarian cancer by identifying SCC-antigen on a multiwalled carbon nanotube-modified dielectrode sensor. *Biotechnol. Appl. Biochem.* **2019**, *66*, 939–944. [CrossRef]
74. Hazan, Z.; Zumeris, J.; Jacob, H.; Raskin, H.; Kratysh, G.; Vishnia, M.; Dror, N.; Barliya, T.; Mandel, M.; Lavie, G. Effective Prevention of Microbial Biofilm Formation on Medical Devices by Low-Energy Surface Acoustic Waves. *Antimicrob. Agents Chemother.* **2006**, *50*, 4144–4152. [CrossRef]
75. Van Oss, C.J.; Giese, R.F. The Hydrophilicity and Hydrophobicity of Clay Minerals. *Clays Clay Miner.* **1995**, *43*, 474–477. [CrossRef]
76. Van Oss, C.J.; Chaudhury, M.K.; Good, R.J. Interfacial Lifshitz-van der Waals and polar interactions in macroscopic systems. *Chem. Rev.* **1988**, *88*, 927–941. [CrossRef]
77. Van Oss, C.J. *Interfacial Forces in Aqueous Media*, 1st ed.; Marcel Dekker Inc.: New York, NY, USA, 1994; p. 452.
78. Gomes, L.; Moreira, J.; Teodósio, J.; Araújo, J.D.P.; Miranda, J.M.; Simões, M.; Melo, L.; Mergulhão, F.J. 96-well microtiter plates for biofouling simulation in biomedical settings. *Biofouling* **2014**, *30*, 535–546. [CrossRef] [PubMed]
79. Moreira, J.M.; Gomes, L.; Araújo, J.D.P.; Miranda, J.M.; Simões, M.; Melo, L.; Mergulhão, F.J. The effect of glucose concentration and shaking conditions on *Escherichia coli* biofilm formation in microtiter plates. *Chem. Eng. Sci.* **2013**, *94*, 192–199. [CrossRef]
80. Teodósio, J.; Simões, M.; Melo, L.; Mergulhão, F.J. Flow cell hydrodynamics and their effects onE. colibiofilm formation under different nutrient conditions and turbulent flow. *Biofouling* **2010**, *27*, 1–11. [CrossRef] [PubMed]
81. Busscher, H.J.; Van Der Mei, H.C. Microbial Adhesion in Flow Displacement Systems. *Clin. Microbiol. Rev.* **2006**, *19*, 127–141. [CrossRef] [PubMed]
82. Mosayyebi, A.; Yue, Q.Y.; Somani, B.K.; Zhang, X.; Manes, C.; Carugo, D. Particle Accumulation in Ureteral Stents Is Governed by Fluid Dynamics: In Vitro Study Using a "Stent-on-Chip" Model. *J. Endourol.* **2018**, *32*, 639–646. [CrossRef]

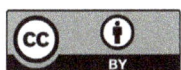

© 2020 by the authors. Licensee MDPI, Basel, Switzerland. This article is an open access article distributed under the terms and conditions of the Creative Commons Attribution (CC BY) license (http://creativecommons.org/licenses/by/4.0/).

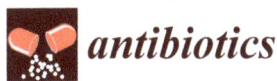

Review

Strategies to Reduce Biofilm Formation in PEEK Materials Applied to Implant Dentistry—A Comprehensive Review

Renata Scheeren Brum [1,*], Luiza Gomes Labes [1], Cláudia Ângela Maziero Volpato [1], César Augusto Magalhães Benfatti [1,*] and Andrea de Lima Pimenta [2,3]

1. Center for Research on Dental Implants (CEPID), Dentistry Department (ODT), Federal University of Santa Catarina (UFSC), Rua Delfino Conti, 1240, Campus Universitário—Trindade, Florianópolis SC 88036-020, Brazil; luiza_labes@hotmail.com (L.G.L.); claudia.m.volpato@ufsc.br (C.Â.M.V.)
2. Integrated Laboratories Technologies (InteLab), Department Chemical Engineering (EQA), Federal University of Santa Catarina (UFSC), Florianópolis SC 88040-970, Brazil; andrea@intelab.ufsc.br
3. Department of Biology, ERRMECe, Université de CergyPontoise, MaisonInternationale de la Recherche, Rue Descartes, CEDEX, 95000 Neuville sur Oise, France
* Correspondence: renatasbrum@live.com (R.S.B.); cesar.benfatti@ufsc.br (C.A.M.B.)

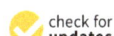

Received: 1 July 2020; Accepted: 15 September 2020; Published: 16 September 2020

Abstract: Polyether-ether-ketone (PEEK) has emerged in Implant Dentistry with a series of short-time applications and as a promising material to substitute definitive dental implants. Several strategies have been investigated to diminish biofilm formation on the PEEK surface aiming to decrease the possibility of related infections. Therefore, a comprehensive review was carried out in order to compare PEEK with materials widely used nowadays in Implant Dentistry, such as titanium and zirconia, placing emphasis on studies investigating its ability to grant or prevent biofilm formation. Most studies failed to reveal significant antimicrobial activity in pure PEEK, while several studies described new strategies to reduce biofilm formation and bacterial colonization on this material. Those include the PEEK sulfonation process, incorporation of therapeutic and bioactive agents in PEEK matrix or on PEEK surface, PEEK coatings and incorporation of reinforcement agents, in order to produce nanocomposites or blends. The two most analyzed surface properties were contact angle and roughness, while the most studied bacteria were *Escherichia coli* and *Staphylococcus aureus*. Despite PEEK's susceptibility to biofilm formation, a great number of strategies discussed in this study were able to improve its antibiofilm and antimicrobial properties.

Keywords: biofilms; biofilm inhibition; dental implants; bacteria; peri-implantitis; polyether-ether-ketone

---

1. Introduction

The diverse microbiome that harbors in the oral cavity plays an important role in health maintenance through the development of the immune response and inhibition of the pathogen colonization [1]. However, under certain circumstances, normal microbiota may be responsible for many oral diseases [2,3]. Oral dysbiosis triggers important changes, reducing the number of beneficial bacteria and favoring the growth of potential pathogens [4]. This is particularly worrying in susceptible individuals affected by periodontitis, a biofilm related disease characterized by alveolar bone resorption, which may lead to tooth mobility and tooth loss [5,6]. In fact, periodontal patients who were rehabilitated with dental implants are more predisposed to develop peri-implant diseases, for which poor plaque control also acts as a primary etiologic factor [7].

In a systematic review carried out in 2017, [8] patient-level data and implant-level data indicated that peri-implantitis was present in 9.25% and 19.83% of analyzed cases, respectively, while mucositis affected 29.48% of patients and 46.83% of implants analyzed [8]. Since there was no consensus on the best treatment protocol [9], biofilm prevention becomes not only desirable but necessary [10]. This can be achieved at the clinical level through favorable implant position and adequate prosthetic design, accompanied by oral hygiene education and regular appointments [10]. Still, at the research level, there is an incessant demand for investigations to develop materials with either antibiofilm or antimicrobial surfaces, or both, through manipulation of surface topographical properties (i.e., contact angle and roughness), or by the incorporation of antibiofilm agents, which can be evaluated through physicochemical analysis [11–14].

Since the demonstration of titanium osseointegration by Branemark et al. (1981) [15], this material has been widely used in Implant Dentistry, revolutionizing oral rehabilitation modalities [16]. However, under certain circumstances, such as therapeutic treatment of peri-implantitis [17] or wear-corrosion, metallic debris is released resulting in prejudicial effects to peri-implant tissues. It had been proved that those metal particles stimulate molecular mechanisms such as enhancement of proinflammatory cytokines and osteoclasts activity, as well as infiltration of inflammatory cells with cytotoxic and genotoxic effects [18]. Hence, there is a growing interest in the development of an alternative material that can be used in dental implants and as implant abutments [19–21].

Within this context, the thermoplastic biocompatible polymer polyether-ether-ketone (PEEK) stands out, with several desired properties to Implant Dentistry improvements, such as mechanical and chemical resistance, stability at high temperatures (enabling sterilization) and natural white pigmentation (favorable for esthetics) [22,23]. Several methods have been studied to establish an effective adhesion of PEEK to resin-matrix composite in restorative dentistry, which is useful to the esthetic of provisional restorations [24]. Moreover, its production process is very versatile, as PEEK is compatible with many reinforcement agents and surface coatings, which can be used to improve its mechanical and biological properties [25–27]. Currently, PEEK is safely used in Implant Dentistry as provisional abutments, healing screws, prosthetic transfers and frameworks [20,23,28]. Nevertheless, as reported by Khonsari et al. [29], there are cases in which PEEK dental implants had been employed in patients and poor osseointegration led to severe infectious complications and subsequent implant loss.

Figure 1 ilustrates the propositions exposed above. In order to develop a PEEK-based dental implant or even to convert the available applications from provisional to definitive (i.e., PEEK-based prosthetic components), additional research is necessary. Therefore, a comprehensive literature review was carried out aiming to investigate available strategies to reduce biofilm formation on PEEK materials for Implant Dentistry applications.

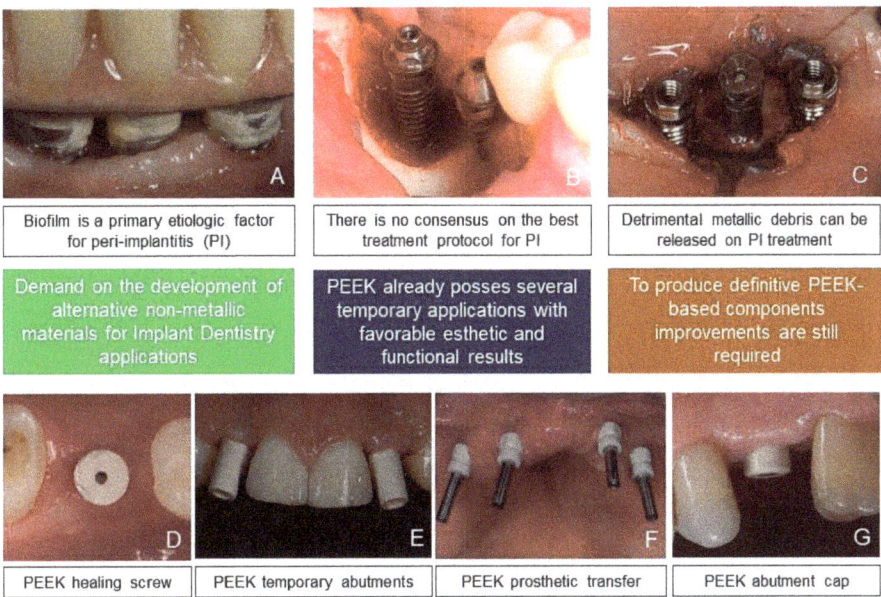

Figure 1. (**A**) Biofilm formation on titanium implants, underneath an implant-supported total prosthesis; (**B**) bone defects around dental implants at posterior lower jaw, a sequel of peri-implantitis; (**C**) metallic debris being released to peri-implant tissues during peri-implantitis treatment (implantoplasty); (**D**) PEEK healing screw (FGM, Brazil); (**E**) PEEK temporary abutments (Straumann, Switzerland) that support esthetic restorations; (**F**) PEEK prosthetic transfers (FGM, Brazil); (**G**) PEEK abutment cap (Straumann, Switzerland).

2. Strategies to Reduce Biofilm Formation in PEEK Materials Applied to Implant Dentistry

A full strategy with inclusion and exclusion criteria, as well as the flow chart of selected studies, are available as Supplementary Data. From a total of 376 studies initially found during the literature search, 33 were chosen for full text reading based on titles. Thereafter, 31 studies fulfilled the inclusion criteria of this review. Tables 1 and 2 reveal comprehensive information on pure and modified PEEK, respectively.

2.1. Study Characteristics

Amongst the included studies, 5 involved in vitro associated to in vivo (animal) investigations, while 26 were restricted to in vitro studies. In vivo (human) studies did not fulfill inclusion criteria of this review. Regarding PEEK modification strategies, 6 studies analyzed pure PEEK compared to other materials [30–35] (e.g., titanium, silicon, gold, silver, zinc oxide, zirconia, silicon nitride) and none of them revealed special antibiofilm or antimicrobial properties of PEEK material. A total of 25 studies used strategies to reduce biofilm and bacterial colonization on PEEK, which were able to successfully confer either antibiofilm or antimicrobial properties, or both, to the material. Regarding applications aimed at the investigated materials, orthopedic, dental and the treatment of bone defects were the most commonly mentioned, followed by the development of biomaterials in general.

Table 1. Descriptive analysis of unmodified PEEK materials [a].

Reference	Materials (Roughness and Contact Angle Values) [b]		Microorganisms		Microbiologic Assay		Biologic Response
1. Barton et al. [30]	Poly(orthoester) (78°); Poly(L-lactic acid) (84°); PEEK (90°); Polysulfone (84°); High molecular weight polyethylene (106°);	✓ ✓ ✓ ✓ ✓	Staphylococcus epidermidis; Pseudomonas aeruginosa; Escherichia coli;	✓ ✓ ✓	Bacteria adhesion with or without hyaluronic acid;	✓	Bacterial adhesion was higher on PEEK than on biodegradable polymers;
2. Bock et al. [31]	PEEK (1.034 nm; 86°); Si$_3$N$_4$ (1094 nm; 28°); Af-Si$_3$N$_4$ (830 nm; 66°); Ox-Si$_3$N$_4$ (745 nm; 8°); N$_2$-Si$_3$N$_4$ (654 nm; 9°); Ti$_6$Al$_4$V (494 nm; 71°);	✓ ✓ ✓ ✓ ✓ ✓	Escherichia coli; Staphylococcus epidermidis;	✓ ✓	Bacterial detachment and counting; average colony forming units (CFU/mm^2)	✓	For both bacteria and at both experimental times biofilm growth was greater on PEEK;
3. Bressan et al. 2017 [32]	Taper cap gold coping; PEEK coping Copings were connected to dental implants;	✓ ✓	Aggregatibacter actinomycetemcomitans; Porphyromonas gingivalis; Fusobacterium nucleatum;	✓ ✓ ✓	Real-time polymerase chain reaction (PCR); Visual assessment;	✓ ✓	No significant differences between groups were identified;
4. Gorth et al. [33]	PEEK (1 nm); Titanium (3 nm); Si$_3$N$_4$ (25 nm) Si$_3$N$_4$ polished (10 nm);	✓ ✓ ✓ ✓	Staphylococcus epidermidis; Pseudomonas aeruginosa; Staphylococcus aureus; Escherichia coli; Enterococcus;	✓ ✓ ✓ ✓ ✓	Bacterial function: crystal violet staining and a Live/Dead assay;	✓	Exponential growth of biofilm was noted on PEEK when exposed to S. epidermidis, S. aureus, P. aeruginosa and E. coli. With the exception of Enterococcus, biofilm formation was lower on titanium compared to PEEK for time periods >48 h. PEEK showed the highest biofilm affinity;

Table 1. *Cont.*

Reference	Materials (Roughness and Contact Angle Values) [b]	Microorganisms	Microbiologic Assay	Biologic Response
5. Hahnel et al. 2015 [34]	✓ Zirconia (0.16 µm); ✓ Titanium (0.17 µm); ✓ PEEK (0.04 µm); ✓ Polymethylmethacrylate—PMMA (0.05 µm);	✓ *Candida albicans*; ✓ *Streptococcus mutans*; ✓ *Actinomyces naeslundii*; ✓ *Streptococcus gordonii*;	✓ Biofilm analysis: MTT-based cell viability assay and Live/Dead BacLight bacterial viability kit solution. ✓ Analysis on fluorescence microscope;	The lowest quantity of adherent viable biomass was identified on the surface of PEEK compared to other groups. After 44 h, biofilms on zirconia yielded the highest value of dead microorganisms and PMMA yielded the lowest value;
6. Webster et al. [35]	✓ Si_3N_4 (39°); ✓ ASTM grade 4 titanium (76°); ✓ PEEK (95°);	✓ *Staphylococcus epidermidis*;	✓ Bacterial infection and bone growth: histologic quantification for the number of bacteria in the implant area and juxtaposed to the implant;	Live bacteria were identified around PEEK (88%) and Ti (21%) implants, while none were observed adjacent to Si_3N_4;

[a] A decrease in free energy favors stability. [b] Contact angle ≥ 90° means that the material is hydrophobic, and <90° means that it is hydrophilic.

Table 2. Descriptive analysis of modified PEEK materials.

Reference	PEEK Modification Strategy	Materials (Roughness and Contact Angle Values)		Microorganisms		Microbiologic Assay	Biologic Response
1. Barkarmo et al. [36]	PEEK blasting;	PEEK (0.57 µm; 70.33°); Blasted PEEK (1.85 µm; 108.36°); Titanium Grade 4 (0.23 µm; 62.43°); Ti$_6$Al$_4$V (0.28 µm; 58.82°);	✓ ✓ ✓ ✓	Streptococcus sanguinis; Streptococcus oralis; Enterococcus faecalis; Streptococcus gordonii;	✓ ✓ ✓ ✓	Modification of the original method of Christensen et al. (1985).	Bacteria showed increased biofilm formation on blasted PEEK (exception: E. faecalis—higher on cp-Ti compared with other materials).
2. Deng et al. [37]	Novel Ag-decorated 3D printed PEEK via catecholamine chemistry;	PEEK scaffolds fabricated layer by layer; PEEK coated with a pDAnanolayer by dopamine solution and immersion in AgNO$_3$ with subsequent UV light treatment;	✓ ✓	Escherichia coli; Staphylococcus aureus;	✓ ✓	Evaluation of bacterial dynamics curves; Antibiofilm formation;	PEEK scaffold pDA-coated and UV-treated had significant contact and release killing capacities. Biofilms were reduced in the presence of silver;
3. Deng et al. [38]	Hierarchically micro/nanoscale produced on PEEK and a simvastatin-PLLA film-tobramycin microspheres delivery system was fabricated;	PEEK; NSPEEK (treatment with mixed acid H$_2$SO$_4$:HNO3); NSP/SIM(1 mm)-PLLA (additional immersion in SIM solution) (93°); NSP/SIM (1 mm)-TOB: additional emulsion 3% of PLLA in CH$_2$Cl$_2$; 0.3% of TOB in ultra-pure water) dropped and spin-coated (84°);	✓ ✓ ✓ ✓	Escherichia coli; Staphylococcus. aureus.	✓ ✓	Agar diffusiontest; Bacteria Adhesion; Antibiofilm Tests; Evaluation through Live/Dead kits, FE-SEM and confocal laser scanning microscopy;	Few bacteria were detected on the NSP/SIM (1 mm)-TOB group, while other groups had plenty of bacteria adhered. PEEK and NSPEEK showed uncontrolled biofilm proliferation, while no biofilm was observed on NSP/SIM (1 mm)-TOB group;

Table 2. Cont.

Reference	PEEK Modification Strategy	Materials (Roughness and Contact Angle Values)	Microorganisms	Microbiologic Assay	Biologic Response
4. Deng et al. [39]	Dual therapy implant coating developed on the 3D micro-/nanoporous sulfonated PEEK via layer-by-layer self-assembly of Ag ions and Zn ions;	✓ SPEEK: sulfonated PEEK (83.75°); ✓ Ag-SPEEK: SPEEK further treated by chitosan solution, and by Ag ion-sodium alginate solution; ✓ Zn-SPEEK: assembling of Zn ion-containing chitosan with pure sodium alginate; ✓ Ag/Zn-SPEEK: Ag-SPEEK further exposed to UV/ozone;	✓ Escherichia coli; ✓ Staphylococcus aureus;	✓ Antibacterial Kinetic Tests; ✓ Determination of CFU; ✓ Bacterial Growth Inhibition Zone Tests; ✓ SEM Characterization of Bacteria;	Ag-SPEEK substrate was superior regarding antibacterial properties against E. coli, while absence of obvious antibacterial effects against S. aureus was observed;
5. Diez-Pascual et al. [40]	Production of nanocomposites via melt-blending, by addition of a carboxylated polymer derivative covalently grafted onto the surface of hydroxyl-terminated ZnO nanoparticles;	✓ PEEK, PEEK/ZnO (nanoparticle content: 1.0); ✓ PEEK/ZnO (2.5); ✓ PEEK/ZnO (5.0); ✓ PEEK/COOH; ✓ PCOZnO, PEEK/PCOZnO (1.0); ✓ PEEK/PCOZnO (2.5); ✓ PEEK/PCOZnO (5.0); ✓ Obs:PCOZnO is PEEK-CO-O-CH$_2$-ZnO;	✓ Escherichia coli; ✓ Staphylococcus. aureus;	✓ CFU/sample calculation;	Nanocomposites with polymer-grafted nanoparticles exhibited superior antibacterial activity against both studied bacteria. This effect increased upon raising nanoparticle content and was stronger on E. coli;
6. Diez-Pascual et al. [41]	Production of biocompatible ternary nanocomposites based on poly PEEK/poly(ether-imide) (PEI) blends reinforced with bioactive titanium dioxide (TiO$_2$) nanoparticles via ultrasonication followed by melt-blending;	✓ TiO$_2$; ✓ PEEK; ✓ PEI; ✓ PEEK/PEI; ✓ PEEK/PEI/ TiO$_2$ (1.0 wt %); ✓ PEEK/PEI/ TiO$_2$ (4.0 wt %); ✓ PEEK/PEI/ TiO$_2$ (8.0 wt %) UV irradiated;	✓ Escherichia coli; ✓ Staphylococcus aureus;	✓ Survival ratio calculation under presence or absence of UV light against bacteria;	The nanoparticles conferred antibacterial action versus tested bacteria in the presence and in the absence of UV light. The highest inhibition was attained at 4.0 wt % nanoparticle concentration;

Table 2. Cont.

Reference	PEEK Modification Strategy	Materials (Roughness and Contact Angle Values)	Microorganisms	Microbiologic Assay	Biologic Response
7. Gan et al. [42]	Nitrogen plasma immersion ion implantation (PIII) on PEEK;	PEEK-C (50.6 nm; 84.5°), ✓ PEEK-I: N$_2$, no voltage, no pulse width and no frequency—90 min (435.9 nm; 19.93°), ✓ PEEK-L: N$_2$, −20 kV of voltage, pulse width of 30 uS, frequency of 1000 W—90 min (443.23 nm; 20.67°), ✓ PEEK-H: N$_2$, −20 kV of voltage, pulse width of 50 uS, frequency of 1000W—90 min (608.4 nm; 17.74°); ✓	Staphylococcus aureus; ✓	Colony-counting and plate-counting methods; ✓	The number of colonies adherents on the PEEK-L and PEEK-H was lower than that on PEEK-C and PEEK-I. Nitrogen PIII using high pulse or low pulse inhibited S. aureus early adhesion on PEEK, which exhibited antibacterial property;
8. He et al. [43]	Drug-loaded (chlorogenic acid, CGA)/grafted peptide (BFP) hydrogel system supported on a sulfonated PEEK (SPEEK) surface, using sodium alginate (SA);	SPEEK (67.75°), ✓ SPEEK@SA (23.33°) ✓ SPEEK@SA-CGA—(30.5°); ✓ SPEEK@SA(CGA)BFP (28.08°); ✓	Escherichia coli; ✓ Staphylococcus aureus; ✓	Evaluation through plate-counting method after inoculation and incubation. ✓	SPEEK and SPEEK@SA did not inhibit E. coli growth. SPEEK@SA(CGA) and SPEEK@SA(CGA)BFP scaffolds had a noticeable antibacterial effect on both tested bacteria;
9. Lu et al. [44]	Dual zinc and oxygen plasma immersion ion implantation (Zn/O-PIII) applied to modify carbon fiber reinforced PEEK (CFRPEEK);	CFRPEEK (66.6°); ✓ CFRPEEK + oxygen plasma immersion ion implantation (Zn/O-PIII) (144.1°); ✓	Escherichia coli; ✓ Staphylococcus. aureus; ✓ Pseudomonas aeruginosa; ✓ Methicillin-resistant Staphylococcus. aureus; ✓ Staphylococcus. epidermidis; ✓ Biofilm-negative Staphylococcus epidermidis; ✓	Antibacterial activity: bacterial counting method; ✓ Morphology of the adhered bacteria: SEM; ✓	S. aureus, MRSA and S. epidermidis reduction on Zn/O-PIII-CFRPEEK is over 95% at 24 h. This group showed no antibacterial effect on S. epidermidis (biofilm-negative strain), E. coli and P. aeruginosa;

Table 2. Cont.

Reference	PEEK Modification Strategy	Materials (Roughness and Contact Angle Values)	Microorganisms	Microbiologic Assay	Biologic Response
10. Montero et al. [45]	PEEK sulfonation treatment to functionalize and embed therapeutical substances (lactam);	✓ Sulphonated-PEEK without lactams embedded; ✓ Sulphonated-PEEK with lactams embedded;	✓ Streptococcus mutans;	✓ Evaluation through plate-counting method after inoculation and incubation (biofilm and planktonic); ✓ Bacterial morphology: SEM;	Planktonic growth showed no significant difference between groups, while biofilm inhibition was found comparing SPEEK with lactams. S. mutans biofilm grew widely separately as agglomerates on SPEEK without lactams, while it could not be detected on SPEEK with lactams;
11. Montero et al. [46]	PEEK sulfonation (SPEEK) on various degrees (SD):62%, G2 68%, G3 90%, G4 75% and G5 69%	✓ SPEEK (50 °C, 1 h, SD: 62%); ✓ SPEEK (50 °C, 1.5 h, SD: 68%); ✓ SPEEK (50 °C, 2 h, SD: 90%); ✓ SPEEK (50 °C, 2.5 h, 75%); ✓ SPEEK (50 °C. 3 h, SD: 69%);	✓ Streptococcus mutans; ✓ Enterococcus faecalis;	✓ Evaluation through plate-counting method after inoculation and incubation (biofilm and planktonic);	SPEEK heated for 3 h was the group with lowest values of planktonic growth,CFU from S. mutans biofilm showed a significant decrease on SPEEK sulfonated for 2, 2.5 and 3 h. E. faecalis showed this reduction only on groups sulfonated for 2.5 and 3 h;
12. Ouyang et al. [47]	Preparation of graphene oxide (GO) modified SPEEK (GO-SPEEK) through dip-coating method;	✓ PEEK (91.2°); ✓ SPEEK (103.9°); ✓ 0.5 GO-SPEEK (57°); ✓ 1 GO-SPEEK (47.7°);	✓ Escherichia coli; ✓ Staphylococcus aureus;	✓ Live/Dead fluorescence imaging (Confocal laser scanning microscope-CLSM evaluation);	0.5 GO-SPEEK and 1 GO-SPEEK groups exhibit proper antibacterial properties against E. coli, but poor against S. aureus;
13. Ouyang et al. [48]	PEEK was sulfonated by concentrated sulfuric acid to fabricate a three-dimensional (3D) network with hydrothermal treatment subsequently;	✓ PEEK (86°); ✓ SPEEK (110°); ✓ SPW25 (110°); ✓ SPW120 (110°);	✓ Escherichia coli; ✓ Staphylococcus aureus;	✓ Incubation according the standard of Luria–Bertani; Bacteria morphology: SEM;	Amounts of E.coli were reduced to nearly 100%, 100%, and 24% on SPEEK, SPW25 and SPW120, respectively. On the same groups S. aureus was reduced by nearly 100%.

Table 2. Cont.

Reference	PEEK Modification Strategy	Materials (Roughness and Contact Angle Values)	Microorganisms	Microbiologic Assay	Biologic Response
14. Rochford et al. [49]	Injection moulded (PO) or machined (PA) PEEK exposed to an oxygen gas plasma in a plasma cleaner;	✓ Injection molded PEEK (PO) (85 nm, 83°); ✓ Injection molded PEEK machined (PA) (536 nm, 73°); ✓ Commercially pure micro-rough titanium (Ti) (530 nm, 68°); ✓ Treated side of sterile Thermanox Txh (7.5 nm, 67°);	✓ Staphylococcus aureus; JAR (bothclinicalisolates) ✓ Staphylococcus epidermidis;	✓ Bacterial adhesion quantification: adhesion chamber biofilm reactor;	Surface modification of PEEK did not lead to a significant change in bacterial adhesion in the preoperative contamination model. In the postoperative contamination model, S. aureus adhesion was increased on the modified surfaces. S. epidermidis adhesion to modified PEEK was lower than to nonmodified PEEK in the postoperative model;
15. Rochford et al. [50]	PEEK films were oxygen plasma treated to increase surface free energy;	✓ PEEK (28 nm, 81°); ✓ PEEK exposed to oxygen gas plasma for 900 s (21 nm, 53°); ✓ PEEK exposed to oxygen gas plasma for 1800 s (15 nm, 51°);	✓ Staphylococcus epidermidis; ✓ Staphylococcus aureus;	✓ Bacterial adhesion was assessed using a parallel plate flow chamber and camera;	There was no significant difference in bacterial adhesion between treated and untreated surfaces;
16. Tateishi et al. [51]	Modified PEEK surface by photoinduced and self-initiated graft polymerization with 2methacryloyloxyethyl phosphorylcholine, under radiation UV;	✓ Untreated PEEK; ✓ PMPC-grafted PEEK;	✓ Escherichia coli;	✓ Number of bacteria adhered on the surface was countered from the SEM images;	SEM revealed adhered bacteria on PEEK, whereas no bacterium was observed on the PMPC-grafted PEEK;

Table 2. Cont.

Reference	PEEK Modification Strategy	Materials (Roughness and Contact Angle Values)	Microorganisms	Microbiologic Assay	Biologic Response
17. Tran et al. [52]	Production of a hybrid coating of titanium dioxide and polydimethylsiloxane (PDMS) to regulate silver releasing;	✓ PEEK (90°), ✓ Coated PEEK in H50 volume and 38.4 µL Ag (H50-38.4) (>120°); ✓ Coated PEEK in H50 volume and 384 µL Ag (H50-384) (>120°); ✓ Coated PEEK in H75 volume and 38.4 µL Ag (H75-38.4) (>120°); ✓ Coated PEEK in H75 volume and 384 µL Ag (H75-384) (>120°); ✓ Coated PEEK in H95 volume and 38.4 µL Ag (H95-38.4) (>120°); ✓ Coated PEEK in H95 volume and 384 µL Ag (H95-384) (>120°);	✓ *Staphylococcus aureus*; ✓ *Staphylococcus epidermidis*;	✓ Antibacterial property: Kirby–Bauer tests; ✓ Biofilm growth: after incubation samples were analyzed by SEM;	Higher Ag loadings resulted in a significant increase in the diameter of the bacteria inhibition zone. On PEEK, a thick and dense biofilm was formed. On H50-38.4, H75-38.4 and H95-38.4 smaller colonies of *S. aureus* were found, while in H50-384, H75-384 and H95-384 no bacterial colonies were found;
18. Ur Rehman et al. [53]	Chitosan/bioactive glass (BG)/lawsone coatings were deposited by electrophoretic deposition (EPD) on polyetheretherketone (PEEK)/BG layers (previously deposited by EPD on 316-L stainless steel);	✓ PEEK/BG (2.2 µm, 100°), ✓ Chitosan/BG/lawsone (1.3 µm, 45°), ✓ Stainless steel chitosan/BG/lawsone and PEEK/BG coated (multilayered);	✓ *Staphylococcus carnosus*;	✓ Inhibition zones were measured using 'ImageJ' analysis;	Chitosan/BG/lawsone and the stainless steel chitosan/BG/lawsone PEEK/BG coated induced inhibition halo against *S. carnosus*. Halo zone was wider for the multilayered group (10 mm vs 4 mm);
19. Wang et al. [54]	Development of a PEEK/nano-fluorohydroxyapatite (PEEK/nano-FHA) biocomposite;	✓ PEEK (83.5°); ✓ PEEK/nano-fluorohydroxyapatite (PEEK/nano-FHA) (71.5°);	✓ *Streptococcus mutans*	✓ Microbial ViabilityAssay Kit; ✓ Biofilm formation assay: LIVE/DEAD BacLight bacterial viability kit and evaluation on CLSM;	PEEK/nano-FHA biocomposite inhibited bacterial adhesion and proliferation, which did not occur with PEEK;

Table 2. Cont.

Reference	PEEK Modification Strategy	Materials (Roughness and Contact Angle Values)	Microorganisms	Microbiologic Assay	Biologic Response
20. Wang et al. [55]	PEEK coated with red and gray selenium nanoparticles through a quick precipitation method;	✓ Red selenium nanoparticles as coatings for PEEK (78.148°); ✓ Grey selenium nanoparticles as coatings for PEEK (76.988°); ✓ PEEK without selenium coatings (68.478°);	✓ *Pseudomonas aeruginosa*;	✓ Bacterial inhibition: crystal violet assays;	Red and gray selenium-coated PEEK significantly inhibited the growth of *P. aeruginosa* compared with uncoated PEEK at all experimental times.
21. Wang et al. [56]	Titanium plasma immersion ion implantation (PIII) technique was applied to modify the carbon-fiber-reinforced polyetheretherketone (CFRPEEK) surface, constructing a unique multilevel TiO$_2$ nanostructure;	✓ CFRPEEK; ✓ CFRPEEK modified with titanium plasma immersion ion implantation (PIII) technique (Ti-120);	✓ *Streptococcus mutans*; ✓ *Fusobacterium nucleatum*; ✓ *Porphyromonas gingivalis*;	✓ Live/Dead BacLight bacteria viability kits and evaluation at confocal laser-scanning microscope; ✓ Morphological-observation: SEM; ✓ Longevity and stability of antibacterial activity;	The TiPIII modified surface can reduced *S. mutans*, *F. nucleatum* and *P. gingivalis* adhesion and growth, directly implicating on death of adhesive bacterial;
22. Xu et al. [57]	PEEK modified surface using dexamethasone plus minocycline-loaded liposomes (Dex/Mino liposomes) bonded by a mussel-inspired polydopamine coating (pDA);	✓ PEEK (22.25 nm, 71°); ✓ PEEK-pDA (53.33 nm, 24°); ✓ PEEK blankliposomes (35.90 nm, 61°);	✓ In vitro: *Streptococcus mutans* and *Porphyromonas gingivalis*;	✓ The Microbial Viability Assay Kit-WST and LIVE/DEAD BacLight Bacterial Viability Kit (CLSM evaluation); ✓ Cell morphology imaging;	Minor releasing from PEEK blank lipossomes surfaces effectively prevented bacterial adhesion and proliferation. The antibacterial efficiency of PEEK blank lipossomes was about 97.4% against *S. mutans*;

Table 2. Cont.

Reference	PEEK Modification Strategy	Materials (Roughness and Contact Angle Values)	Microorganisms	Microbiologic Assay	Biologic Response
23. Yan et al. [58]	A mussel inspired self-polymerized polydopamine (PDA) with silver nanoparticles (AgNPs) incorporated and silk fibroin (SF)/ gentamicin sulfate (GS) coating was constructed upon porous PEEK surface;	✓ PEEK (65°); ✓ SPEEK (81°); ✓ SP-PDA (49°); ✓ SP-PDA-Ag (without UV); ✓ SP-PDA-Ag (46°); ✓ SP-PDA-Ag/GS-Silk (56°);	✓ Staphylococcus aureus; ✓ Escherichia coli;	✓ Antibacterial assay: Plate-counting method; ✓ Bacterial morphology: SEM;	SP-PDA-Ag/GS-Silk showed reliable antibacterial capacity against S. aureus and E. coli. It was observed smoothly adhered, proliferated and aggregated bacteria on PEEK, SPEEK and SP-PDA groups;
24. Yuan et al. [59]	Mouse beta-defensin-14 (MBD-14) was immobilized on the PEEK surface with 3D porous structure through sulfonation process;	✓ PEEK—polished, ✓ SP—sulfonated PEEK hydrothermally treated at 120 °C for 4 h (109.11°), ✓ SP-MBD2-SP loaded with 10 uL of solution containing 2 ug/mL MBD-14 (73.40°), ✓ SP-MBD5—SP loaded with 10 uL of solution containing 5 ug/mL MBD-14 (68.25°), ✓ SP-MBD10—SP loaded with 10 uL of solution containing 10 ug/mL MBD-14 (64.80°);	✓ Staphylococcus aureus; ✓ Pseudomonas aeruginosa;	✓ Agar diffusion assay: National Standard of China GB/T 2738-2012 protocol; ✓ Bacterial morphology: SEM; ✓ Antibacterial longevity;	SP-MBD with different MBD-14 solutions could effectively kill S. aureus and P. aeruginosa; PEEK with MBD-14 exercised durable and broad-spectrum antibacterial activity;
25. Zhang et al. [60]	Macro-microporous bone implants of nano-bioglass (nBG) and polyetheretherketone (PK) composite (mBPC) were fabricated;	✓ Macroporous-microporous nBG/PK composites (mBPC) with the nBG contents of 30 wt %, PK withoutnBG (mPK), ✓ Macroporous nBG / PK (BPC) compounds with 30% by weight of nBG, ✓ Thiol (HK) loaded in mBPC (dmBPC);	✓ Staphylococcus aureus;	✓ The number of CFUs on medium and on biofilm was counted; ✓ Antibacterial activity: LIVE/DEAD Bac light Bacteria Viability Kits (evaluation at CLSM);	Thiol (HK) loaded in mBPC (dmBPC) inhibited S. aureus growth and no viable bacteria were found. The presence of higher bacteria number on macro-microporous nBG/PK composites indicated stimulation of bacterial growth/ adhesion;

2.2. Available Strategies to Reduce Biofilm Formation on PEEK Materials

Strategies are summarized and illustrated at Figure 2 and are listed as follows:

(a) PEEK sulfonation process, which can be employed either to produce a 3D network on polymer surface [39], or to embed therapeutic compounds (e.g., lactams [45,46], mouse beta-defensin [59]). Further surface treatments were also employed after the sulfonation process, such as chlorogenic acid/grafting peptide [43], graphene oxide coating [61] and hydrothermal treatment [48].

(b) Incorporation of therapeutic and/or bioactive agents in the PEEK matrix or on the PEEK surface, such as simvastatin-PLLA [39]; Ag and Zn ions [37,39,40,58], dexamethasone plus minocycline-loaded liposomes [57], bioactive titanium dioxide (TiO2) [52], 2-methacryloyloxyethyl phosphorylcholine [51] and titanium plasma [56].

(c) PEEK coatings, such as the hybrid coating of titanium dioxide and polydimethylsiloxane [52]; chitosan/bioactive glass/lawsone [53], red and gray selenium nanoparticles [56], mussel-inspired polydopamine with silver nanoparticles incorporated and silk fibroin gentamicin sulfate [57,58].

(d) Incorporation of reinforcement agents to produce nanocomposites and/or blends (carbonylated PEEK grafted to ZnO45, PEEK/poly-ether-imide blends [41], carbon fiber reinforced PEEK further treated with oxygen plasma [44], PEEK/nano-fluorohydroxyapatite [54], nano-bioglass/PEEK [60]).

2.3. Microbiological Analysis

The most commonly investigated bacteria were *Escherichia coli* and *Staphylococcus aureus*, but other microorganisms such as *Streptococcus sanguinis*, *Streptococcus oralis*, *Streptococcus faecalis*, *Streptococcus gordonni*, *Streptococcus epidermidis*, *Pseudomonas aeruginosa*, *Aggregatibacter actinomycetemcomitans*, *Porphyromonas gingivalis*, *Fusobacterium nucleatum*, *Enterococcus faecalis*, *Candida albicans*, *Actinomyces naeslundii*, *Streptococcus mutans* and *Staphylococcus epidermidis* were also studied. Microbiological analysis was very heterogenic, and several methods were used, which are summarized in Tables 1 and 2. Among the included methods, it should be highlighted that the most recurrent ones were plate-counting, for the determination of average colony forming units (CFU/mm^2); Real-Time Polymerase Chain Reaction (RT-PCR) and Live/Dead cells analysis, followed by FE-SEM and confocal laser scanning microscopy; bacterial growth inhibition zone tests; crystal violet assays; longevity and stability of antibacterial activity and agar diffusion assay.

2.4. Physicochemical and Topographical Characterization

With the exception of 7 papers [32,37,40,41,45,56,60], all the other studies analyzed surface topographical aspects, such as either or both contact angle and surface roughness. The physicochemical and additional characterization of included papers was achieved by energy-dispersive X-ray spectroscopy (EDX), X-ray photoelectron spectroscopy (XPS), porosity evaluation through drainage method, dynamic differential scanning calorimetry (DSC), X-ray diffractograms (XRD), Hydrogen nuclear magnetic resonance (^{1}H-NMR), thermogravimetric analysis (TGA), Fourier-transform infrared spectroscopy (FTIR) and UV spectrophotometer.

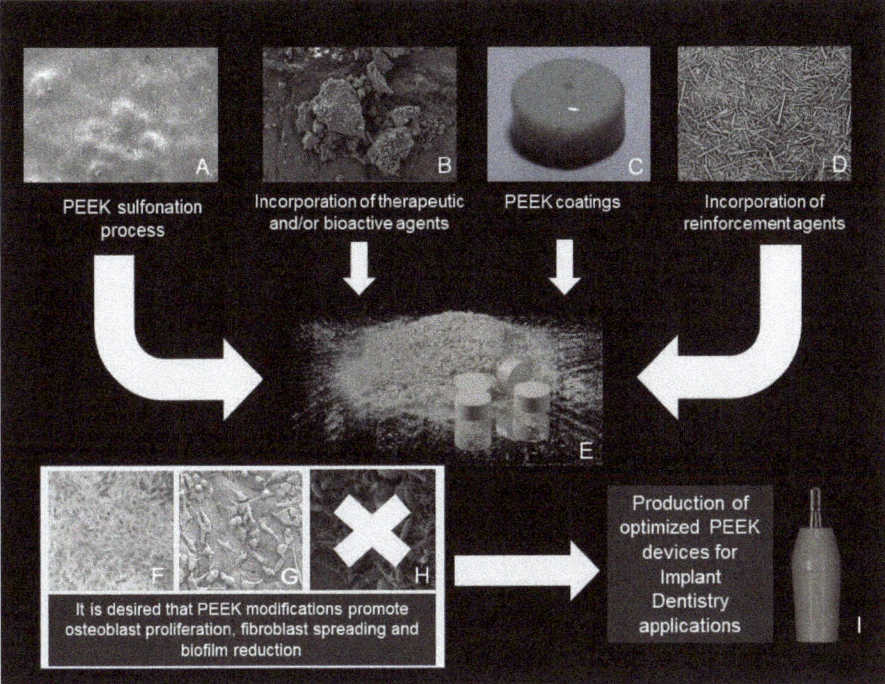

Figure 2. Summary of some available strategies to improve PEEK biological properties. (**A**) SEM image of a sulfonated PEEK membrane; (**B**) SEM image of bioglass particles; (**C**) photography of PEEK coated with adhesive film; (**D**) SEM image of natural amorphous silica fibers; (**E**) photography of PEEK powder and PEEK cylinders manufactured through compression molding; (**F,G**) SEM images of MC3T3 osteoblasts on zirconia surface; L929 fibroblasts on PEEK surface; (**H**) undesired biofilm formation on material surface; (**I**) PEEK provisional abutment (Straumann, Switzerland).

3. Discussion

Investigations have demonstrated that peri-implantitis is a heterogeneous infection, in which periodontopathogens and opportunistic microorganisms act simultaneously [62–64]. Moreover, the disease has been associated to specific immunological alterations on peri-implant crevicular fluid levels of proinflammatory, anti-inflammatory and osteoclastogenesis-related chemokines [65]. Several studies analyzed in this review [30–35] investigated biofilm and antimicrobial properties of pure PEEK, demonstrating that the polymer is susceptible to biofilm colonization. Within a context in which PEEK clinical applications in Implant Dentistry are increasing [28], strategies to modify its surface to enhance its antimicrobial/antibiofilm properties are crucial.

It becomes even more important to improve PEEK materials with the above-mentioned properties when considering that biofilms are organized polymicrobial communities that offer bacteria protection against environmental factors and antibiotic treatments [66,67]. In vitro analysis of submucosal biofilm samples of 120 peri-implantitis sites revealed that 71.7% exhibited bacterial pathogens resistance to one or more of tested antibiotics (clindamycin, amoxicillin, doxycycline or metronidazole) [68]. Therefore, the identification of compounds capable of inhibiting biofilm formation or disrupt biofilm organization emerges as an attractive alternative to avoid peri-implant related infections [69,70]. It is important to notice that this approach is not expected to completely eliminate biofilm formation, but it is a very effective way of modifying oral ecology instead, reducing the number of pathogenic bacteria and favoring the growth of mutualistic species. By doing so, the host organism is provided with just the necessary advantage to defeat the pathogens using its own resources.

Additionally, it is important to analyze PEEK surface properties and its influence on biologic systems. For example, the PEEK hydrophobic surface associated to its bio inertness is a major concern when prospecting for the expansion of its application in Implant Dentistry [28,71], as this type of surface typically reduces cellular adhesion and does not promote osseointegration [22]. Numerous modifications have been proposed to overcome those limitations, such as blending with bioactive particles such as titanium dioxide, hydroxyapatite and fluorapatite [72–74]. Interestingly, the present review exposed that some of those strategies showed the favorable additional effect of reducing biofilm formation [41,44,54]. For example, a very promising candidate to replace metallic implants is carbon fiber reinforced PEEK (CFRPEEK) [75], which has similar elastic modulus to the human cortical bone [22]. One of the studies included in this review [44] proposed a dual zinc and oxygen plasma immersion ion implantation to modify CFRPEEK. Despite the fact that this strategy made the surface far more hydrophobic (contact angle shifted from 66.6° to 144.1° after surface modification), it also improved both osteogenic and antibacterial activities, as evaluated through MC3T3-E1 and rat bone mesenchymal stem cell development and through *Staphylococcus aureus*, MRSA and *Staphylococcus epidermidis* inhibition [44]. Those findings provide positive perspectives of the development of PEEK surfaces enhanced with bioactive and antibiofilm properties, which is favorable for PEEK-based dental implant development.

Bone cell activity on the PEEK surface is very important to achieve proper osseointegration on dental implants, but considering that an imperative application for PEEK in Implant Dentistry is as implant abutments [76], the gingival sealing must be analyzed as well, since it provides protection to implants against infections by potential pathogens [10]. Among the studies included in this review describing strategies for PEEK modification through the incorporation of antibiofilm agents, the embedding of lactams through the PEEK sulfonation process is worth mentioning [45]. Lactams are compounds analogous to furanones, which were initially isolated from the algae *Delisea pulchra*, and had been proved to be effective against *Streptococus mutans* biofilms [77]. An in vitro study [26] demonstrated that PEEK sulfonation positively interferes with the ability of fibroblasts L929 to spread over the surface of the material [26]. This corroborates previous indications that PEEK sulfonation is a suitable process for the development of modified PEEK abutments with embedded antibiofilm compounds.

In addition to the mentioned in vitro studies indicating these strategies as promising approaches to develop clinical materials biofilm resistant, an in vivo (human) investigation also revealed that PEEK healing abutments did not affect important parameters of peri-implant health, such as marginal bone loss and soft tissue recession, during a three-month evaluation period [78]. Therefore, it seems plausible to associate PEEK inherent favorable properties with adequate strategies to maximize its biological properties and consequently achieve even better clinical outcomes in the near future.

4. Conclusions

Within the scope of the present review, it may be concluded that pure PEEK is susceptible to biofilm formation and that several strategies presented here are able to significantly improve its antibiofilm and antimicrobial properties. Those strategies include the PEEK sulfonation process, incorporation of therapeutic and/or bioactive agents in the PEEK matrix or on the PEEK surface, PEEK coatings and incorporation of reinforcement agents to produce nanocomposites and/or blends. Since the use of PEEK in Implant Dentistry is increasing, those modifications are necessary in order to enable patients to benefit from these new materials which present great potential to prevent infections. Therefore, it is expected that further in vivo studies, both in animals and humans, will make available PEEK-based dental implants and improved implant abutments for clinical practice applications.

Author Contributions: R.S.B.—Conceptualization, formal analysis, investigation, methodology, writing—original draft preparation; L.G.L.—validation, formal analysis, investigation; C.Â.M.V.—conceptualization, data curation, visualization, supervision; C.A.M.B.—conceptualization, resources, visualization, project administration; A.d.L.P.—conceptualization, writing—review and editing, supervision. All authors have read and agreed to the published version of the manuscript.

Funding: This project was supported by a grant from the ITI Foundation, Switzerland.

Acknowledgments: Authors express their gratitude to CAPES and FAPEU in Brazil. Additionally, authors are grateful to Felipe Ouriques, Bruna Barbosa Côrrea, Mario Eduardo Escobar-Ramos, Maria Elisa Galarraga-Vinueza, Mariane Beatriz Sordi and Patrícia Rabelo Monich due to their collaboration on images that enabled the creation of the present figures. Authors are also thankful to Camila Rodrigues de Souza due to her efforts in the language review.

Conflicts of Interest: The authors declare no conflict of interest.

References

1. Huttenhower, C.; Gevers, D.; Knight, R.; Abubucker, S.; Badger, J.H.; Chinwalla, A.T.; Creasy, H.H.; Earl, A.M.; FitzGerald, M.G.; Fulton, R.; et al. Structure, function and diversity of the healthy human microbiome. *Nature* **2012**, *486*, 207–214. [CrossRef]
2. Takahashi, N.; Nycad, B. The role of bacteria in the caries process: Ecological perspectives. *J. Dent. Res.* **2011**, *90*, 294–303. [CrossRef] [PubMed]
3. Coventry, J.; Griffiths, G.; Scully, C.; Tonetti, M. ABC of oral health: Periodontal disease. *BMJ* **2000**, *321*, 36–39. [CrossRef] [PubMed]
4. Sharma, N.; Bhatia, S.; Sodhi, A.S.; Batra, N. Oral microbiome and health. *AIMS Microbiol.* **2018**, *4*, 42–66. [CrossRef] [PubMed]
5. Jepsen, S.; Caton, J.G.; Albandar, J.M.; Bissada, N.F.; Bouchard, P.; Cortellini, P.; Demirel, K.; Sanctis, M.; Ercoli, C.; Fan, J.; et al. Periodontal manifestations of systemic diseases and developmental and acquired conditions: Consensus report of workgroup 3 of the 2017 World Workshop on the Classification of Periodontal and Peri-Implant Diseases and Conditions. *J. Periodontol.* **2018**, *89*, 237–248. [CrossRef] [PubMed]
6. Socransky, S.S.; Haffajee, A.D.; Cugini, M.A.; Smith, C.; Kent, R.L., Jr. Microbial complexes in subgingival plaque. *J. Clin. Periodontol.* **1998**, *25*, 134–144. [CrossRef]
7. Berglundh, T.; Armitage, G.; Araujo, M.G.; Avila-Ortiz, G.; Blanco, J.; Camargo, P.M.; Chen, S.; Cochran, D.; Derks, J.; Figuero, E.; et al. Peri-implant diseases and conditions: Consensus report of workgroup 4 of the 2017 world workshop on the classification of periodontal and peri-implant diseases and conditions. *J. Clin. Periodontol.* **2018**, *45*, 286–291. [CrossRef] [PubMed]
8. Lee, C.; Huang, Y.; Zhu, L.; Weltman, R. Prevalences of peri-implantitis and peri-implant mucositis: Systematic review and meta-Analysis. *J. Dent.* **2017**. [CrossRef]
9. Robertson, K.; Shahbazian, T.; Macleod, S. Treatment of peri-implantitis and the failing implant. *Dent. Clin. N. Am.* **2015**, *59*, 329–343. [CrossRef]
10. Berglundh, T.; Jepsen, S.; Stadlinger, B.; Terheyden, H. Peri-implantitis and its prevention. *Clin. Oral Implant. Res.* **2019**, *30*, 150–155. [CrossRef]
11. Bollenl, C.M.L.; Lambrechts, P.; Quirynen, M. Comparison of surface roughness of oral hard materials to the threshold surface roughness for bacterial plaque retention: A review of the literature. *Den. Mater.* **1997**, *13*, 258–269. [CrossRef]
12. Falde, E.J.; Yohe, S.T.; Colson, Y.L.; Grinstaff, M.W. Superhydrophobic materials for biomedical applications. *Biomaterials* **2016**, *104*, 87–103. [CrossRef] [PubMed]
13. Nedeljkovic, I.; Munck, J.; Ungureanu, A.; Slomka, V.; Bartic, C.; Vananroye, A.; Clasen, C.; Teughels, W.; van Meerbeek, B.; van Landuyt, K.L. Biofilm-induced changes to the composite surface. *J. Dent.* **2017**, *63*, 36–43. [CrossRef] [PubMed]
14. Guéhennec, L.L.; Soueidan, A.; Layrolle, P.; Amouriq, Y. Surface treatments of titanium dental implants for rapid osseointegration. *Den. Mater.* **2007**, *23*, 844–854. [CrossRef] [PubMed]
15. Albrektsson, T.; Brånemark, P.I.; Hansson, H.A.; Lindström, J. Osseointegrated titanium implants. Requirements for ensuring a long-lasting, direct bone-to-implant anchorage in man. *Acta Orthop. Scand* **1981**, *52*, 155–170. [CrossRef]

16. Buser, D.; Sennerby, L.; Bruyn, H. Modern implant dentistry based on osseointegration: 50 years of progress, current trends and open questions. *Periodontol. 2000* **2017**, *73*, 7–21. [CrossRef]
17. Bianchini, M.A.; Galarraga-Vinueza, M.E.; Apaza-Bedoya, K.; Souza, J.M.; Magini, R.S.; Schwarz, F. Two to six-year disease resolution and marginal bone stability rates of a modified resective-implantoplasty therapy in 32 peri-implantitis cases. *Clin. Implant. Dent. Relat. Res.* **2019**, *21*, 758–765. [CrossRef]
18. Oliveira, M.N.; Schunemann, W.V.H.; Mathew, M.T.; Henriques, B.; Magini, R.S.; Teughels, W.; Souza, J.M. Can degradation products released from dental implants affect peri-implant tissues? *J. Periodontal. Res.* **2017**, *53*, 1–11. [CrossRef]
19. Hu, M.; Chen, J.; Pei, X.; Han, J.; Wang, J. Network meta-analysis of survival rate and complications in implant-supported single crowns with different abutment materials. *J. Dent.* **2019**, *88*, 103115. [CrossRef]
20. Schwitalla, A.; Muller, W.D. PEEK dental implants: A review of the literature. *J. Oral Implant.* **2012**, *39*, 743–749. [CrossRef]
21. Depprich, R.; Naujoks, C.; Ommerborn, M.; Schwarz, F.; Kübler, N.R.; Handschel, J. Current findings regarding zirconia implants. *Clin. Implant. Dent. Relat. Res.* **2012**, *16*, 124–137. [CrossRef] [PubMed]
22. Kurtz, S.M.; Devine, J.N. PEEK biomaterials in trauma, orthopedic, and spinal implants. *Biomaterials* **2007**, *28*, 4845–4869. [CrossRef] [PubMed]
23. Agustín-Panadero, R.; Serra-Pastor, B.; Roig-Vanaclocha, A.; Román-Rodriguez, J.; Fons-Font, A. Mechanical behavior of provisional implant prosthetic abutments. *Med. Oral Patol. Oral Cir. Bucal.* **2015**, *20*, 94–102. [CrossRef] [PubMed]
24. Escobar, M.; Henriques, B.; Fredel, M.C.; Silva, F.S.; Özcan, M.; Souza, J.M. Adhesion of PEEK to resin-matrix composites used in dentistry: A short review on surface modification and bond strength. *J. Adhes. Sci. Technol.* **2019**, 1241–1252. [CrossRef]
25. Monich, P.R.; Berti, F.V.; Porto, L.M.; Henriques, B.; Oliveira, A.P.N.; Fredel, M.C.; Souza, J.M. Physicochemical and biological assessment of PEEK composites embedding natural amorphous silica fibers for biomedical applications. *Mater. Sci. Eng. C Mater. Biol. Appl.* **2017**, *79*, 354–362. [CrossRef] [PubMed]
26. Brum, R.S.; Monich, P.R.; Berti, F.; Fredel, M.C.; Porto, L.M.; Benfatti, C.A.M.; Souza, J.M. On the sulphonated PEEK for implant dentistry: Biological and physicochemical assessment. *Mater. Chem. Phys.* **2019**, *223*, 542–547. [CrossRef]
27. Brum, R.S.; Monich, P.R.; Fredel, M.C.; Contri, G.; Ramoa, S.D.S.; Magini, R.S.; Benfatti, C.A.M. Polymer coatings based on sulfonated-poly-ether-ether-ketone films for implant dentistry applications. *J. Mater. Sci. Mater. Med.* **2018**, *29*, 132. [CrossRef]
28. Najeeb, S.; Zafar, M.S.; Khurshid, Z.; Siddiqui, F. Applications of polyetheretherketone (PEEK) in oral implantology and prosthodontics. *J. Prosthodont. Res.* **2016**, *60*, 12–19. [CrossRef]
29. Khonsari, R.H.; Berthier, P.; Rouillonc, T.; Perrina, J.; Corre, P. Severe infectious complications after PEEK-derived implant placement: Report of three cases. *J. Oral Maxillofac. Surg. Med. Pathol.* **2014**, *26*, 477–482. [CrossRef]
30. Barton, A.J.; Sagers, R.D.; Pitt, W.G. Bacterial adhesion to orthopedic implant polymers. *J. Biomed. Mater. Res.* **1996**, *30*, 403–410. [CrossRef]
31. Bock, R.M.; Jones, E.N.; Ray, D.R.; Bal, B.S.; Pezzotti, G.; Bryan, J.; McEntire, B.J. Bacteriostatic behavior of surface modulated silicon nitride in comparison to polyetheretherketone and titanium. *J. Biomed. Mater. Res. A* **2017**, *105*, 1521–1534. [CrossRef] [PubMed]
32. Bressan, E.; Stocchero, M.; Jimbo, R.; Rosati, C.; Fanti, E.; Tomasi, C.; Lops, D. Microbial leakage at morse taper conometric prosthetic connection: An in vitro investigation. *Implant. Dent.* **2017**, *26*, 756–761. [CrossRef] [PubMed]
33. Gorth, D.J.; Puckett, S.; Ercan, B.; Webster, T.J.; Rahaman, M.; Bal, B.S. Decreased bacteria activity on $Si_{(3)}N_{(4)}$ surfaces compared with PEEK or titanium. *Int. J. Nanomed.* **2012**, *7*, 4829–4840. [CrossRef]
34. Hahnel, S.; Wieser, A.; Lang, R.; Rosentritt, M. Biofilm formation on the surface of modern implant abutment materials. *Clin. Oral Implant. Res.* **2015**, *26*, 1297–1301. [CrossRef]
35. Webster, T.J.; Patel, A.A.; Rahaman, M.N.; Bal, B.S. Anti-infective and osteointegration properties of silicon nitride, poly(ether ether ketone), and titanium implants. *Acta Biomater.* **2012**, *8*, 4447–4454. [CrossRef]
36. Barkarmo, S.; Longhorn, D.; Leer, K.; Johansson, C.B.; Stenport, V.; Franco-Tabares, S.; Kuehne, S.A.; Sammons, R. Biofilm formation on polyetheretherketone and titanium surfaces. *Clin. Exp. Dent. Res.* **2019**, *5*, 427–437. [CrossRef]

37. Deng, L.; Deng, Y.; Xie, K. AgNPs-decorated 3D printed PEEK implant for infection control and bone repair. *Colloids Surf. B Biointerfaces* **2017**, *160*, 483–492. [CrossRef]
38. Deng, L.; He, X.; Xie, K.; Xie, L.; Deng, Y. Dual therapy coating on micro/nanoscale porous polyetheretherketone to eradicate biofilms and accelerate bone tissue repair. *Macromol. Biosci.* **2019**, *19*, 1800376. [CrossRef]
39. Deng, Y.; Yang, L.; Huang, X.; Chen, J.; Shi, X.; Yang, W.; Hong, M.; Wang, Y.; Dargusch, M.S.; Chen, Z. Dual Ag/ZnO-Decorated Micro-/nanoporoussulfonatedpolyetheretherketone with superior antibacterial capability and biocompatibility via layer-by-layer self-assembly strategy. *Macromol. Biosci.* **2018**, *18*, 1800028. [CrossRef]
40. Diez-Pascual, A.M.; Diez-Vicente, A.L. Development of nanocomposites reinforced with carboxylated poly(ether ether ketone) grafted to zinc oxide with superior antibacterial properties. *ACS Appl. Mater. Interfaces* **2014**, *6*, 3729–3741. [CrossRef]
41. Diez-Pascual, A.M.; Diez-Vicente, A.L. Nano-TiO$_2$ reinforced PEEK/PEI blends as biomaterials for load-bearing implant applications. *ACS Appl. Mater. Interfaces* **2015**, *7*, 5561–5573. [CrossRef] [PubMed]
42. Gan, K.; Liu, H.; Jiang, L.; Liu, X.; Song, X.; Niu, D.; Chen, T.; Liu, C. Bioactivity and antibacterial effect of nitrogen plasma immersion ion implantation on polyetheretherketone. *Dent. Mater.* **2016**, *32*, 263–274. [CrossRef] [PubMed]
43. He, X.; Deng, Y.; Yu, Y.; Lyu, H.; Liao, L. Drug-loaded/grafted peptide-modified porous PEEK to promote bone tissue repair and eliminate bacteria. *Colloids Surf. B Biointerfaces* **2019**, *181*, 767–777. [CrossRef] [PubMed]
44. Lu, T.; Li, J.; Qian, S.; Cao, H.; Ning, C.; Liu, X. Enhanced osteogenic and selective antibacterial activities on micro-/nano-structured carbon fiber reinforced polyetheretherketone. *J. Mater. Chem. B* **2016**, *4*. [CrossRef]
45. Montero, J.F.; Barbosa, L.C.; Pereira, U.A.; Barra, G.M.; Fredel, M.C.; Benfatti, C.A.M.; Magini, R.S.; Pimenta, A.L.; Souza, J.M. Chemical, microscopic, and microbiological analysis of a functionalized poly-ether-ether-ketone-embedding antibiofilm compounds. *J. Biomed. Mater. Res. A* **2016**, *104*, 3015–3020. [CrossRef]
46. Montero, J.F.; Tajiri, H.A.; Barra, G.M.; Fredel, M.F.; Benfatti, C.A.M.; Magini, R.S.; Pimenta, A.L.; Souza, J.M. Biofilm behavior on sulfonated poly(ether-ether-ketone) (sPEEK). *Mater. Sci. Eng. C Mater. Biol. Appl.* **2017**, *70*, 456–460. [CrossRef]
47. Ouyang, L.; Deng, Y.; Yang, L.; Shi, X.; Dong, T.; Tai, Y.; Yang, W.; Chen, Z. Graphene-oxide-decorated microporous polyetheretherketone with superior antibacterial capability and in vitro osteogenesis for orthopedic implant. *Macromol. Biosci.* **2018**, *18*. [CrossRef]
48. Ouyang, L.; Zhao, Y.; Jin, G.; Lu, T.; Li, J.; Qiao, Y.; Ning, C.; Zhang, X.; Chu, P.K.; Liu, X. Influence of sulfur content on bone formation and antibacterial ability of sulfonated PEEK. *Biomaterials* **2016**, *83*, 115–126. [CrossRef] [PubMed]
49. Rochford, E.T.J.; Poulsson, A.H.C.; Varela, S.J.; Richards, R.G.; Moriarty, T.F. Bacterial adhesion to orthopaedic implant materials and a novel oxygen plasma modified PEEK surface. *Colloids Surf. B Biointerfaces* **2014**, *113*, 213–222. [CrossRef] [PubMed]
50. Rochford, E.T.J.; Subbiahdoss, G.; Moriarty, T.F.; Poulsson, A.H.; van der Mei, H.C.; Busscher, H.J.; Richards, R.G. An in vitro investigation of bacteria-osteoblast competition on oxygen plasma-modified PEEK. *J. Biomed. Mater. Res. A* **2014**, *102*, 4427–4434. [CrossRef]
51. Tateishi, T.; Kyomoto, M.; Kakinoki, S.; Yamaoka, T.; Ishihara, K. Reduced platelets and bacteria adhesion on poly(ether ether ketone) by photoinduced and self-initiated graft polymerization of 2-methacryloyloxyethyl phosphorylcholine. *J. Biomed. Mater. Res. A* **2014**, *102*, 1342–1349. [CrossRef] [PubMed]
52. Tran, N.; Kelley, M.N.; Tran, P.A.; Garcia, D.R.; Jarrel, J.D.; Hayda, R.A.; Born, C.T. Silver doped titanium oxide-PDMS hybrid coating inhibits *Staphylococcus aureus* and *Staphylococcus epidermidis* growth on PEEK. *Mater. Sci. Eng. C Mater. Biol. Appl.* **2015**, *49*, 201–209. [CrossRef] [PubMed]
53. Rehman, M.A.; Ferraris, S.; Goldmann, W.H.; Perero, S.; Bastan, F.E.; Nawaz, Q.; di Confiengo, G.G.; Ferraris, M.; Boccaccini, A.R. Antibacterial and bioactive coatings based on radio frequency co-sputtering of silver nanocluster-silica coatings on PEEK/bioactive glass layers obtained by electrophoretic deposition. *ACS Appl. Mater. Interfaces* **2017**, *9*, 32489–32497. [CrossRef] [PubMed]
54. Wang, L.; Shu He, S.; Wu, X.; Liang, S.; Mu, Z.; Wei, J.; Deng, F.; Deng, Y.; Wei, S. Polyetheretherketone/nano-fluorohydroxyapatite composite with antimicrobial activity and osseointegration properties. *Biomaterials* **2014**, *35*, 6758–6775. [CrossRef]

55. Wang, Q.; Jaramillo, A.M.; Pavon, J.J.; Webster, T.J. Red selenium nanoparticles and gray selenium nanorods as antibacterial coatings for PEEK medical devices. *J. Biomed. Mater. Res. B Appl. Biomater.* **2016**, *104*, 1352–1358. [CrossRef]
56. Wang, X.; Lu, T.; Wen, J.; Xu, L.; Zeng, D.; Wu, Q.; Cao, L.; Lin, S.; Liu, X.; Jiang, X. Selective responses of human gingival fibroblasts and bacteria on carbon fiber reinforced polyetheretherketone with multilevel nanostructured TiO_2. *Biomaterials* **2016**, *83*, 207–218. [CrossRef]
57. Xu, X.; Li, Y.; Wang, L.; Li, Y.; Pan, J.; Fu, X.; Luo, Z.; Sui, Y.; Zhang, S.; Wang, L.; et al. Triple-functional polyetheretherketone surface with enhanced bacteriostasis and anti-inflammatory and osseointegrative properties for implant application. *Biomaterials* **2019**, *212*, 98–114. [CrossRef]
58. Yan, J.; Zhou, W.; Jia, Z.; Xiong, P.; Li, Y.; Wang, P.; Li, Q.; Cheng, Y.; Zheng, Y. Endowing polyetheretherketone with synergistic bactericidal effects and improved osteogenic ability. *Acta Biomater.* **2018**, *79*, 216–229. [CrossRef]
59. Yuan, X.; Ouyang, L.; Luo, Y.; Sun, Z.; Yang, C.; Wang, J.; Liu, X.; Zhang, Z. Multifunctional sulfonated polyetheretherketone coating with beta-defensin-14 for yielding durable and broad-spectrum antibacterial activity and osseointegration. *Acta Biomater.* **2019**, *86*, 323–337. [CrossRef]
60. Zhang, J.; Wei, W.; Yang, L.; Pan, Y.; Wang, X.; Wang, T.; Tang, S.; Yao, Y.; Hong, H.; Wei, J. Stimulation of cell responses and bone ingrowth into macro-microporous implants of nano-bioglass/polyetheretherketone composite and enhanced antibacterial activity by release of hinokitiol. *Colloids Surf. B Biointerfaces* **2018**, *164*, 347–357. [CrossRef]
61. Ouyang, L.; Qi, M.; Wang, S.; Tu, S.; Li, B.; Deng, Y.; Yang, W. Osteogenesis and antibacterial activity of graphene oxide and dexamethasone coatings on porous polyetheretherketone via polydopamine-assisted chemistry. *Coatings* **2018**, *8*, 203. [CrossRef]
62. Schwarz, F.; Derks, J.; Monje, A.; Wang, H. Peri-implantitis. *J. Clin. Periodontol.* **2018**, *45*, 246–266. [CrossRef]
63. Rakic, M.; Grusovin, M.G.; Canullo, L. The microbiologic profile associated with peri-implantitis in humans: A systematic review. *Int. J. Oral Maxillofac. Implant.* **2016**, *31*, 359–368. [CrossRef] [PubMed]
64. Padial-Molina, M.; Lopez-Martinez, J.; O'Valle, F.; Galindo-Moreno, P. Microbial profiles and detection techniques in peri-implant diseases: A systematic review. *J. Oral Maxillofac. Res.* **2016**, *7*, e10. [CrossRef]
65. Faot, F.; Nascimento, G.G.; Bielemann, A.M.; Campao, T.D.; Leite, F.R.; Quirynen, M. Can peri-implant crevicular fluid assist in the diagnosis of peri-implantitis? A systematic review and meta-analysis. *J. Periodontol.* **2015**, *86*, 631–645. [CrossRef]
66. Teughels, W.; Assche, N.V.; Sliepen, I.; Quirynen, M. Effect of material characteristics and/or surface topography on biofilm development. *Clin. Oral Implant. Res.* **2006**, *17*, 68–81. [CrossRef]
67. Ceri, H.; Olson, M.E.; Stremick, C.; Read, R.R.; Morck, D.; Buret, A. The Calgary biofilm device: New technology for rapid determination of antibiotic susceptibilities of bacterial biofilms. *J. Clin. Microbiol.* **1999**, *37*, 1771–1776. [CrossRef]
68. Rams, T.E.; Degener, J.E.; van Winkelhoff, A.J. Antibiotic resistance in human peri-implantitis microbiota. *Clin. Oral Implant. Res.* **2014**, *25*, 82–90. [CrossRef] [PubMed]
69. Natrah, F.M.I.; Kenmegne, M.M.; Wiyoto, W.; Sorgeloos, P.; Bossier, P.; Defoirdt, T. Effects of micro-algae commonly used in aquaculture on acyl-homoserine lactone quorum sensing. *Aquaculture* **2011**, *317*, 53–57. [CrossRef]
70. Hentzer, M.; Givskov, M. Pharmacological inhibition of quorum sensing for the treatment of chronic bacterial infections. *J. Clin. Investig.* **2003**, *112*, 1300–1307. [CrossRef]
71. Katzer, A.; Marquardt, H.; Westendorf, J.; Wening, J.V.; von Foerster, G. Polyetheretherketone cytotoxicity and mutagenicity in vitro. *Biomaterials* **2002**, *23*, 1749–1759. [CrossRef]
72. Suska, F.; Omar, O.; Emanuelsson, L.; Taylor, M.; Gruner, P.; Kinbrum, A.; Hunt, D.; Hunt, T.; Taylor, A.; Palmquist, A. Enhancement of CRF-PEEK osseointegration by plasma-sprayed hydroxyapatite: A rabbit model. *J. Biomater. Appl.* **2014**, *29*, 234–242. [CrossRef] [PubMed]
73. Bakar, M.S.A.; Cheng, M.H.W.; Tang, S.M.; Yu, S.C.; Liao, K.; Tan, C.T.; Khor, K.A.; Cheang, P. Tensile properties, tension-tension fatigue and biological response of polyetheretherketone-hydroxyapatite composites for load-bearing orthopedic implants. *Biomaterials* **2003**, *24*, 2245–2250. [CrossRef]
74. Rabiei, A.; Sandukas, S. Processing and evaluation of bioactive coatings on polymeric implants. *J. Biomed. Mater. Res. A* **2013**, *101*, 2621–2629. [CrossRef]

75. Lee, W.; Koak, J.; Lim, Y.; Kim, S.; Kwon, H.; Kim, M. Stress shielding and fatigue limits of poly-ether-ether-ketone dental implants. *J. Biomed. Mater. Res. B Appl. Biomater.* **2012**, *100*, 1044–1052. [CrossRef]
76. Mishra, S.; Chowdhary, R. PEEK materials as an alternative to titanium in dental implants: A systematic review. *Clin. Implant. Dent. Relat. Res.* **2018**. [CrossRef]
77. Sordi, M.B.; Moreira, T.A.; Montero, J.F.D.; Barbosa, L.C.; Benfatti, C.A.M.; Magini, R.S.; Pimenta, A.L.; Souza, J.C.M. Effect of γ-lactones and γ-lactams compounds on *Streptococcus mutans* biofilms. *J. Appl. Oral Sci.* **2018**, *26*, e20170065. [CrossRef]
78. Koutouzis, T.; Richardson, J.; Lundgren, T. Comparative soft and hard tissue responses to titanium and polymer healing abutments. *J. Oral Implant.* **2011**, *37*, 174–182. [CrossRef]

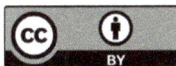

© 2020 by the authors. Licensee MDPI, Basel, Switzerland. This article is an open access article distributed under the terms and conditions of the Creative Commons Attribution (CC BY) license (http://creativecommons.org/licenses/by/4.0/).

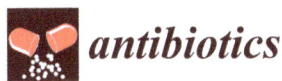

Review

Insights into Host–Pathogen Interactions in Biofilm-Infected Wounds Reveal Possibilities for New Treatment Strategies

Hannah Trøstrup [1],*, Anne Sofie Boe Laulund [2] and Claus Moser [2]

1. Department of Plastic Surgery and Breast Surgery, Zealand University Hospital, 4000 Roskilde, Denmark
2. Department of Clinical Microbiology, Copenhagen University Hospital, 2200 Copenhagen, Denmark; annesofielaulund@gmail.com (A.S.B.L.); moser@dadlnet.dk (C.M.)
* Correspondence: htroestrup@gmail.com; Tel.: +45-4632-3200

Received: 3 June 2020; Accepted: 7 July 2020; Published: 10 July 2020

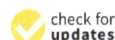

Abstract: Normal wound healing occurs in three phases—the inflammatory, the proliferative, and the remodeling phase. Chronic wounds are, for unknown reasons, arrested in the inflammatory phase. Bacterial biofilms may cause chronicity by arresting healing in the inflammatory state by mechanisms not fully understood. *Pseudomonas aeruginosa*, a common wound pathogen with remarkable abilities in avoiding host defense and developing microbial resistance by biofilm formation, is detrimental to wound healing in clinical studies. The host response towards *P. aeruginosa* biofilm-infection in chronic wounds and impact on wound healing is discussed and compared to our own results in a chronic murine wound model. The impact of *P. aeruginosa* biofilms can be described by determining alterations in the inflammatory response, growth factor profile, and count of leukocytes in blood. *P. aeruginosa* biofilms are capable of reducing the host response to the infection, despite a continuously sustained inflammatory reaction and resulting local tissue damage. A recent observation of in vivo synergism between immunomodulatory and antimicrobial S100A8/A9 and ciprofloxacin suggests its possible future therapeutic potential.

Keywords: biofilm; chronic wounds; host response; S100A8/A9

---

1. Introduction

Normal wound healing is a complicated, tightly regulated process in which a proliferative phase succeeds inflammation. The inflammatory phase lasts for approximately 48 h and is characterized by the influx of polymorphonuclear leucocytes (PMNs) and macrophages to the wound bed. The phagocytosis carried out by these immune cells prevents bacterial infection. This phase is followed by angiogenesis and the secretion of growth factors by fibroblasts and macrophages and, subsequently, the formation of a provisional extracellular matrix in a time span of approximately one week. Tissue remodeling will occur for the next one month to a year [1].

A chronic wound is one which fails to heal spontaneously within three months [2]. The reasons for the recalcitrance of some wounds are unclear, but emerging evidence point to a key role of *Pseudomonas aeruginosa* biofilm causing low-grade infection locally and causing a prolonged inflammatory state [3].

Predisposing factors for developing wound chronicity include chronic or acute infections, age, venous or arterial insufficiency, diabetes, neuropathy, renal impairment, malignancy, lymphedema, trauma, rheumatologic or other autoimmune conditions, pressure over a prominent bone, and immune suppression [4]. Venous leg ulcers, the most common type of non-healing ulcers, constitute 50–70% of all chronic ulcers and are caused by increased hydrostatic pressure due to venous insufficiency. *P. aeruginosa* infection is found in approximately 50% of venous leg ulcers. Although predominant in chronic venous ulcers, *P. aeruginosa* also challenges additional ulcers [5,6]. In the so-called post antibiotic era, *P. aeruginosa* is one of the predominant pathogens involved in burn wound infections, as these wounds are rapidly colonized after the skin's natural barrier is damaged by thermal injury [7].

Clinical studies are often blurred by the heterogeneity of the etiology of wounds enrolled. Other studies may be limited due to the small number of wounds assessed. Comparing chronic venous leg ulcer fluids to acute wounds fluids, divergent results were found depending on the type of control wound chosen [8]. Superficial venous insufficiency can be managed by surgical intervention or split skin transplant in the case of non-healing wounds, although this is often challenged by *P. aeruginosa* biofilm infection [9]. The use of topical growth factors such as platelet-derived growth factor (PDGF) or allografts which release growth factors or the promotion of angiogenesis might be beneficial to healing in diabetic patients [10]. Similar results may be obtained by the wound application of autologous patches, constituting of leucocytes, thrombocytes, and fibrin generated from the patient's own blood by special centrifugation [11]. Such application was shown to improve the healing of hard-to-heal diabetic ulcers as compared to the standard of care [12], and gives hope for new treatment approaches. However, the lack of basic knowledge of the causes of wound chronicity hinders truly successful medical treatment and ultimately worsens the prognosis for these patients. Chronic wounds can lead to devastating situations such as amputations and even death due to sepsis. There is a silent epidemic of biofilm-infected wounds, and now is the time for the thorough investigation of the underlying pathophysiological mechanisms of wound chronicity [13].

Translational medicine based on in vitro experiments and, more importantly, representative in vivo models can be used in the search for insights into the pathophysiology of host/pathogen interactions in chronic biofilm-infected wounds. Although Kadam and colleagues in 2019 showed that the number of publications concerning chronic wounds overall were increasing, a substantial paucity remains in publications on the basic science regarding the chronic wound microenvironment—i.e., on development of suitable laboratory model systems [14].

In the present review, we therefore discuss the impact of *P. aeruginosa* biofilm on the local and systemic host response from clinical and animal experimental observations and the current literature. Observations in mouse models will be considered for this review. With this background, implications for clinical wound healing are discussed and, finally, whether immunomodulatory topical treatment with the antimicrobial peptide, S100A8/A9, could be an adjuvant therapy strategy in chronic biofilm infections is also discussed.

2. Host/Pathogen Interactions in Chronic Wounds and Implications for Wound Healing

2.1. Bacteriology

Normal wound healing occurs in three phases—the inflammatory, the proliferative, and the remodeling phase. Chronic wounds are arrested in the inflammatory phase [15]. The immunogenicity of bacterial biofilms may be the explanation for stalled wound healing. Multiple bacterial species reside in the chronic wound environment. Most common are *Staphylococcus aureus*, the *Enterococcus* species, and *P. aeruginosa* [16,17]. *P. aeruginosa* is an opportunistic Gram-negative rod. The biofilm mode of growth is well described for this bacterium [18]. Bacterial subpopulations in the biofilms are metabolically less active. Adaptive and intrinsic mechanisms, such as the production of enzymes which are able to inactivate some antibiotics or by modifying cell permeability through efflux pumps, cause a thousand-fold resistance compared to planktonic bacteria, all in order to secure microbial survival [19].

A quantitative analysis of the cellular response towards biofilms in chronic wounds revealed that *P. aeruginosa* attracts more PMNs than *S. aureus* [20], which makes it an excellent choice for the assessment of host/pathogen interaction. *P. aeruginosa* biofilms are in human chronic wounds located in the subcutaneous fatty tissue [5,6], preventing their detection by standard wound swabbing techniques.

The majority of studies investigating the mechanisms of *P. aeruginosa* to avoid clearance and progress to a chronic infection are from patients with cystic fibrosis (CF) and lung infections. In particular, the regular sampling of CF sputum has enabled such studies which, to our best knowledge, have not been performed with chronic wounds [21]. The relatively high intrinsic antibiotic resistance and ubiquitous nature of *P. aeruginosa* as well as its well-known ability to develop further antibiotic resistance mechanisms is an important cause for the colonization of the wounds and the lack of standard antibiotic effect.

In the development of chronic infections, *P. aeruginosa* circumvents the early host defense by mechanisms that are not understood. Several metabolic changes—not virulence factors per se—of *P. aeruginosa* also occurs in establishing the chronic infection. One mechanism is by the secretion of elastase, which digests human thrombin and ultimately succeeds in preventing Toll-like receptor dimerization, thus avoiding host response [22]. Other ways to attenuate the host response is by rhamnolipid production, thereby impairing calcium-regulated pathways and protein kinase C activation [23], and complement inhibition by biofilm matrix exopolysaccharides [24] and LPS (smooth colony types) [25]. The Type III secretion system is another way to impair the innate immune response [26].

Furthermore, it has been described how *P. aeruginosa* transcription factors repress flagellar and pili genes and stress response regulator genes [27]. Especially flagellas can be strong stimulators of immune responses and have been used as a vaccine candidate [28]. The increased production of extracellular polysaccharides will be mentioned below. It has also been suggested that the well-developed ability of *P. aeruginosa* to adapt and generate subclones results in an insurance effect of the population and thereby the infection [29].

2.2. Experimental Models of Chronic Pseudomonas aeruginosa Biofilm Wound Infections

Experimental models comprise in vitro systems—e.g., cell cultures and in vivo animal models. Of the two, animal models are closer to the human wounds, as complex interactions between the host response and pathogens are present. Furthermore, in vivo models allow for clinically relevant endpoints. Rodents are the most commonly used in these settings. The use of larger animals such as pigs is often stated as providing a more human-like skin [30]. In contrast to the rodent's dense layer of hair, thin dermis, and panniculus carnosus, pigs have a thick epidermis, well-developed rete-ridges, dermal papillary bodies, abundant subdermal adipose tissue, and similar dermal collagen and orientation and distribution of blood vessels in the dermis [31]. Rodents have an obvious wound contraction as wound closure, whereas pigs have a human-like healing dominated by epithelialization and similar turnover time [32]. Pigs can also encompass several wounds, numerous different topical treatments or infectious challenges, and have biopsies taken [33]. Despite these advantages, pigs have heterogenic skin anatomy, the costs are high, and need for space is challenging. Furthermore, it is extremely challenging to avoid the unintended colonization of the pigs' wounds, and there exist only sparse reagents for the evaluation of host responses [34]. Still, rodents reveal several similar healing mechanisms to humans and are the most used species in wound research, albeit with different approaches and set ups [35–37]. Wounds are often incisional full thickness or burn wounds, although several additional strategies to generate the necessary initial skin defect have been described [38–40].

The host–pathogen interplay in a chronic wound environment in the presence of *P. aeruginosa* biofilm infection can be assessed in a representative murine wound model. This model described below will be used for comparison throughout this paper. A pre-formed biofilm with alginate-embedded *P. aeruginosa* was injected subcutaneously beneath a full-thickness burn wound [41] on the back of anesthetized, shaved, immunologically diverse inbred strains of mice to explore the local and systemic host response [42]. Immediately post injury, the wounds are brown and homogenous. At day 2–3, they progress to resolution by peripheral detachment and the appearance of a red, vascularized healing area (Figure 1). The peripheral healing area can be compared to the necrotic central area of the wound.

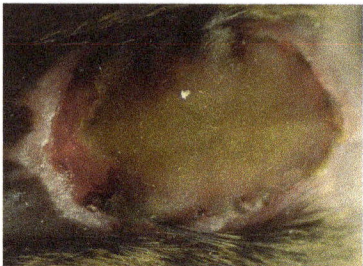

Figure 1. The appearance of an infected burn wound on a C3H/HeN mouse in the proliferative state of healing, approximately 7 days after infection (data not published). Note the peripheral healing red compartment and the central necrotic compartment.

The advantages of this model as compared to other established mouse wound models are the presence of a refractory, full-thickness skin necrosis and a long-lasting, exclusively local biofilm infection, with no systemic dissemination of bacteria. A shortcoming is that murine skin heals primarily by contraction, which could be circumvented by the use of splinting (see below, Section 3).

2.3. Host Response to Pseudomonas aeruginosa Biofilm Wound Infection

The mouse model has been successful for research groups studying chronic wounds and biofilms. For instance, the impact of the course of infection and the impact of biofilm on the bacteriology, histopathology, local and systemic host response, and consequences for wound healing in two different inbred mouse strains have been assessed in one strain susceptible to *P. aeruginosa* biofilm infection (BALB/c) and one relatively resistant (C3H/HeN) in a chronic *P. aeruginosa* lung infection model [43] and in a chronic wound model [42]. The BALB/c mouse strain with an established chronic *P. aeruginosa* biofilm infection is considered to be most representative of a chronic venous leg ulcer due to the increased lack of infectious control, in addition to an arrested healing process (see below). Using those two mouse strains, it was possible to evaluate the improved outcome of novel treatment strategies in the relatively susceptible BALB/c mouse strain. Accordingly, it was possible to investigate the factors suspected to be important for the aggravated course of the biofilm infection using the relatively resistant C3H/HeN mouse strain.

The host response towards *P. aeruginosa* wound infection can be characterized in a wound model by the following approaches:

1. Quantitative bacteriology and visualization of the bacteria and inflammatory cells in close proximity to the biofilm, located in the hypodermis.
2. Proinflammatory cytokines and neutrophil chemoattractant profiling.
3. Alterations in the growth factor profile in the proliferative state of healing.
4. The impact of the biofilm-mediated recruitment of PMNs from the bone marrow to the blood.

Using the setup with the two inbred mouse strains, we showed how the host factor profile is correlated to the outcome of *P. aeruginosa* biofilm infection in a chronic wound. In the natural course of infection, a lack of infection resolution in the susceptible mouse strain, BALB/C, was observed as compared to the resistant strain, C3H/HeN. The BALB/c mice had more *P. aeruginosa* biofilm in their wounds than the C3H/HeN mice at day four. The biofilms were in all samples located in the hypodermis of the skin [42]. No clearance of biofilm infection was observed.

Important differences in the chronic *P. aeruginosa* biofilm infection in the two mouse strains are provided in Table 1.

Table 1. Host response to *Pseudomonas aeruginosa* biofilm wound infection in two immunologically diverse mouse strains.

C3H/HeN	BALB/c
Resistant towards infection	Susceptible to infection
Faster infection control	Aggravated inflammatory IL-1β response
	No infection control
Faster wound closure	Delayed wound closure

Infected wounds display an inflammatory influx of PMNs and mononuclear cells (MNs) in response to bacterial infection [41]. Interestingly, the *P. aeruginosa* biofilm arrested BALB/c wounds in an acute, PMN-dominated inflammatory state [42], which is also described in human wounds [3]. An inflammatory infiltrate adjacent to the biofilms is visualized in the hypodermis of infected wounds (Figure 2).

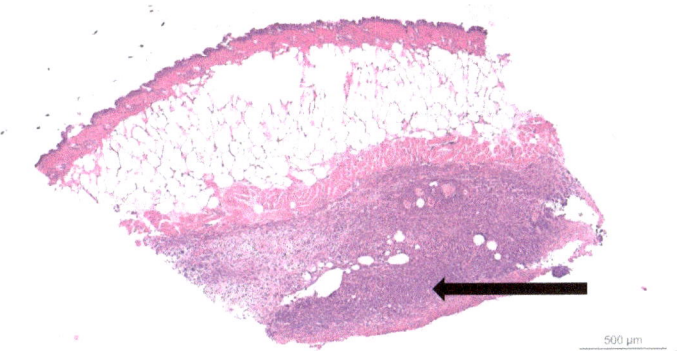

Figure 2. A representative hematoxylin and eosin-stained slide of a *Pseudomonas aeruginosa* biofilm-infected murine wound 7 days after infection (data not published). Note the darker purple inflammatory infiltrate containing leucocytes just below the panniculus carnosus in the hypodermis (black arrow).

2.4. Perturbation of Local Proinflammatory Cytokine and Growth Factor Profile by Pseudomonas aeruginosa Biofilm

The *P. aeruginosa* biofilm infection initially elicits a marked host response in wounds due to the virulence of *P. aeruginosa*. Virulence factors include lipopolysaccharide (LPS) and the most important exopolysaccharide, alginate, and protease production [44]. It has been suggested that *P. aeruginosa* secretes factors to dampen the local host response [23,26,45,46]. Accordingly, we observed and reported how the *P. aeruginosa* biofilm infection suppresses local neutrophil markers (S100A8/A9 and chemoattractants such as Keratinocyte-derived chemokine (KC) and the PMN mobilizer Granulocyte-colony stimulating factor (G-CSF)) in murine wounds, especially in susceptible mice. This induces a steady state, which may impair wound healing in a chronic course [47]. The local suppression of PMN-related markers in the presence of *P. aeruginosa* biofilm could be ascribed to the induction of a rapid necrotic killing of PMNs produced by these bacteria [48]. These observations are in accordance with our own research on suppressed S100A8/A9 in non-healing human wounds (a topic that is further discussed in a following section).

Furthermore, BALB/c mice are representative of a chronic wound model, as their wounds are arrested in the inflammatory phase of wound healing, expressing continuously high levels of Interleukin-1β (IL-1β) besides the lack of ability to gain infection control [42]. IL-1β, expressed by monocytes, is used as a marker for general inflammation caused by infection [49].

Growth factors essential in wound healing are vascular endothelial growth factor (VEGF), PDGF, and fibroblast growth factor (FGF), which are secreted by fibroblasts and macrophages in the proliferative phase of wound healing [50]. The wound growth factor profile is altered by the *P. aeruginosa* biofilm and correlated to the wound compartment and to the host defense profile [51]. VEGF is an angiogenic factor induced in human macrophages in hypoxic tissue or other situations of cell stress [52]. Being an endothelial cell mitogen, it contributes to neovascularization during wound healing. Furthermore, it has proinflammatory potential. It perpetuates local inflammation by PMN recruitment due to increasing vascular permeability [53]. The suppression of VEGF in necrotic tissue observed centrally in infected murine wounds could imply a reason for the topical growth factor substitution of this protein in clinical wound research. However, the proteolytic degradation of VEGF has been reported [54]. This may be the reason for the lack of clinical success in the use of topical growth factors in chronic wounds, since the prevalent proteolytic activity of the wound bed would presumably degrade the topically applied VEGF [55].

Excessive amounts of VEGF act as a chemoattractant to *P. aeruginosa*, thereby exacerbating the infection [56]. Thus, the levels of VEGF were assessed using the chronic wound model in a setup where the host factor production was estimated and compared in the peripheral, healing part of the wound to the central non-healing and necrotic part of the wound. The *P. aeruginosa* biofilm infection induced VEGF protein levels by a factor 3 to 4 in the healing peripheral parts of murine wounds (Figure 3), thereby establishing the infection [51]. In a clinical study, we described a positive correlation between the levels of lipopolysaccharide and VEGF protein levels in wound fluids [57]. The expression of VEGF is strongly stimulated by tissue hypoxia, which is observed in the infectious environment caused by the oxygen consumption by the PMNs in respiratory bursts as well as the aerobic respiration of *P. aeruginosa* [58,59]. The insufficient supply of oxygen impairs wound healing and is the rationale for the therapeutic use of hyperbaric oxygen [60]. Furthermore, hypoxia impairs keratinocyte migration and proliferation in human chronic venous leg ulcers [61].

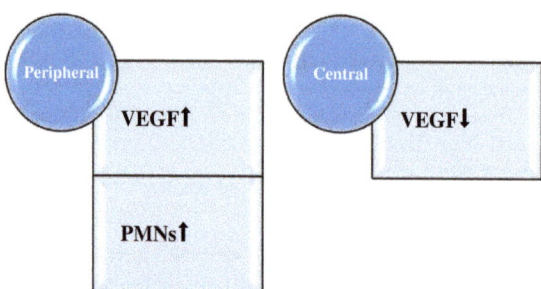

Figure 3. *Pseudomonas aeruginosa* biofilm increases vascular endothelial growth factor (VEGF) in the peripheral, healing compartments of the wounds, which also contain more polymorphonuclear cells as compared to the central compartment. Centrally, VEGF is suppressed.

2.5. Systemic Impact of Pseudomonas aeruginosa Biofilm Infection in Animal Models of Chronic Wounds

Whereas G-CSF is the most important mobilizer of PMNs from the bone marrow, KC is an important chemoattractant for the extravasation of PMNs from the blood to the wound bed [62]. KC remained elevated in serum from BALB/c mice [42]. This may be an expression of the host response trying to recruit further immunoactive leukocytes to the chronic biofilm infected wound. Regarding the cellular systemic reaction to the infection in the response to *P. aeruginosa* biofilm, more PMNs are mobilized in the blood of susceptible BALB/c mice as compared to C3H/HeN mice [42]. The findings support that C3H/HeN mice have a more efficient immune reaction to the infection than the BALB/c mice, as a faster reduction in leukocytes was observed in the peripheral blood from C3H/HeN mice.; the total white blood cell count (WBC) and PMN count in the blood decreases more rapidly in the

C3H/HeN strain. Interestingly, Sroussi and colleagues reported an inhibitory effect of S100A8 and A9 on neutrophil migration in vitro [63]. This observation is in accordance with our finding that topical treatment with S100A8/A9 for 5 days dampened the PMN count in blood from infected BALB/c mice [64].

2.6. Impact of Pseudomonas aeruginosa Biofilm on Murine Wound Healing

P. aeruginosa biofilm affects the host response by causing delayed wound healing [47]. The perturbation of host response causes significant tissue damage to the skin, thereby hindering wound resolution. With the use of translational research—e.g., by animal chronic wound models—important factors for healing have been revealed. In clinically relevant animal models—e.g., Zhao et al. [65]—*P. aeruginosa* biofilm infection delayed wound healing in diabetic mice. Accordingly, Watters et al. demonstrated a lack of infection resolution and impaired wound healing by the infliction of full-thickness surgical excision wounds on diabetic mice backs, inoculated with *P. aeruginosa* PAO1 to each wound [66]. The fact that mice heal predominantly by contraction and less by the emergence of granulation tissue as in humans is addressed by Ahn and Mustoe, who developed a wound model using a rabbit ear. In this model, the underlying cartilage functions as a splint, thereby circumventing the wound contraction [67]. Although other models exist, it should be highlighted that mouse models can reveal important healing parameters.

Wound healing can be evaluated by the digital planimetric assessment [68] of the reduction in the total wound area, by the size of necrosis and subsequent analysis ImageJ® [69–71]. Interestingly, infected susceptible BALB/c mice are delayed healers compared to C3H/HeN mice, since the C3H/HeN mouse strain reached a reduced wound size and a reduced area of the central necrosis as compared to the BALB/c mouse strain [47,51]. Actually, and in accordance with this, Li et al. described BALB/c genetically as slow healers compared to C3H/HeN mice, who were characterized as intermediate healers [72]. Those observations support the use of the BALB/c mouse strain as a model of chronic wounds and poor healing.

3. Topical Intervention on *Pseudomonas aeruginosa* Biofilm-Infected Wounds through Mouse Models

Evidence of clinically effective treatment modalities is surprisingly scarce. The chronic biofilm formation is an efficient mechanism against host response and antibiotic treatment [73]. Enzymes capable of degrading the biofilm are thus an interesting suggestion. Indeed, Fleming and Rumbaugh recently showed how glycoside hydrolases disperse biofilms. In addition, they augmented the efficacy of Meropenem towards *P. aeruginosa* infection in a full thickness murine wound model [74]. Further studies of the clinical implications are awaited.

Another approach describes the advantages of naturally occurring antimicrobial peptides (AMPs), which protect the skin from bacterial invasion [75]. In previous studies, it was shown that S100A8/A9 RNA and protein levels are upregulated in the epidermis of acute murine as well as human wounds [76]. Furthermore, chronic human wounds lack S100A8/A9 [57,77]. S100A8/A9, also known as Calprotectin, is a calcium-binding, heterodimeric protein, constituting 40–60% of the cytosol of PMNs and 5% of monocytes. It is an alarmin, a constitutively available endogenous molecule. It is released from dead or necrotic cells upon tissue damage [78]. In a non-healing wound setting, mesenchymal stem cells were subjected to human recombinant S100A8/A9 accelerated healing of murine full-thickness wounds [79]. In a paper on *P. aeruginosa*-induced keratitis, the authors discuss the role of S100A8/A9 in the host defense towards *P. aeruginosa* infections in vivo, as the genes for S100A8/A9 seem to be the most highly upregulated by bacterial flagellin exposure. Flagellin is a ligand of the Toll-like receptor which is able to recognize pathogen-associated molecular patterns to initiate immune responses. The upregulation of such genes results in a flagellin-induced protection, whereas the functional blocking of both peptides increased the susceptibility to *P. aeruginosa* infection [80]. In another model of murine fungal keratitis, 1 µg of recombinant S100A8/A9 injection into the corneas of S100A9$^{-/-}$ mice restored the ability to inhibit the hyphal growth of *Aspergillus fumigatus* 24 h post infection [81]. Both those studies support the existence of the direct antimicrobial activity of S100A8/A9, at least in the planktonic state.

Topical recombinant S100A8/A9 injected underneath the wounds of *P. aeruginosa*-biofilm infected wounds in BALB/c mice ameliorated local wound infection after 5 days of treatment [64]. In a later study, S100A8/A9 augmented the effect of 1 mg of systemic ciprofloxacin in the same model of chronic biofilm-infected wounds in BALB/c mice [82]. When S100A8/A9 was combined with systemic ciprofloxacin, the bacterial load was lowered significantly, even after 3 days of therapy, and the levels of the individual S100A8 and S100A9 was further increased. Besides being a consequence of the topical therapy, the S100A8/A9 increase is interpreted as a surrogate marker of promoted wound healing. Interestingly, no in vitro synergistic effect between S100A8/A9 and ciprofloxacin was shown. This emphasizes that the synergistic ciprofloxacin potentiating effect of S100A8/A9 is highly dependent on host cells and further underlines the importance of using representative animal models, if it is not possible to proceed directly to clinical trials. The clinical implication in a non-healing wound setting of the synergistic S100A8/A9 effect is further stressed due to the relatively poor penetration of antibiotics to a skin focus, even with a biofilm infection—adding an antibiotic augmenting compound could potentially compensate for this phenomenon. The results presented directly point towards clinical testing and possible new therapeutic approaches. Whether the combination therapy of S100A8/A9 and ciprofloxacin will prevent the development of bacterial resistance and improve wound healing is currently being investigated.

S100A8/A9 may be released by active phagocytes, acting as a dose-dependent switch by initially stimulating phagocytosis, but in higher concentrations terminating neutrophil recruitment, acting more as an anti-inflammatory agent. Thus, one could speculate that the lack of S100A8/A9 is an expression of a chronic infection: The host defense is incapable of resolving the local infection, as PMNs are efficiently recruited from the blood to the site of infection but are counteracted by the close proximity to the biofilms. A major challenge in the use of S100A8/A9 as an adjuvant to ordinary antimicrobial treatment is the challenge of the dose-dependent effect, as the dual effects of alarmins are known [78]. The growth factor potential of these innate host response proteins depends on release, dose, and context as they may mediate repair after injury [76]. Human and animal model observations strongly indicate that the S100A8/A9 response is perturbed and inappropriate in chronic wounds. Further studies are warranted to describe the pathophysiological impact of the multifaceted role of S100A8/A9 on biofilm-infected wounds. Of course, the lack of permission to use S100A8/A9 clinically has to be solved, but promising results may promote a solution to this challenge.

4. Conclusions

Chronic wounds are arrested in the inflammatory phase of wound healing for reasons that are unknown. Host/pathogen interaction is ultimately detrimental to wound healing. *P. aeruginosa* biofilm affects wound healing negatively via alterations in host defense mechanisms; PMNs are initially recruited to the site of infection. S100A8/A9, KC, and G–CSF are locally dampened by *P. aeruginosa* biofilm, which establishes chronicity. In the chronic state, the PMNs proceed into a quiescent phase, unable to resolve the infection. Loops of these distorted pathways cause high levels of local tissue damage and contribute further to wound development (see Figure 4). The wound environment is characterized by high proinflammatory IL-1β and proangiogenic VEGF, although the latter seems repressed by the biofilm or the central necrosis. Still, the inflammation is inappropriate and lacks the resolution of the infection due to the attenuation of phagocytic cell activity, despite the continuous recruitment of such cells. This may play a pivotal role in the modulation of the tissue repair response to infection by inducing premature cellular senescence [83].

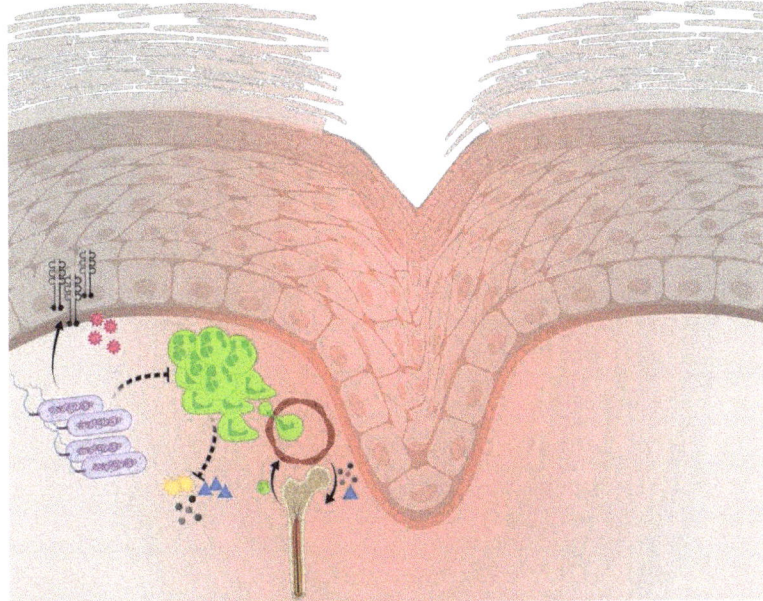

Figure 4. The hypothesis of the host/pathogen interaction between biofilm (Gram-negative rods in biofilm aggregates, left) and incoming polymorphonuclear neutrophils (green large cells, right). The biofilm causes increased levels of interleukin-1β (black dimers) and vascular endothelial growth factor in the wound periphery (pink spiky balls), and it inhibits neutrophil activity, reflected by reduced levels of S100A8/A9 (yellow stars), Keratinocyte-derived Chemokine (blue triangles), and Granulocyte-Colony Stimulating Factor (black dots). Full arrows: promotion; dotted arrows: inhibition. This figure was created with Biorender.com.

The restoration of normal PMN activity holds a potential for the adjunctive therapy of wound chronicity. The impact of *P. aeruginosa* biofilm and the host defense interaction on wound fibroblasts and keratinocytes, crucial to wound healing, are also areas of great importance and deserve further investigation.

Overall, due to the risk of surgical intervention or even amputation, there is a need to assess the basic science of wound chronicity and rethink strategies to combat the biofilms in chronic wounds. In order to substantiate a role for the use of topical antimicrobial peptides or other local interventional therapies, biofilms should be taken into consideration. This includes regimes with sufficient antibiotic doses, combination antibiotic therapy targeting different niches of the biofilms, topical treatment being considered, and the use of antibiotics with a good penetration of the skin; prolonged or repeated treatments might be beneficial. In addition, correct sampling should be used—biopsies are preferable to swabs. The gold standard level of proof would be a randomized, controlled study in groups of patients with venous leg ulcers and arterial or diabetic ulcers. Confounding factors should be minimized, and patient homogeneity could ensure group compatibility and improve the internal strength of such clinical studies.

All the procedures performed in studies involving animals were in accordance with the ethical standards of the institution or practice at which the studies were conducted (approved by the Animal Ethics Committee of Denmark (2010/561-1766).

Author Contributions: Conceptualization, H.T. and C.M.; methodology, H.T., A.S.B.L., and C.M.; validation, formal analysis, and investigation, H.T., A.S.B.L. and C.M.; writing—original draft preparation: H.T.; writing—review and editing, H.T., A.S.B.L. and C.M., supervision, C.M. All authors have read and agreed to the published version of the manuscript.

Funding: This research received no external funding. CM is funded by the Novo Nordic Foundation, Borregaard Clinical Scientist Fellowship NNF17OC0025074. Anne Sofie Boe Laulund is funded by the Research Foundation of Rigshospitalet, Denmark.

Conflicts of Interest: The authors declare no conflict of interest.

References

1. Gurtner, G.C.; Werner, S.; Barrandon, Y.; Longaker, M.T. Wound repair and regeneration. *Nature* **2008**, *453*, 314–321. [CrossRef]
2. Saltmarche, A.E. Low level laser therapy for healing acute and chronic wounds—The extendicare experience. *Int. Wound J.* **2008**, *5*, 351–360. [CrossRef] [PubMed]
3. Bjarnsholt, T.; Kirketerp-Møller, K.K.; Jensen, P.Ø.; Madsen, K.G.; Phipps, R.; Krogfeldt, K.; Høiby, N.; Givskov, M. Why chronic wounds will not heal: A novel hypothesis. *Wound Repair Regen.* **2008**, *16*, 2–10. [CrossRef]
4. Trøstrup, H.; Bjarnsholt, T.; Kirketerp-Møller, K.; Høiby, N.; Moser, C. What is new in the understanding of nonhealing wounds. Epidemiology, pathophysiology and therapies. *Ulcers* **2013**, *2013*, 625934. [CrossRef]
5. Kirketerp-Møller, K.; Jensen, P.Ø.; Fazli, M.; Madsen, K.G.; Pedersen, J.; Moser, C.; Tolker-Nielsen, T.; Høiby, N.; Givskov, M.; Bjarnsholt, T. Distribution, organization, and ecology of bacteria in chronic wounds. *J. Clin. Microbiol.* **2008**, *46*, 2717–2722. [CrossRef] [PubMed]
6. Fazli, M.; Bjarnsholt, T.; Kirketerp-Møller, K.; Jørgensen, B.; Andersen, A.S.; Krogfelt, K.A.; Givskov, M.; Tolker-Nielsen, T. Nonrandom distribution of *Pseudomonas aeruginosa* and *Staphylococcus aureus* in chronic wounds. *J. Clin. Microbiol.* **2009**, *47*, 4084–4089. [CrossRef] [PubMed]
7. Church, D.; Elsayed, S.; Reid, O.; Winston, B.; Lindsay, R. Burn Wound Infections. *Clin. Microbiol. Rev.* **2006**, *19*, 403–434. [CrossRef]
8. Subramaniam, K.; Pech, C.M.; Stacey, M.C.; Wallace, H.J. Induction of MMP-1, MMP-3 and TIMP-1 in normal dermal fibroblasts by chronic venous leg ulcer wound fluid. *Int. Wound J.* **2008**, *5*, 79–86. [CrossRef]
9. Høgsberg, T.; Bjarnsholt, T.; Thomsen, J.S.; Kirketerp-Møller, K. Succes rate of split-thickness skin grafting of chronic venous leg ulcers depends on the presence of *Pseudomonas aeruginosa*: A retrospective study. *PLoS ONE* **2011**, *6*, e20492. [CrossRef]
10. Jeffcoate, W.J.; Harding, K.G. Diabetic foot ulcers. *Lancet* **2003**, *361*, 1545–1551. [CrossRef]
11. Thomsen, K.; Trøstrup, H.; Christophersen, L.; Lundquist, R.; Høiby, N.; Moser, C. The phagocytic fitness of leukopatches may impact the healing of chronic wounds. *Clin. Exp. Immunol.* **2016**, *184*, 368–377. [CrossRef] [PubMed]
12. Game, F.; Jeffcoate, W.; Tarnow, L.; Jacobsen, J.L.; Whitham, D.J.; Harrison, E.F.; Ellender, S.J.; Fitzsimmons, D.; Löndahl, M. LeucoPatch system for the management of hard-to-heal diabetic foot ulcers in the UK, Denmark, and Sweden: An observer-masked, randomised controlled trial. *Lancet Diabetes Endocrinol.* **2018**, *6*, 870–878. [CrossRef]
13. Zhao, R.; Liang, H.; Clarke, E.; Jackson, C.; Xue, M. Inflammation in chronic wounds. *Int. J. Mol. Sci.* **2016**, *17*, 2085. [CrossRef] [PubMed]
14. Kadam, S.; Nadkarni, S.; Lele, J.; Sakhalkar, S.; Mokashi, P.; Kaushik, K.S. Bioengineered platforms for chronic wound infection studies: How can we make them more human-relevant? *Front. Bioeng. Biotechnol.* **2019**, *7*, 418. [CrossRef] [PubMed]
15. Falanga, V. Classifications for wound bed preparation and stimulation of chronic wounds. *Wound Repair Regen.* **2000**, *8*, 347–352.
16. Gjødsbøl, K.; Christensen, J.J.; Karlsmark, T.; Jørgensen, B.; Klein, B.M.; Krogfeldt, K.A. Multiple bacterial species reside in chronic wounds: A longitudinal study. *Int. Wound J.* **2006**, *3*, 225–231.
17. Thomsen, T.R.; Aasholm, M.S.; Rudkjøbing, V.B.; Saunders, A.M.; Bjarnsholt, T.; Givskov, M.; Kirketerp-Møller, K.; Nielsen, P.H. The bacteriology of chronic venous leg ulcers examined by culture-independent molecular methods. *Wound Repair Regen.* **2010**, *18*, 38–49. [CrossRef]

18. Costerton, J.W.; Stewart, P.S.; Greenberg, E.P. Bacterial biofilms: A common cause of persistent infections. *Science* **1999**, *284*, 1318–1322. [CrossRef]
19. Parrino, B.; Schillaci, D.; Carnevale, I.; Giovanetti, E.; Diana, P.; Cirrincione, G.; Cascioferro, S. Synthetic small molecules as anti-biofilm agents in the struggle against antibiotic resistance. *Eur. J. Med. Chem.* **2019**, *161*, 154–178. [CrossRef]
20. Fazli, M.; Bjarnsholt, T.; Kirketerp-Møller, K.; Jørgensen, A.; Andersen, C.B.; Givskov, M.; Tolker-Nielsen, T. Quantitative analysis of the cellular inflammatory response against biofilm bacteria in chronic wounds. *Wound Repair Regen.* **2011**, *19*, 387–391. [CrossRef]
21. Folkesson, A.; Jelsbak, L.; Yang, L.; Johansen, H.K.; Ciofu, O.; Høiby, N.; Molin, S. Adaptation of *Pseudomonas aeruginosa* to the cystic fibrosis airway: An evolutionary perspective. *Nat. Rev. Microbiol.* **2012**, *10*, 841–851. [CrossRef] [PubMed]
22. Van der Plas, M.J.; Bhongir, R.K.; Kjellström, S.; Siller, H.; Kasetty, G.; Morgelin, M.; Schmidtchen, A. *Pseudomonas aeruginosa* elastase cleaves a C-terminal peptide from human thrombin that inhibits host inflammatory responses. *Nat. Commun.* **2016**, *7*, 11567. [CrossRef] [PubMed]
23. Dössel, J.; Meyer-Hoffert, U.; Schröder, J.-M.; Gerstel, U. Pseudomonas aeruginosa- derived rhamnolipids subvert the host inate immune response through manipulation of the human beta-defensin-2 expression. *Cell. Microbiol.* **2012**, *14*, 1364–1375. [CrossRef] [PubMed]
24. Mishra, M.; Byrd, M.S.; Sergeant, S.; Azad, A.K.; Parsek, M.R.; McPhail, L.; Schlesinger, L.S.; Wozniak, D.J. Pseudomonas aeruginosa Psl polysaccharide reduces neutrophil phagocytosis and the oxidative response by limiting complement-mediated opsonization. *Cell. Microbiol.* **2012**, *14*, 95–106. [CrossRef] [PubMed]
25. Schiller, N.L.; Joiner, K.A. Interaction of complement with serum-sensitive and serum-resistant strains of *Pseudomonas aeruginosa*. *Infect. Immun.* **1986**, *54*, 689–694. [CrossRef]
26. Hauser, A.R. The type III secretion system of Pseudomonas aeruginosa: Infection by injection. *Nat. Rev. Microbiol.* **2009**, *7*, 654–665. [CrossRef] [PubMed]
27. Southley-Pillig, C.J.; Davies, D.G.; Sauer, K. Characterization of temporal protein production in Pseudomonas aeruginosa biofilms. *J. Bacteriol.* **2005**, *187*, 8114–8126. [CrossRef] [PubMed]
28. Döring, G.; Flume, P.; Heijerman, H.; Elborn, J.S.; Consensus Study Group. Treatment of lung infection in patients with cystic fibrosis: Current and future strategies. *J. Cyst. Fibros.* **2012**, *11*, 461–479. [CrossRef] [PubMed]
29. Boles, B.R.; Thoendel, M.; Singh, P.K. Self-generated diversity produces 'insurance effects' in biofilm communities. *Proc. Natl. Acad. Sci. USA* **2004**, *101*, 16630–16635. [CrossRef] [PubMed]
30. Davidson, J. Animal models for wound repair. *Arch. Dermatol. Res.* **1998**, *290*, S1–S11. [CrossRef]
31. Sullivan, T.P.; Eaglstein, W.H.; Davis, S.C.; Mertz, P. The pig as a model for human wound healing. *Wound Repair Regen.* **2001**, *9*, 66–76. [CrossRef] [PubMed]
32. Gloag, E.S.; Marshall, C.W.; Snyder, D.; Lewin, G.R.; Harris, J.S.; Santos-Lopez, A.; Chaney, S.B.; Whiteley, M.; Cooper, V.S.; Wozniak, D.J. *Pseudomonas aeruginosa* interstrain dynamics and selection of hyperbiofilm mutants during a chronic infection. *mBio* **2019**, *10*, e01698-19. [CrossRef] [PubMed]
33. Masella, P.C.; Balent, E.M.; Carlson, T.L.; Lee, K.W.; Pierce, L.M. Evaluation of six split-thickness skin graft donor-site dressing materials in a swine model. *Plast. Reconstr. Surg. Glob. Open* **2013**, *1*, e84. [CrossRef] [PubMed]
34. Seaton, M.; Hocking, A.; Gibran, N.S. Porcine models of cutaneous wound healing. *ILAR J.* **2015**, *56*, 127–138. [CrossRef]
35. Pletzer, D.; Mansour, S.C.; Wuerth, K.; Rahanjam, N.; Hancock, R.E.W. New mouse model for chronic infections by gram-negative bacteria enabling the study of anti-infective efficacy and host-microbe interactions. *MBio* **2017**, *8*. [CrossRef] [PubMed]
36. Sweere, J.M.; Ishak, H.; Sunkari, V.; Bach, M.S.; Manasherob, R.; Yadava, K.; Ruppert, S.M.; Sen, C.K.; Balaji, S.; Keswani, S.G.; et al. The Immune Response to Chronic Pseudomonas aeruginosa Wound Infection in Immunocompetent Mice. *Adv. Wound Care* **2020**, *9*, 35–47. [CrossRef] [PubMed]
37. Dalton, T.; Dowd, S.E.; Wolcott, R.D.; Sun, Y.; Watters, C.; Griswold, J.A.; Rumbaugh, K.P. An in vivo polymicrobial biofilm wound infection model to study interspecies interactions. *PLoS ONE* **2011**, *6*, e27317. [CrossRef]

38. Asada, M.; Nakagami, G.; Minematsu, T.; Nagase, T.; Akase, T.; Huang, L.; Yoshimura, K.; Sanada, H. Novel models for bacterial colonization and infection of full-thickness wounds in rats. *Wound Repair Regen.* **2012**, *20*, 601–610. [CrossRef]
39. Nakagami, G.; Morohoshi, T.; Ikeda, T.; Ohta, Y.; Sagara, H.; Huang, L.; Nagase, T.; Sugama, J.; Sanada, H. Contribution of quorum sensing to the virulence of Pseudomonas aeruginosa in pressure ulcer infection in rats. *Wound Repair Regen.* **2011**, *19*, 214–222. [CrossRef]
40. Rashid, M.H.; Rumbaugh, K.; Passador, L.; Davies, D.G.; Hamood, A.N.; Iglewski, B.H.; Kornberg, A. Polyphosphate kinase is essential for biofilm development, quorum sensing, and virulence of Pseudomonas aeruginosa. *Proc. Natl. Acad. Sci. USA* **2000**, *97*, 9636–9641. [CrossRef]
41. Calum, H.; Moser, C.; Jensen, P.Ø.; Christophersen, L.; Malling, D.S.; van Gennip, M.; Bjarnsholt, T.; Hougen, H.-P.; Givskov, M.; Jacobsen, G.K.; et al. Thermal injury induces impaired function in polymorphonuclear neutrophil granulocytes and reduced control of burn wound infection. *Clin. Exp. Immunol.* **2009**, *156*, 102–110. [CrossRef] [PubMed]
42. Trøstrup, H.; Thomsen, K.; Christophersen, L.; Hougen, H.-P.; Bjarnsholt, T.; Jensen, P.Ø.; Kirkby, N.; Calum, H.; Høiby, N.; Moser, C. *Pseudomonas aeruginosa* Biofilm Aggravates Skin Inflammatory Response in BALB/c Mice in a Novel Chronic Wound Model. *Wound Rep. Reg.* **2013**, *21*, 292–299. [CrossRef] [PubMed]
43. Moser, C.; Johansen, H.K.; Song, Z.; Hougen, H.-P.; Rygaard, J.; Høiby, N. Chronic *Pseudomonas aeruginosa* lung infection is more severe in Th2 responding BALB/c mice compared to Th1 responding C3H/HeN mice. *APMIS* **1997**, *105*, 838–842. [CrossRef] [PubMed]
44. Rumbaugh, K.P.; Griswold, J.A.; Iglewski, B.H.; Hamood, A.N. Contribution of quorum sensing to the virulence of *Pseudomonas aeruginosa* in bund wound infections. *Infect. Immune.* **1999**, *67*, 5854–5862. [CrossRef]
45. Wolcott, R.D.; Rhoads, D.D.; Dowd, S.E. Biofilms and chronic wound inflammation. *J Wound Care* **2008**, *17*, 333–341. [CrossRef]
46. Kharazmi, A.; Nielsen, H. Inhibition of human monocyte chemotaxis and chemiluminiscence by Pseudomonas aeruginosa elastase. *APMIS* **1991**, *99*, 93–95. [CrossRef]
47. Trøstrup, H.; Lerche, C.J.; Christophersen, L.J.; Thomsen, K.; Jensen, P.Ø.; Hougen, H.-P.; Høiby, N.; Moser, C. Chronic *Pseudomonas aeruginosa* Biofilm Infection Impairs Murine S100A8/A9 and Neutrophil Effector Cytokines—Implications for Delayed Wound Closure? *Pathog. Dis.* **2017**, *75*, ftx068. [CrossRef]
48. Jensen, P.Ø.; Bjarnsholt, T.; Phipps, R.; Rasmussen, T.B.; Calum, H.; Christoffersen, L.; Moser, C.; Williams, P.; Pressler, T.; Givskov, M.; et al. Rapid necrotic killing of polymorphonuclear leukocytes is caused by quorum-sensing-controlled production of rhamnolipid by *Pseudomonas aeruginosa*. *Microbiology* **2007**, *153 Pt 5*, 1329–1338. [CrossRef]
49. Hsi, E.D.; Remick, D.G. Monocytes are the major producers of interleukin-1 beta in an ex vivo model of local cytokine production. *J. Interferon Cytokine Res.* **1995**, *15*, 89–94. [CrossRef]
50. Grazul-Bilska, A.T.; Johnson, M.L.; Bilski, J.J.; Redmer, D.A.; Reynolds, L.P.; Abdullah, A.; Abdullah, K.M. Wound healing: The role of growth factors. *Drugs Today* **2003**, *39*, 787–800. [CrossRef]
51. Trøstrup, H.; Lerche, C.J.; Christophersen, L.J.; Thomsen, K.; Jensen, P.Ø.; Hougen, H.-P.; Høiby, N.; Moser, C. *Pseudomonas aeruginosa* Biofilm Hampers Murine Central Wound Healing by Suppression of Vascular Endothelial Growth Factor. *Int. Wound J.* **2018**, *15*, 123–132. [CrossRef] [PubMed]
52. Ramakrishnan, S.; Anand, V.; Roy, S. Vascular endothelial growth factor signaling in hypoxia and inflammation. *J. Neuroimmune Pharmacol.* **2014**, *9*, 142–160. [CrossRef] [PubMed]
53. Bates, D.O.; Curry, F.E. Vascular endothelial growth factor increases hydraulic conductivity of isolated perfused microvessels. *Am J Physiol.* **1996**, *271 Pt 2*, H2520–H2528. [CrossRef]
54. Lauer, G.; Sollberg, S.; Cole, M.; Flamme, I.; Stürzebecher, J.; Mann, K.; Krieg, T.; Eming, S.A. Expression and proteolysis of vascular endothelial growth factor is increased in chronic wounds. *J. Investig. Dermatol.* **2000**, *115*, 12–18. [CrossRef] [PubMed]
55. Barrientos, S.; Brem, H.; Stojadinovic, O.; Tomic-Canic, M. Clinical application of growth factors and cytokines in wound healing. *Wound Repair Regen.* **2014**, *22*, 569–578. [CrossRef]
56. Birkenhauer, E.; Neethirajan, S. A double-edged sword: The role of VEGF in wound repair and chemoattraction of opportunist pathogens. *Int. J. Mol. Sci.* **2015**, *16*, 7159–7172. [CrossRef]
57. Trøstrup, H.; Holstein, P.; Christophersen, L.; Jørgensen, B.; Karlsmark, T.; Høiby, N.; Moser, C.; Ågren, M.S. S100A8/A9 is an important host defence mediator in neuropathic foot ulcers in patients with type 2 diabetes mellitus. *Arch. Dermatol. Res.* **2016**, *308*, 347–355. [CrossRef]

58. Detmar, M.; Brown, L.F.; Berse, B.; Jackman, R.W.; Elicker, B.M.; Dvorak, H.F.; Claffey, K.P. Hypoxia regulates the expresssion of vascular permeability factoe/vascular endothelial growth factor (VPF/VEGF) and its receptors in human skin. *J. Investig. Derm.* **1997**, *108*, 263–268. [CrossRef]
59. James, G.A.; Zhao, A.G.; Usui, M.; Underwood, R.A.; Nguyen, H.; Beyenal, H.; deLancey Pulcini, E.; Agostinho Hunt, A.; Bernstein, H.C.; Fleckman, P.; et al. Microsensor and transcriptomic signatures of oxygen depletion in biofilms associated with chronic wounds. *Wound Repair Regen.* **2016**, *24*, 373–383. [CrossRef]
60. Tibbles, P.M.; Edelsberg, J.S. Hyperbaric-oxygen therapy. *N. Engl. J. Med.* **1996**, *334*, 1642–1648. [CrossRef] [PubMed]
61. Schreml, S.; Meier, R.J.; Kirschbaum, M.; Kong, S.C.; Gehmert, S.; Felthaus, O.; Küchler, S.; Sharpe, J.R.; Wöltje, K.; Weiß, K.T.; et al. Luminescent dual sensors reveal extracellular pH-gradients and hypoxia on chronic wounds that disrupt epidermal repair. *Theranostics* **2014**, *4*, 721–735. [CrossRef] [PubMed]
62. Armstrong, D.A.; Major, J.A.; Chudyk, A.; Hamilton, T.A. Neutrophil chemoattractant genes KC and MIP-2 are expressedin different cell populations at sites of surgical injury. *J. Leukoc. Biol.* **2004**, *75*, 641–648. [CrossRef] [PubMed]
63. Sroussi, H.Y.; Berline, J.; Palefsky, J.M. Oxidation of methionine 63 and 83 regulates the effect of S100A9 on the migration of neutrophils in vitro. *J. Leukoc. Biol.* **2007**, *81*, 818–824. [CrossRef] [PubMed]
64. Trøstrup, H.; Lerche, C.J.; Christophersen, L.; Jensen, P.Ø.; Høiby, N.; Moser, C. Immune Modulating Topical S100A8/A9 Inhibits Growth of *Pseudomonas aeruginosa* and Mitigates Biofilm Infection in Chronic Wounds. *Int. J. Mol. Sci.* **2017**, *18*, 1359. [CrossRef]
65. Zhao, G.; Hochwalt, P.C.; Usui, M.L.; Underwood, R.A.; Singh, P.K.; James, G.A.; Stewart, P.S.; Fleckman, P.; Olerud, J.E. Delayed wound healing in diabetic (db/db) mice with *Pseudomonas aeruginosa* biofilm challenge: A model for the study of chronic wounds. *Wound Repair Regen.* **2010**, *18*, 467–477. [CrossRef]
66. Watters, C.; DeLeon, K.; Trivedi, U.; Griswold, J.A.; Lyte, M.; Hampel, K.J.; Wargo, M.J.; Rumbaugh, K.P. *Pseudomonas aeruginosa* biofilms perturb wound resolution and antibiotic tolerance in diabetic mice. *Med. Microbiol. Immunol.* **2013**, *202*, 131–141. [CrossRef]
67. Ahn, S.T.; Mustoe, T.A. effects of ischemia on ulcer wound healing: A new model in the rabbit ear. *Ann. Plast. Surg.* **1990**, *24*, 17. [CrossRef]
68. Chang, A.C.; Dearman, B.; Greenwood, J.E. A comparison of wound area measurement techniques: Visitrak versus photography. *Eplasty* **2011**, *11*, e18.
69. Jeffcoate, W.J.; Musgrove, A.J.; Lincoln, N.B. Using Image J to document healing in ulcers of the foot in diabetes. *Int. Wound J.* **2017**, *14*, 1137–1139. [CrossRef]
70. Aragón- Sanchez, J.; Quintana-Marrero, Y.; Aragón-Hernandez, C.; Hernández-Herero, M.J. Image J: A free, easy, and reliable method to measure leg ulcers using digital pictures. *Int. J. Low. Extrem. Wounds* **2017**, *16*, 269–273. [CrossRef]
71. Nunes, J.P.S.; Dias, A.A.M. ImageJ macros for the user-friendly analysis of soft-agar and wound healing assays. *Biotechniques* **2017**, *62*, 175–179. [PubMed]
72. Li, X.; Gu, W.; Masinde, G.; Hamilton-Ulland, M.; Xu, S.; Mohan, S.; Baylink, D.J. Genetic control of the rate of wound healing in mice. *Heredity* **2001**, *86 Pt 6*, 668–674. [CrossRef]
73. Moser, C.; Pedersen, H.T.; Lerche, C.J.; Kolpen, M.; Line, L.; Thomsen, K.; Høiby, N.; Jensen, P.Ø. Biofilms and host response—Helpful or harmful. *APMIS* **2017**, *125*, 320–338. [CrossRef] [PubMed]
74. Fleming, D.; Rumbaugh, K. The consequences of biofilm dispersal on the host. *Sci. Rep.* **2018**, *8*, 10738. [CrossRef] [PubMed]
75. Percival, S.L.; Emanuel, C.; Cutting, K.F.; Williams, D.W. Microbiology of the skin and the role of biofilms in infection. *Int. Wound J.* **2012**, *9*, 14–32. [CrossRef] [PubMed]
76. Thorey, I.S.; Roth, J.; Regenbogen, J.; Halle, J.P.; Bittner, M.; Vogl, T.; Kaesler, S.; Bugnon, P.; Reitmaier, B.; Durka, S.; et al. The Ca^{2+}-binding proteins S100A8 and S100A9 are encoded by novel injury regulated genes. *J. Biol. Chem.* **2001**, *276*, 35818–35825. [CrossRef]
77. Trøstrup, H.; Lundquist, R.; Christensen, L.H.; Jørgensen, L.N.; Karlsmark, T.; Haab, B.B.; Ågren, M.S. S100A8/A9 deficiency in nonhealing venous leg ulcers uncovered by multiplexed antibody microarray profiling. *Br. J. Dermatol.* **2011**, *165*, 292–301. [CrossRef]
78. Chan, J.K.; Roth, J.; Oppenheim, J.J.; Tracey, K.J.; Vogl, T.; Feldmann, M.; Horwood, N.; Nanchahal, J. Alarmins: Awaiting a clinical response. *J. Clin. Investig.* **2012**, *122*, 2711–2719. [CrossRef]

79. Basu, A.; Munir, S.; Mulaw, M.A.; Singh, K.; Crisan, D.; Sindrilaru, A.; Treiber, N.; Wlaschek, M.; Huber-Lang, M.; Gebhard, F.; et al. A Novel S100A8/A9 induced fingerprint of mesenchymal stem cells associated with enhanced wound healing. *Sci. Rep.* **2018**, *8*, 10214. [CrossRef]
80. Gao, N.; Sang Yoon, G.; Liu, X.; Mi, X.; Chen, W.; Standiford, T.J.; Yu, F.S. Genome-wide transcriptional analysis of differentially expressed genes in flagellin-pretreated mouse corneal epithelial cells in response to *Pseudomonas aeruginosa*: Involvement of S100A8/A9. *Mucosal Immunol.* **2013**, *6*, 993–1005. [CrossRef]
81. Clark, H.L.; Jhingran, A.; Sun, Y.; Vareechon, C.; de Jesus Carrion, S.; Skaar, E.P.; Chazin, W.J.; Calera, J.A.; Hohl, T.M.; Pearlman, E. Zinc and manganese chelation by neutrophil S100A8/A9 (Calprotectin) limits extracellular *Aspergillus fumigatus* hyphal growth and corneal infection. *J. Immunol.* **2016**, *196*, 336–344. [CrossRef] [PubMed]
82. Laulund, A.S.B.; Trøstrup, H.; Lerche, C.J.; Thomsen, K.; Christophersen, L.; Calum, H.; Høiby, N.; Moser, C. Synergistic effect of immunomodulatory S100A8/A9 and ciprofloxacin against *Pseudomonas aeruginosa* biofilm in a murine chronic wound model. *Pathog. Dis.* **2019**, *22*, ftz027. [CrossRef] [PubMed]
83. Glaros, T.; Larsen, M.; Li, L. Macrophages and fibroblasts during inflammation, tissue damage and organ injury. *Front. Biosci.* **2009**, *14*, 3988–3993. [CrossRef] [PubMed]

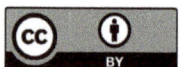 © 2020 by the authors. Licensee MDPI, Basel, Switzerland. This article is an open access article distributed under the terms and conditions of the Creative Commons Attribution (CC BY) license (http://creativecommons.org/licenses/by/4.0/).

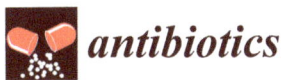

Perspective

Bacteriophage Therapy for Clinical Biofilm Infections: Parameters That Influence Treatment Protocols and Current Treatment Approaches

James B. Doub

Division of Infectious Diseases, University of Maryland School of Medicine, Baltimore, MD 21201, USA; jdoub@ihv.umaryland.edu

Received: 30 September 2020; Accepted: 10 November 2020; Published: 12 November 2020

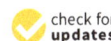

Abstract: Biofilm infections are extremely difficult to treat, which is secondary to the inability of conventional antibiotics to eradicate biofilms. Consequently, current definitive treatment of biofilm infections requires complete removal of the infected hardware. This causes significant morbidity and mortality to patients and therefore novel therapeutics are needed to cure these infections without removal of the infected hardware. Bacteriophages have intrinsic properties that could be advantageous in the treatment of clinical biofilm infections, but limited knowledge is known about the proper use of bacteriophage therapy in vivo. Currently titers and duration of bacteriophage therapy are the main parameters that are evaluated when devising bacteriophage protocols. Herein, several other important parameters are discussed which if standardized could allow for more effective and reproducible treatment protocols to be formulated. In addition, these parameters are correlated with the current clinical approaches being evaluated in the treatment of clinical biofilm infections.

Keywords: biofilm; bacteriophage therapy; prosthesis related infections; hardware infections; left ventricular assist devices

1. Introduction

When bacteria attach to surfaces they can form an extracellular matrix comprised of proteins, polysaccharides, extracellular DNA and water [1–5]. The extracellular matrix and the bacteria that reside within this matrix are what comprise biofilms. Contrary to planktonic bacteria that are free floating, biofilm bacteria are sessile. Bacteria in these sessile states have drastically different characteristics than planktonic bacteria causing conventional antibiotics to have limited ability to eradicate biofilms [1–5]. This stems from the reduced metabolic activity of biofilm bacteria and the architecture of biofilm itself [1]. The minimal inhibitory concentration of antibiotics to biofilm bacteria can be up to 1000 times that of planktonic bacteria [1]. Therefore to definitively cure these infections surgical removal of all the hardware (Figure 1) that harbor biofilms, in combination with prolonged systemic antibiotic therapy, is required. However, this causes significant morbidity and mortality to the patients who suffer from these infections. As a result, new antimicrobial methods are needed that can treat these biofilm infections without removal of the hardware. Bacteriophages might be such an adjuvant therapeutic.

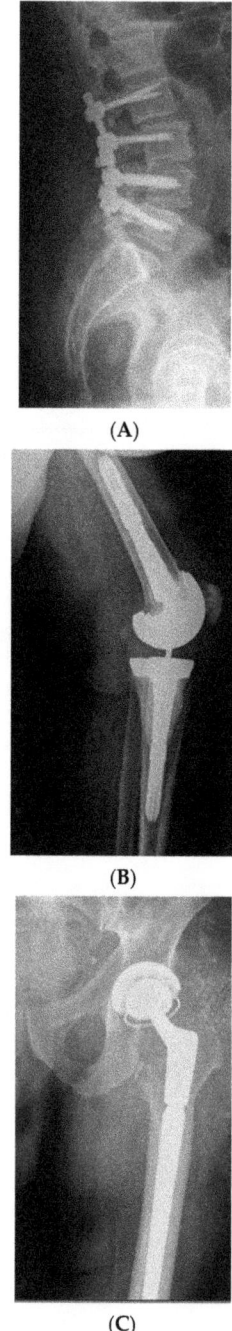

Figure 1. Examples of a few types of "hardware" that once infected require removal for definitive cure of these biofilm infections. (**A**) A lumbar posterior spinal rods and pedicle screw construct. (**B**) Total knee arthroplasty with long stem femoral and tibial components. (**C**) Total hip arthroplasty.

1.1. Bacteriophages

Bacteriophages are viruses with a very narrow spectrum of activity to only certain strains of a certain bacterial species. Infection of human cells has not been observed and therefore bacteriophages are attractive therapeutics to use in bacterial infections [6,7]. These viruses can either be lytic or lysogenic. Lytic bacteriophages hold the most promise in treating infections given their ability to lyse bacteria. Lysogenic bacteriophages incorporate into bacterial DNA and do not induce bacterial lysis until reactivated at a later time, making them not advantageous in the treatment of infections. In nature, the majority of bacteria live in sessile states associated with biofilms and through evolution bacteriophages have coevolved to be able to infect and lyse bacteria inside biofilms [6,7].

1.2. Bacteriophage Activity in Biofilms

In order to eradicate a clinical biofilm, an effective agent must be able to penetrate the biofilm and kill the bacteria that are present in various metabolic states while also degrading the biofilm extracellular matrix. Bacteriophages possess these abilities, but are not motile agents [6,7]. Therefore if bacteriophages can establish an infection within a biofilm, high rates of replication can occur given the high densities of biofilm bacteria in a structured space [8]. Bacteriophages even retain lytic activity against reduced metabolically active bacteria [9,10]. In the deepest regions of a biofilm, bacteria known as persister cells are semi-dormant [11]. All conventional therapeutics have limited activity to persister cells [11]. However, bacteriophages have the ability to infect persister cells and then lyse these bacteria once they become metabolically active again [12].

Bacteriophages also can enzymatically degrade the biofilm extracellular matrix thus allowing for dissemination within the biofilm. This occurs through use of endolysins and depolymerases [13,14]. Enodolysins are enzymes produced by bacteriophages to weaken the bacterial cell wall allowing for lysis to occur releasing their progeny [13]. Endolysins also have activity in degrading the extracellular matrix [13]. Depolymerases are enzymes attached to some bacteriophages that can also degrade the biofilm matrix in functionally different ways to endolysins [13]. Unique to bacteriophages is their ability to self-replicate and increase their own concentrations. This occurs when bacteriophage induced bacterial lysis causes release of progeny into the local environment to infect other bacterial cells. In the confined space of a biofilm this could be advantageous allowing for bacteriophages to infect biofilm bacteria and slowly degrade the biofilm [6]. However bacteriophages are not motile agents and finding biofilm bacteria may be an arduous undertaking if not directly applied to the biofilm.

Several preclinical animal studies support the use of bacteriophage therapy in clinical biofilm infections [15–23]. These studies show that local administrations of bacteriophages to the site of biofilm infections result in biofilm reduction [15–23]. In addition, these studies show that, without local administration of bacteriophage therapy, reduction in biofilms on hardware is not significantly reduced [19]. One of the most relevant preclinical studies was conducted by Morris et al. [19]. Rats were implanted with replica orthopedic prosthetics and then infected with *Staphylococcus aureus*. A total of 3 weeks later rats were given intraperitoneal bacteriophage therapy for 3 days. Results show synergistic activity of bacteriophage therapy with vancomycin in local infected tissues but no statistical reductions in biofilm burden on infected prosthetic material [19]. These findings support other preclinical testing that direct instilment of bacteriophage therapy to the site of biofilm infection is needed to achieve significant biofilm reduction. The intrinsic abilities of bacteriophages and results of animal studies support evaluation of bacteriophages in the treatment of clinical biofilm infections. However bacteriophages are not like conventional antibiotics and several parameters need to be understood before using this therapeutic in vivo.

2. Parameters that Impact Treatment Protocols

Unlike conventional antibiotics, bacteriophage therapy is not a one size fits all antimicrobial therapeutic. Rather a bacteriophage that has robust activity to a clinical isolate of a specific bacterial species may have widely different activity or no activity to another clinical isolate of the same bacterial species. Many other aspects of bacteriophage therapy are poorly understood and not standardized, making creation of treatment protocols an arduous undertaking. At the present time, standardization of protocols can only be achieved with respect to bacteriophage titers and duration of therapy. However, this limits bacteriophage therapy to be used similarly to conventional antibiotics and does not incorporate many other parameters that need to be considered to devise advantageous, reproducible treatment protocols. Herein several additional important parameters are discussed.

2.1. Current "Susceptibility" Testing

At the present time, bacteriophage therapy requires a clinical isolate to be tested against either a library of individual bacteriophages or to a set cocktail of bacteriophages to ensure susceptibility. Given the narrow spectrum of activity, even with the use of bacteriophage cocktails, susceptibility testing is warranted. There is no proverbial gold standard of susceptibility testing and no standardized "breakpoints" are available to determine if a bacteriophage has adequate activity to be used clinically. Therefore, it is vital to understand how in vitro susceptibility testing is conducted to be able to extrapolate these findings to in vivo use. Testing for phage susceptibility usually includes two methods.

(1) Bacterial growth inhibition or "Phagogram": This is conducted when a clinical bacterial isolate is grown in vitro and then inoculated into wells of a 96-microwell plate. The concentration of bacteria in each well is standardized. Then several different bacteriophages (or cocktails) that have potential activity are applied to the wells and monitored for 24 to 48 h to compare growth inhibition to positive controls (Figure 2). It should be noted that the multiplicity of infection (MOI) is usually 100:1. This means bacteriophages outnumber the bacteria 100 to 1. Bacteriophages that inhibit growth of bacteria for durations longer then the positive control are considered candidates. However, no standardized time durations have been established for what is considered long enough growth inhibition to be used in vivo.

(2) Formation of plaques: Once candidate bacteriophages are determined based on growth inhibition, the ability to form plaques on lawns of the bacterial isolate are then conducted. This usually is conducted with double agar overlay plaque assays.

Bacteriophages that form plaques and can inhibit bacterial growth are considered potential therapeutic options. Complicating this testing is that different MOIs can have drastically different growth inhibition durations. For instance an MOI of 100 might inhibit growth for 24 h while an MOI of 10 for the same bacteriophage might not inhibit growth at all. Figure 1 reinforces this for a *Staphylococcus epidermidis* clinical isolate in which PM448, PM472, PM421 have different growth inhibition durations for different MOIs of 100 and 10. This has ramifications when treating biofilm infections as reproducing the high MOI seen in vitro may not occur unless direct bacteriophage application is applied to biofilms. This can also have implications for resistance formation which will be discussed below.

Another important implication of this testing is the lack of standardization with respect to the duration of growth inhibition. A bacteriophage that inhibits growth for 48 h likely has different therapeutic potential compared to a different bacteriophage that only inhibits growth for 8 h. In correlation, different in vivo bacterial metabolic states may require different levels of growth inhibition. For instance, biofilm bacteria are less metabolically active then planktonic bacteria and therefore less in vitro growth inhibition might be needed compared to if bacteriophage therapy is being used to treat a planktonic infection. No standardized growth inhibition duration has been proposed, thereby exposing treatment protocols to potential reproducibility issues. To improve reproducibility, it may be important to standardize what is considered adequate growth inhibition depending on how a bacteriophage therapy is going to be used (intravenously vs. directly applied to biofilms). It should also be mentioned that "susceptibility" testing is usually only conducted against planktonic bacteria. Routine testing for a bacteriophage's ability to remove in vitro biofilms is usually not conducted.

However, in the treatment of biofilm infections, determining the ability of a candidate bacteriophage (or cocktail) to reduce in vitro biofilms should be considered as an additional susceptibility testing step once adequate growth inhibition and formation of plaques has been proven.

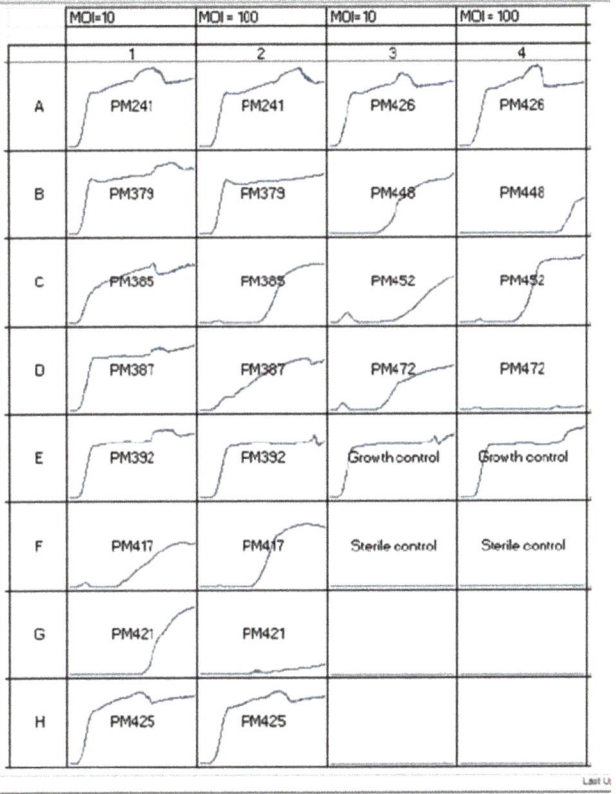

Figure 2. Bacterial growth inhibition curves or "Phagogram" for a compassionate use *Staphylococcus epidermidis* case in a recalcitrant prosthetic joint infection. Different bacteriophages are indicated by PM241-PM472. MOI refers to multiplicity of infection. Growth control is the bacterial isolate with no bacteriophages. Each box has time on the *x*-axis from 0 to 48 h. This figure shows how growth inhibition testing is conducted to determine potential bacteriophage candidates (PM448, PM472, and PM421). This figure also shows how different MOIs can cause different growth inhibition durations as seen with bacteriophages: PM448, PM472, and PM421.

2.2. Pharmacology

The main routes of phage administration that are being investigated in western medicine for the treatment of biofilm infections are local administration directly applied to the infected hardware and intravenous therapy. Eastern European studies have had limited success with topical or oral phage therapies in the treatment of biofilm infections and therefore little interest is present for these methods beyond topical application for burns and wounds [24–26]. Given the novelty of this therapeutic there is a paucity of data with respect to pharmacokinetics of local administration of bacteriophage therapy to biofilms. No data are present to suggest how long locally administrated bacteriophage reside at the infection site, how much is systemically absorbed or the safety of this approach. On the other hand, intravenous bacteriophage therapy has been more widely used and data are present to help guide treatment protocols. Therefore discussion about simple pharmacokinetics is limited to intravenous use.

Distribution: Bacteriophages are expected to be diluted in the whole body volume when given intravenously [27]. In numerous animal studies the titers of bacteriophages after intravenous infusions can be reduced 100–100,000-fold within 30 min of infusion [27]. Animal studies have shown distribution to various other organs including but not limited to heart, lungs, brain, skeletal muscle, bone marrow, and genitourinary tract [27]. However there are no data on intravenous bacteriophage therapy distribution to joints, spinal hardware, Left ventricular assist devices (LVADs) or other spaces that could have poor vascularization.

Metabolism: This is the chemical modification of bacteriophage therapy to reduce its activity. With bacteriophage therapy this occurs mainly through inactivation by the human immune system by neutralizing antibodies [28]. Neutralizing antibody responses have occurred with all forms of bacteriophage administration and this is a theoretical concern for long duration bacteriophage therapies [28,29].

Elimination: Elimination occurs mainly through hepatic clearance. In 1969, using a T4 bacteriophage, Inchley demonstrated that the liver phagocytosed and eliminated more than 99% of the bacteriophages within 30 min after systemic administration [30]. Other studies have supported this extensive hepatic elimination [30–33]. In one compassionate use case, 50 min after intravenous administration no bacteriophage could be detected in patient's serum [34].

Based on these data, intravenous bacteriophage therapies are likely to have significant reduction in titers, secondary to volume of distribution and hepatic elimination. Therefore, achieving MOIs similar to what occurs with in vitro susceptibility testing may be difficult. With the use of bacteriophage therapy applied directly to biofilm infections, MOIs may be similar to what was observed with in vitro susceptibility testing. However, limited pharmacological data have been found to help direct dosing, duration or safety of local bacteriophage administration.

2.3. Safety

Unbeknownst to most, humans are exposed to low titers of bacteriophages on a continual basis [35]. Eastern European medicine has used bacteriophage therapy for close to 100 years with few significant adverse reactions being reported [36]. However, given the extensive hepatic clearance, western medicine is entertaining the use of high titers (greater than 10^9) of intravenous bacteriophage therapy and direct injection of high titers of bacteriophages directly to biofilm infections. Limited safety studies have been conducted using these techniques beyond a phase 1 clinical trial evaluating a three-bacteriophage cocktail with titers of 1×10^9 plaque-forming unit (PFU) twice a day for 14 days to *Staphylococcus aureus* bacteremia [37].

While intravenous bacteriophage therapy has been used in the past with limited adverse events, recent compassionate use cases have shown two adverse events [38,39]. One occurred in the treatment of chronic pseudomonas left ventricular assist device (LVAD) infection in which no success occurred with low titers of intravenous bacteriophage therapy and subsequent bacteriophage therapy with high titers of 1×10^{11} PFU induced fever, shortness of breath and wheezing [38]. These symptoms resolved with supportive medical care but continued with repeat dosing with the same titers. When titers were diluted to 1×10^{10} PFU, the authors document that no adverse events occurred [38]. Endotoxin units were well below the United States Food and Drug Administration approved limit. In the other case, a significant transaminitis occurred after three doses of daily intravenous bacteriophage therapy with titers of 2.7×10^9 PFU in the treatment of a recalcitrant methicillin-resistant *Staphylococcus aureus* prosthetic joint infection. No causative etiology other than bacteriophage therapy could be found [39]. After cessation of bacteriophage therapy liver function returned to normal after 14 days. These two cases suggest that an upper limit may exist with respect to the titers that can be intravenously infused without exposing patients to potential adverse events. However only further safety trials with high titers given intravenously or directly to sites of biofilm infections will be able to assess safety and if there is a ceiling for the amount of titers that can be given.

2.4. Resistance Development

With longer bacteriophage therapies, concern arises for the development of resistance. Resistance usually occurs from bacterial modifications of cell surface receptors or down regulation of receptors used in phage–bacteria attachment [40,41]. Other means of resistance can occur through adaptive systems such as the CRISPR–Cas9 system that cleaves phage DNA thus not allowing for progeny phage to be created [40]. Means to overcome or prevent resistance from occurring include use of cocktails of bacteriophages and bacteriophage substitutions. Bacteriophage cocktails are a group of different bacteriophages that theoretically use different attachment receptors. Therefore, if resistance develops to one receptor, the cocktail should continue to be effective. A recent study showed the frequency of spontaneous induction of resistance to a cocktail of three *Staphylococcus aureus* bacteriophages was no greater than 3×10^{-9} [42]. Bacteriophage substitutions are simply changing therapy to a different bacteriophage that has lytic activity to the bacterium.

Bacteriophage resistance can occur rapidly causing formation of resistant variants that are immune to further bacteriophage infection [41]. This could impede effectiveness of bacteriophage therapy but resistance may also come at a cost to the bacterium especially when antimicrobial agents are present [41]. Moreover, bacteriophage-resistant bacteria often lack important surface features that are responsible for bacterial virulence [41]. Nonetheless resistance is an important factor that should be accounted for especially with prolonged bacteriophage treatments. In a case series of 10 intravenous bacteriophage only cases, resistance occurred in a significant portion of patients and required bacteriophage substitutions [38]. Resistance development is dependent on complex interplays of MOIs, growth inhibition durations and other bacteriophage–bacteria interactions [41]. Therefore resistance might develop rapidly or slower depending on these complex interactions. Determining in vitro resistance development to a clinical isolate is not routinely conducted, but could be easily assessed with susceptibility testing by evaluating the bacterial overgrowth for resistant variants. Resistance development is an important parameter that can have ramifications on efficacy and reproducibility of treatment protocols. Therefore it might be prudent to routinely test for and standardize what an acceptable level of in vitro resistance development is for different infectious processes to reduce further problems of reproducibility and improve efficacy of treatment protocols.

2.5. Synergistic or Antagonistic Activity with Antibiotics

While resistance is an important parameter so is compatibility with systemic antibiotics which may have synergistic or antagonistic activity with bacteriophage therapy. Theoretically, antibiotics that inhibit protein synthesis (rifampin, tetracyclines, linezolid and others) can inhibit phage gene expression and therefore be antagonistic [43]. Antibiotics that inhibit cell wall synthesis inhibitors such as beta-lactams are potentially more synergistic [43]. These findings have been reinforced in numerous in vitro studies [43]. It has also been documented that concentrations of antibiotics also have important ramification of synergistic or antagonistic activity with higher antibiotic concentrations tending to be more antagonistic compared to lower concentrations which tend to be more synergistic [43]. It is interesting that in vivo studies have shown more synergistic activity of antibiotics with bacteriophage therapy then antagonism [15–23]. Spatial and temporal interactions of antibiotics and bacteriophages in vivo likely account for this synergistic activity [43]. It should be reinforced that biofilm bacteria reside where there is poor vascularization and therefore very low concentrations of systemic antibiotics may make phage–antibiotic compatibility less of an issue in vivo [43]. Testing for in vitro for phage–antibiotic compatibility is not commonly conducted. As with resistance development and susceptibility testing, it may be prudent to ensure bacteriophage–antibiotic compatibility with the systemic antibiotics that are planned to be used thus allowing for more reproducible treatment protocols.

2.6. Clinical Biofilms

In vitro bacteriophage biofilm studies are traditionally conducted in static environments. These studies are usually devoid of human plasma proteins, lack in vivo stressors and normally remove planktonic infections before experiments are conducted. However, in vivo, planktonic infections overly clinical biofilm infections and are what causes the majority of the symptoms that patient's experience. Without eradicating these planktonic bacteria, bacteriophage therapy protocols will have to account for the planktonic infection and the biofilm infection. This adds complexity to the use of bacteriophage therapy and potentially further hinders reproducibility given the heterogeneity of these planktonic infections.

Other clinical factors that should be considered include: stability of infected hardware and importance of manual debridement of biofilms. Stability of hardware must be assessed to ensure retaining these materials is possible. This is usually conducted by imaging but manual inspection and manipulation is the most advantageous way to assess the ability to retain these materials. Manual debridement of biofilms has also been shown to be synergistic with respect to bacteriophage activity in biofilms [16,17]. This synergistic activity is likely a result of better bacteriophage penetration into biofilm and exposing biofilm bacteria to bacteriophages [16,17].

2.7. Conclusions

The parameters discussed show that currently bacteriophage therapy is not a therapeutic that can be used similarly to conventional antibiotics. In addition relying mainly on bacteriophage's ability to self-replicate is unlikely to be beneficial beyond isolated case reports given the complexity of these other parameters. Rather thoughtful consideration of many parameters needs to be considered to devise effective, reproducible treatment protocols. Most of these parameters discussed are intertwined but standardization is lacking. Given the heterogeneity of these parameters glaring issues of reproducibility are present at this nascent stage of bacteriophage therapy. To reduce these reproducibility issues standardizing some of these parameters might be needed which include: minimal duration of growth inhibition, resistance testing, bacteriophage–antibiotic compatibility and ensuring in vitro bacteriophage biofilm activity. This may allow for more rigorous testing of reproducible protocols to therefore definitively determine if this therapeutic has efficacy in treating clinical biofilm infections.

3. Current Theoretical Bacteriophage Protocols for Chronic Biofilm Infections

Many recent compassionate use cases have been conducted recently to treat clinical biofilm infections (prosthetic joint infections, LVAD infections, vascular graft infections and others). Two main approaches are being used in western medicine which include: intravenous bacteriophage therapy and the use of surgical interventions to directly inject bacteriophages to site of the biofilm. Table 1 discusses the advantages and disadvantages to each approach in relation to the parameters discussed above. Both approaches involve adjuvant bacteriophage therapy in combination with standard of care systemic antibiotics. Further review of recent case reports with respect to the different approaches is discussed here.

3.1. Case Studies of Intravenous Bacteriophage Therapy in Biofilm Infections

Intravenous bacteriophage therapy has been attempted to treat prosthetic joint infections, ventricular assist devices, vascular graft infections and other hardware infections [38,44–46]. In one case series, the authors describe the use of bacteriophage therapy for two *Pseudomonas* LVAD infections with prolonged intravenous bacteriophage therapies with unsuccessful outcomes [38]. The same author also treated a *Staphylococcus aureus* LVAD infection with intravenous bacteriophage therapy and the was documented as a success, but the patient continued to have culture positive *Staphylococcus aureus* infection at the time of LVAD explant, suggesting the inability of intravenous bacteriophage therapy to eradicate the biofilm infection [38,44]. Another case report treated a *Klebsiella pneumonia* prosthetic joint infection with 8 weeks of intravenous bacteriophage therapy with improvement of symptoms [45]. However the patient remains on chronic indefinite oral suppression antibiotics, limiting the ability to assess if eradication of the clinical biofilm was achieved.

Intravenous bacteriophage therapy is optically attractive in that no surgery is needed. However at the present time no case report has definitively shown the ability to eradicate clinical biofilms with this approach. The theoretical concern with intravenous bacteriophage therapy alone is the entrapment of bacteriophages in the planktonic infection limiting exposure of bacteriophages to the biofilm bacteria. In correlation, bacteriophages are extensively cleared by the liver and in vivo biofilms are usually poorly vascularized. Therefore achieving theoretical MOIs seen with in vitro "susceptibility" testing requires very high titers of infused bacteriophages. These high titers may be limited by potential adverse reactions [38,39]. Further complicating intravenous only therapies is the need for prolonged durations driven by limited bacteriophages reaching their bacterial biofilm targets thereby leading to the development of resistance and neutralizing antibodies. These variables when combined cause numerous confounding variables that may cause significant issues of reproducibility at this nascent stage of bacteriophage therapy.

Table 1. Advantages and disadvantages of intravenous and direct injection of bacteriophage therapy for clinical biofilm infections.

	Direct Bacteriophage Therapy in Correlation with Surgical Interventions	Intravenous Bacteriophage Therapy
Advantages	Potentially shorter course with less risk of resistance and neutralizing antibodies occurring Direct injection of high titers to biofilm thereby achieving theoretical MOIs similarly to in vitro testing Removes majority of planktonic infection Ensures hardware salvageable Ensures no other pathogens present Allows for manual scrubbing of biofilm	Circumvent surgery and risks of general anesthesia No wounds created that thus no risk for further infections No confounders with proving efficacy either it works or does not work
Disadvantages	Risks of Anesthesia Risks of poor wound healing Chance for introduction of another pathogen during surgical interventions	Have to treat both planktonic and biofilm infection Limited ability to achieve MOIs that were tested with in vitro testing Limited identification of all pathogens involved to match to bacteriophage therapy Unable to assess prosthesis stability beyond radiographic findings Longer therapy with higher risk of resistance and neutralizing antibodies occurring

3.2. Case Studies of Direct Injection of Bacteriophages to Biofilms with Surgical Intervention

The addition of bacteriophage therapy with debridement and irrigation surgeries is the other approach that has been used in several case studies [38,47–50]. This approach involves injection of high titers of bacteriophage phages directly at the site of the biofilm infection thereby circumventing hepatic clearance. The goal of this approach is to potentially cure these infections without need for removal of the hardware. However the risks of a surgical procedure are present and therefore this approach is optically less desirable.

There have been several compassionate use case reports that have shown successful eradication of biofilm infections which include: chronic orthopedic hardware infections, LVAD infection, vascular graft infection, cardiothoracic surgery infections [38,47–50]. In these case reports different durations of bacteriophage therapy were used. Some cases only required single doses given at the time of surgery while others used drains to continually instill bacteriophage therapy for 7 to 10 days. All cases described no recurrence of bacterial infections while patients were off antimicrobial therapies thereby showing eradication of bacterial biofilms. However with surgical debridement, successful eradication of bacterial biofilm is confounded by the uncertainty of whether it was bacteriophage therapy that was the reason for clearance or if it was the surgical intervention itself. This questioning occurs because success occurs with these surgical debridement procedures without adjuvant bacteriophage therapy albeit at low rates. In addition, limited data are present to help direct safety, appropriate dosing and durations of directly administered bacteriophage therapies but this approach may allow for more standardized reproducible protocols.

4. Conclusions

Many aspects of bacteriophage therapy allow this therapeutic to be an attractive adjuvant therapeutic in the treatment of biofilm infections but much work is needed before definitive efficacy trials are to be conducted. The various parameters discussed here should allow researchers to be more cognizant of the current inherent limitations of bacteriophage therapy. However, given the heterogeneity of these parameters, projected issues of reproducibility are glaring. Therefore, standardizing some of these parameters is warranted to formulate reproducible protocols that will allow for rigorous testing of this therapeutic in the treatment of biofilm infections.

Funding: This research received no external funding.

Acknowledgments: Phagomed are acknowledged for providing and authorization of the use of Figure 2.

Conflicts of Interest: The authors declare no conflict of interest.

References

1. Mah, T.F.; O'Toole, G.A. Mechanisms of biofilm resistance to antimicrobial agents. *Trends Microbiol.* **2001**, *9*, 34–39. [CrossRef]
2. Wille, J.; Coenye, T. Biofilm dispersion: The key to biofilm eradication or opening Pandora's box? *Biofilm* **2020**, *2*, 100027. [CrossRef]
3. Stewart, P.S. Antimicrobial Tolerance in Biofilms. *Microbiol. Spectr.* **2015**, *3*. [CrossRef] [PubMed]
4. Van Acker, H.; Van Dijck, P.; Coenye, T. Molecular mechanisms of antimicrobial tolerance and resistance in bacterial and fungal biofilms. *Trends Microbiol.* **2014**, *22*, 326–333. [CrossRef] [PubMed]
5. Kaplan, J.B. Biofilm dispersal: Mechanisms, clinical implications, and potential therapeutic uses. *J. Dent. Res.* **2010**, *89*, 205–218. [CrossRef]
6. Abedon, S.T. Ecology of Anti-Biofilm Agents II: Bacteriophage Exploitation and Biocontrol of Biofilm Bacteria. *Pharmaceuticals* **2015**, *8*, 559–589. [CrossRef]
7. Hanlon, G.W. Bacteriophages: An appraisal of their role in the treatment of bacterial infections. *Int. J. Antimicrob. Agents* **2007**, *30*, 118–128. [CrossRef]
8. Hadas, H.; Einav, M.; Fishov, I.; Zaritsky, A. Bacteriophage T4 development depends on the physiology of its host Escherichia coli. *Microbiology* **1997**, *143*, 179–185. [CrossRef]
9. Doolittle, M.M.; Cooney, J.J.; Caldwell, D.E. Tracing the interaction of bacteriophage with bacterial biofilms using fluorescent and chromogenic probes. *J. Ind. Microbiol.* **1996**, *16*, 331–341. [CrossRef]
10. Lewis, K. Persister cells. *Annu. Rev. Microbiol.* **2010**, *64*, 357–372. [CrossRef]
11. Pearl, S.; Gabay, C.; Kishony, R.; Oppenheim, A.; Balaban, N.Q. Nongenetic individuality in the host-phage interaction. *PLoS Biol.* **2008**, *6*, e120. [CrossRef] [PubMed]
12. Chan, B.K.; Abedon, S.T. Bacteriophages and their enzymes in biofilm control. *Curr. Pharm. Des.* **2015**, *21*, 85–99. [CrossRef] [PubMed]
13. Tait, K.; Skillman, L.C.; Sutherland, I.W. The efficacy of bacteriophage as a method of biofilm eradication. *Biofouling* **2002**, *18*, 305–311. [CrossRef]
14. Yilmaz, C.; Colak, M.; Yilmaz, B.C.; Ersoz, G.; Kutateladze, M.; Gozlugol, M. Bacteriophage therapy in implant-related infections: An experimental study. *J. Bone Jt. Surg. Am.* **2013**, *95*, 117–125. [CrossRef]

15. Chaudhry, W.N.; Concepción-Acevedo, J.; Park, T.; Andleeb, S.; Bull, J.J.; Levin, B.R. Synergy and Order Effects of Antibiotics and Phages in Killing Pseudomonas aeruginosa Biofilms. *PLoS ONE* **2017**, *12*, e0168615. [CrossRef]
16. Mendes, J.J.; Leandro, C.; Corte-Real, S.; Barbosa, R.; Cavaco-Silva, P.; Melo-Cristino, J.; Górski, A.; Garcia, M. Wound healing potential of topical bacteriophage therapy on diabetic cutaneous wounds. *Wound Repair Regen.* **2013**, *21*, 595–603. [CrossRef]
17. Kaur, S.; Harjai, K.; Chhibber, S. Bacteriophage mediated killing of Staphylococcus aureus in vitro on orthopaedic K wires in presence of linezolid prevents implant colonization. *PLoS ONE* **2014**, *9*, e90411. [CrossRef]
18. Morris, J.L.; Letson, H.L.; Elliott, L.; Grant, A.L.; Wilkinson, M.; Hazratwala, K.; McEwen, P. Evaluation of bacteriophage as an adjunct therapy for treatment of peri-prosthetic joint infection caused by Staphylococcus aureus. *PLoS ONE* **2019**, *14*, e0226574. [CrossRef]
19. Cobb, L.H.; Park, J.; Swanson, E.A.; Beard, M.C.; McCabe, E.M.; Rourke, A.S.; Seo, K.S.; Olivier, A.K.; Priddy, L.B. CRISPR-Cas9 modified bacteriophage for treatment of Staphylococcus aureus induced osteomyelitis and soft tissue infection. *PLoS ONE* **2019**, *14*, e0220421. [CrossRef]
20. Ibrahim, O.; Sarhan, S.; Salih, S. Activity of Isolated Staphylococcal Bacteriophage in Treatment of Experimentally Induced Chronic Osteomyelitis in Rabbits. *Adv. Anim. Vet. Sci.* **2016**, *4*, 593–603. [CrossRef]
21. Kishor, C.; Mishra, R.R.; Saraf, S.K.; Kumar, M.; Srivastav, A.K.; Nath, G. Phage therapy of staphylococcal chronic osteomyelitis in experimental animal model. *Indian J. Med. Res.* **2016**, *143*, 87–94. [PubMed]
22. Wroe, J.; Johnson, C.; Garcia, A. Bacteriophage delivering hydrogels reduce biofilm formation in vitro and infection in vivo. *J. Biomed. Mater. Res. A* **2020**, *108*, 39–49. [CrossRef] [PubMed]
23. Międzybrodzki, R.; Borysowski, J.; Weber-Dąbrowska, B.; Fortuna, W.; Letkiewicz, S.; Szufnarowski, K.; Pawełczyk, Z.; Rogóż, P.; Kłak, M.; Wojtasik, E.; et al. Clinical aspects of phage therapy. *Adv. Virus Res.* **2012**, *83*, 73–121.
24. Jault, P.; Leclerc, T.; Jennes, S.; Pirnay, J.P.; Que, Y.-A.; Resch, G.; Rousseau, A.F.; Ravat, F.; Carsin, H.; Floch, R.L.; et al. Efficacy and tolerability of a cocktail of bacteriophages to treat burn wounds infected by Pseudomonas aeruginosa (PhagoBurn): A randomised, controlled, double-blind phase 1/2 trial. *Lancet Infect. Dis.* **2019**, *19*, 35–45. [CrossRef]
25. Rhoads, D.D.; Wolcott, R.D.; Kuskowski, M.A.; Wolcott, B.M.; Ward, L.S.; Sulakvelidze, A. Bacteriophage therapy of venous leg ulcers in humans: Results of a phase I safety trial. *J. Wound Care* **2009**, *18*, 237–243. [CrossRef] [PubMed]
26. Dąbrowska, K. Phage therapy: What factors shape phage pharmacokinetics and bioavailability? Systematic and critical review. *Med. Res. Rev.* **2019**, *39*, 2000–2025. [CrossRef] [PubMed]
27. Jerne, N.K.; Avegno, P. The development of the phage-inactivating properties of serum during the course of specific immunization of an animal: Reversible and irreversible inactivation. *J. Immunol.* **1956**, *76*, 200–208.
28. Łusiak-Szelachowska, M.; Zaczek, M.; Weber-Dąbrowska, B.; Międzybrodzki, R.; Kłak, M.; Fortuna, W.; Letkiewicz, S.; Rogóż, P.; Szufnarowski, K.; Jończyk-Matysiak, E.; et al. Phage neutralization by sera of patients receiving phage therapy. *Viral. Immunol.* **2014**, *27*, 295–304. [CrossRef]
29. Inchley, C.J. The actvity of mouse Kupffer cells following intravenous injection of T4 bacteriophage. *Clin. Exp. Immunol.* **1969**, *5*, 173–187.
30. Jonczyk-Matysiak, E.; Weber-Dabrowska, B.; Owczarek, B.; Międzybrodzki, B.; Łusiak-Szelachowska, M.; Łodej, N.; Górski, A. Phage-phagocyte interactions and their implications for phage application as therapeutics. *Viruses* **2017**, *9*, 150. [CrossRef]
31. Nelstrop, A.E.; Taylor, G.; Collard, P. Studies on phagocytosis. II. in vitro phagocytosis by macrophages. *Immunology* **1968**, *14*, 339–346. [PubMed]
32. Reynaud, A.; Cloastre, L.; Bernard, J.; Laveran, H.; Ackermann, H.-W.; Licois, D.; Joly, B. Characteristics and diffusion in the rabbit of a phage for Escherichia coli 0103. Attempts to use this phage for therapy. *Vet. Microbiol.* **1992**, *30*, 203–212. [CrossRef]
33. LaVergne, S.; Hamilton, T.; Biswas, B.; Kumaraswamy, M.; Schooley, R.T.; Wooten, D. Phage Therapy for a Multidrug-Resistant Acinetobacter baumannii Craniectomy Site Infection. *Open Forum. Infect. Dis.* **2018**, *5*, ofy064. [CrossRef] [PubMed]
34. Górski, A.; Weber-Dabrowska, B. The potential role of endogenous bacteriophages in controlling invading pathogens. *Cell. Mol. Life Sci.* **2005**, *62*, 511–519. [CrossRef] [PubMed]

35. Sulakvelidze, A.; Alavidze, Z.; Morris, J.G., Jr. Bacteriophage therapy. *Antimicrob. Agents Chemother.* **2001**, *45*, 649–659. [CrossRef]
36. Petrovic Fabijan, A.; Lin, R.C.Y.; Ho, J.; Maddocks, S.; Zakour, N.L.B.; Iredell, J.R.; Westmead Bacteriophage Therapy Team. Safety of bacteriophage therapy in severe Staphylococcus aureus infection. *Nat. Microbiol.* **2020**, *5*, 465–472. [CrossRef]
37. Aslam, S.; Lampley, E.; Wooten, D.; Karris, M.; Benson, C.; Strathdee, S.; Schooley, R.T. Lessons Learned from First Ten Consecutive Cases of Intravenous Bacteriophage Therapy to Treat Multidrug Resistant Bacterial Infections at a Single Center in the US. *Open Forum. Infect. Dis.* **2020**, *7*, ofaa389. [CrossRef]
38. Doub, J.B.; Ng, V.Y.; Johnson, A.J.; Slomka, M.; Fackler, J.; Horne, B.; Brownstein, M.J.; Henry, M.; Malagon, F.; Biswas, B. Salvage Bacteriophage Therapy for a Chronic MRSA Prosthetic Joint Infection. *Antibiotics* **2020**, *9*, 241. [CrossRef]
39. Jackson, S.A.; McKenzie, R.E.; Fagerlund, R.D.; Kieper, S.N.; Fineran, P.C.; Brouns, S.J. CRISPR-Cas: Adapting to change. *Science* **2017**, *356*, eaal5056. [CrossRef]
40. Oechslin, F. Resistance Development to Bacteriophages Occurring during Bacteriophage Therapy. *Viruses* **2018**, *10*, 351. [CrossRef]
41. Lehman, S.M.; Mearns, G.; Rankin, D.; Cole, R.A.; Smrekar, F.; Branston, S.D.; Morales, S. Design and Preclinical Development of a Phage Product for the Treatment of Antibiotic-Resistant Staphylococcus aureus Infections. *Viruses* **2019**, *11*, 88. [CrossRef] [PubMed]
42. Abedon, S.T. Phage-Antibiotic Combination Treatments: Antagonistic Impacts of Antibiotics on the Pharmacodynamics of Phage Therapy? *Antibiotics* **2019**, *8*, 182. [CrossRef] [PubMed]
43. Aslam, S.; Pretorius, V.; Lehman, S.M.; Morales, S.; Schooley, R.T. Novel bacteriophage therapy for treatment of left ventricular assist device infection. *J. Heart Lung Transpl.* **2019**, *38*, 475–476. [CrossRef] [PubMed]
44. Cano, E.J.; Caflisch, K.M.; Bollyky, P.L.; Van Belleghem, J.D.; Patel, R.; Fackler, J.; Brownstein, M.J.; Horne, B.; Biswas, B.; Henry, M.; et al. Phage Therapy for Limb-threatening Prosthetic Knee Klebsiella pneumoniae Infection: Case Report and In Vitro Characterization of Anti-biofilm Activity. *Clin. Infect. Dis.* **2020**, ciaa705. [CrossRef] [PubMed]
45. Duplessis, C.; Stockelman, M.; Hamilton, T.; Merril, G.; Brownstein, M.; Bishop-lilly, K.; Schooley, R.; Henry, M.; Horne, B.; Sisson, B.M.; et al. A Case Series of Emergency Investigational New Drug Applications for Bacteriophages Treating Recalcitrant Multi-drug Resistant Bacterial Infections: Confirmed Safety and a Signal of Efficacy. *J. Intensive Crit. Care* **2019**, *5*, 11.
46. Ferry, T.; Leboucher, G.; Fevre, C.; Herry, Y.; Conrad, A.; Josse, J.; Batailler, C.; Chidiac, C.; Medina, M.; Lustig, S.; et al. Salvage Debridement, Antibiotics and Implant Retention ("DAIR") With Local Injection of a Selected Cocktail of Bacteriophages: Is It an Option for an Elderly Patient With Relapsing Staphylococcus aureus Prosthetic-Joint Infection? *Open Forum. Infect. Dis.* **2018**, *5*, ofy269. [CrossRef]
47. Onsea, J.; Soentjens, P.; Djebara, S.; Merabishvili, M.; Depypere, M.; Spriet, I.; De Munter, P.; Debaveye, Y.; Nijs, S.; Vanderschot, P.; et al. Bacteriophage Application for Difficult-to-treat Musculoskeletal Infections: Development of a Standardized Multidisciplinary Treatment Protocol. *Viruses* **2019**, *11*, 891. [CrossRef]
48. Rubalskii, E.; Ruemke, S.; Salmoukas, C.; Boyle, E.C.; Warnecke, G.; Tudorache, I.; Shrestha, M.; Schmitto, J.D.; Martens, M.A.; Rojas, S.V.; et al. Bacteriophage Therapy for Critical Infections Related to Cardiothoracic Surgery. *Antibiotics* **2020**, *9*, 232. [CrossRef]
49. Tkhilaishvili, T.; Winkler, T.; Müller, M.; Perka, C.; Trampuz, A. Bacteriophages as Adjuvant to Antibiotics for the Treatment of Periprosthetic Joint Infection Caused by Multidrug-Resistant Pseudomonas aeruginosa. *Antimicrob. Agents Chemother.* **2019**, *64*, e00924-19. [CrossRef]
50. Mulzer, J.; Trampuz, A.; Potapov, E.V. Treatment of chronic left ventricular assist device infection with local application of bacteriophages. *Eur. J. Cardio-Thorac. Surg.* **2020**, *57*, 1003–1004. [CrossRef]

Publisher's Note: MDPI stays neutral with regard to jurisdictional claims in published maps and institutional affiliations.

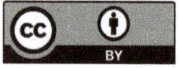

© 2020 by the author. Licensee MDPI, Basel, Switzerland. This article is an open access article distributed under the terms and conditions of the Creative Commons Attribution (CC BY) license (http://creativecommons.org/licenses/by/4.0/).

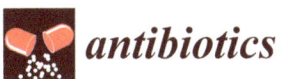

Article

Bacteriophage Cocktail-Mediated Inhibition of *Pseudomonas aeruginosa* Biofilm on Endotracheal Tube Surface

Viviane C. Oliveira [1,2], Ana P. Macedo [2], Luís D. R. Melo [3], Sílvio B. Santos [3], Paula R. S. Hermann [1,4], Cláudia H. Silva-Lovato [2], Helena F. O. Paranhos [2], Denise Andrade [1] and Evandro Watanabe [1,5,*]

[1] Human Exposome and Infectious Diseases Network—HEID, School of Nursing of Ribeirão Preto, University of São Paulo, Bandeirantes Avenue 3900, Ribeirão Preto, São Paulo 14040-904, Brazil; vivianecassia@usp.br (V.C.O.); paularegina@unb.br (P.R.S.H.); dandrade@eerp.usp.br (D.A.)

[2] Department of Dental Materials and Prostheses, School of Dentistry of Ribeirão Preto, University of São Paulo, Café Avenue S/N, Ribeirão Preto, São Paulo 14040-904, Brazil; anapaula@forp.usp.br (A.P.M.); chl@forp.usp.br (C.H.S.-L.); helenpar@forp.usp.br (H.F.O.P.)

[3] Centre of Biological Engineering—CEB, University of Minho, 4710-057 Braga, Portugal; lmelo@deb.uminho.pt (L.D.R.M.); silviosantos@deb.uminho.pt (S.B.S.)

[4] Department of Nursing, University of Brasília, Distrito Federal, Brasília 72220-275, Brazil

[5] Department of Restorative Dentistry, School of Dentistry of Ribeirão Preto, University of São Paulo, Café Avenue S/N, Ribeirão Preto, São Paulo 14040-904, Brazil

* Correspondence: ewatanabe@forp.usp.br; Tel.: +55-16-3315-4078

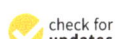

Citation: Oliveira, V.C.; Macedo, A.P.; Melo, L.D.R.; Santos, S.B.; Hermann, P.R.S.; Silva-Lovato, C.H.; Paranhos, H.F.O.; Andrade, D.; Watanabe, E. Bacteriophage Cocktail-Mediated Inhibition of *Pseudomonas aeruginosa* Biofilm on Endotracheal Tube Surface. *Antibiotics* **2021**, *10*, 78. https://doi.org/10.3390/antibiotics10010078

Received: 1 December 2020
Accepted: 12 January 2021
Published: 15 January 2021

Publisher's Note: MDPI stays neutral with regard to jurisdictional claims in published maps and institutional affiliations.

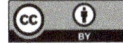

Copyright: © 2021 by the authors. Licensee MDPI, Basel, Switzerland. This article is an open access article distributed under the terms and conditions of the Creative Commons Attribution (CC BY) license (https://creativecommons.org/licenses/by/4.0/).

Abstract: Although different strategies to control biofilm formation on endotracheal tubes have been proposed, there are scarce scientific data on applying phages for both removing and preventing *Pseudomonas aeruginosa* biofilms on the device surface. Here, the anti-biofilm capacity of five bacteriophages was evaluated by a high content screening assay. We observed that biofilms were significantly reduced after phage treatment, especially in multidrug-resistant strains. Considering the anti-biofilm screens, two phages were selected as cocktail components, and the cocktail's ability to prevent colonization of the endotracheal tube surface was tested in a dynamic biofilm model. Phage-coated tubes were challenged with different *P. aeruginosa* strains. The biofilm growth was monitored from 24 to 168 h by colony forming unit counting, metabolic activity assessment, and biofilm morphology observation. The phage cocktail promoted differences of bacterial colonization; nonetheless, the action was strain dependent. Phage cocktail coating did not promote substantial changes in metabolic activity. Scanning electron microscopy revealed a higher concentration of biofilm cells in control, while tower-like structures could be observed on phage cocktail-coated tubes. These results demonstrate that with the development of new coating strategies, phage therapy has potential in controlling the endotracheal tube-associated biofilm.

Keywords: bacteriophage; biofilm; *Pseudomonas aeruginosa*; endotracheal tube

1. Introduction

Ventilator-associated pneumonia (VAP) is a serious concern in critically ill patients occurring within the 48 h period following endotracheal intubation. The current COVID-19 pandemic is a predisposing factor for VAP, since it often requires mechanical ventilation, thus increasing the incidence and relevance of this infection [1]. VAP frequently involves high morbidity and excessive healthcare costs, and its incidence increases with the duration of ventilation [2–4]. The role of the endotracheal tube-associated biofilms in VAP etiology has been largely discussed. Commonly, biofilms on the device surface appear rapidly after intubation, promote a global covering of the internal side, and remain attached even after suctioning [2,5]. These biofilms represent a persistent source of pathogenic bacteria that can invade the lower airways, colonizing the lungs and causing VAP [6].

Strategies for biofilm growth inhibition on the endotracheal tube (ET) surface involve mainly suction systems [7], mucus shavers [8], and antimicrobial coatings [9–12]. Regarding biofilm removal, well-established strategies were not previously described in scientific literature, and direct administration of aerosolized antibiotics [13], cationic peptides [14], and ionized gas [15] have been suggested to control mature biofilm. Nonetheless, the available methods for both inhibiting and removing biofilm are not widely effective in controlling the microorganism layers on the ET surface, and innovative approaches to treat or prevent this contamination source should be investigated.

Even though the ET colonization is polymicrobial, the aerobic nosocomial bacterium *Pseudomonas aeruginosa* has been suggested to play a dominant role in the infection etiology [5,16,17]. In addition, *P. aeruginosa* has shown an enhanced ability to form huge biofilms and to develop antibiotic resistance, which in turn can be considered factors that ensure persistent infection [18,19]. Efforts have been made to reduce complications associated with *P. aeruginosa* colonization in artificial airways; nonetheless, none of them seem to be largely effective [3,20,21].

Considering the successful use of phage therapy in the treatment of *P. aeruginosa* acute respiratory infection in animal models [22], the use of phages is a promising and challenging alternative to deal with the ET-associated biofilms, mainly those formed by antibiotic-resistant strains. The advantages of using phage therapy involve low damage to the host microbiota, ability to self-replicate in the presence of host cells, host specificity, rapid selection and characterization, and low cost [23]. Aiming at treating acute infections caused by nosocomial pathogens, Aleshkin et al. reported that intragastric administration of a phage cocktail in patients with mechanical ventilation promoted an important reduction in bacterial burden [24]. Furthermore, the anti-biofilm activity of recently characterized new phages was demonstrated in vitro in an ET-associated *P. aeruginosa* biofilm model [25]. The authors demonstrated an extensive lytic activity with multidrug-resistant *P. aeruginosa* biofilm, suggesting that the new phages might be considered as good candidates for therapeutic studies [25]. Although encouraging results have revealed the anti-biofilm effect of the phage therapy, the action of immobilized phages on the ET surface, to control biofilm development, is unclear.

Along these lines, it is essential to clarify whether phages could be used for both controlling and preventing ET-associated *P. aeruginosa* biofilm. In the present study, anti-biofilm activity of five recently characterized phages was evaluated by a high content screening assay. Subsequently, two phages were selected as cocktail components and applied as a preventive strategy to inhibit bacteria colonization in a dynamic biofilm model simulating endotracheal intubation. The null hypothesis of this study was that there is no difference in *P. aeruginosa* biofilm when challenged with bacteriophages.

2. Results

2.1. Screening Phages for Anti-Biofilm Activity

An initial screening was performed to select phages with stronger anti-biofilm activity. Biofilm-covered areas showed a significant reduction after phage treatment in 4/15 *P. aeruginosa* strains (Table S1), in which three were classified previously as multidrug-resistant [25]. Biofilm areas of four other *P. aeruginosa* strains were lower, but the difference was not significant. Even though phage infectivity had been previously determined, seven *P. aeruginosa* strains were not affected by the phage treatment. The analysis of the biofilm-covered areas indicated a statistically significant difference ($p < 0.05$) between phage-treated and control; however, statistically significant differences were not observed among the five different phages (Figure 1A). Therefore, based on the broader lytic spectrum of the phages with multidrug-resistant strains; the efficiency of plating and genomic differences, reported by Oliveira et al. [25]; and the anti-biofilm activity presented here (Figure 1B–G), the phages vB_PaeM_USP_2 and vB_PaeM_USP_18 were selected to compose a cocktail in the assays involving dynamic biofilm growth on the ET surface.

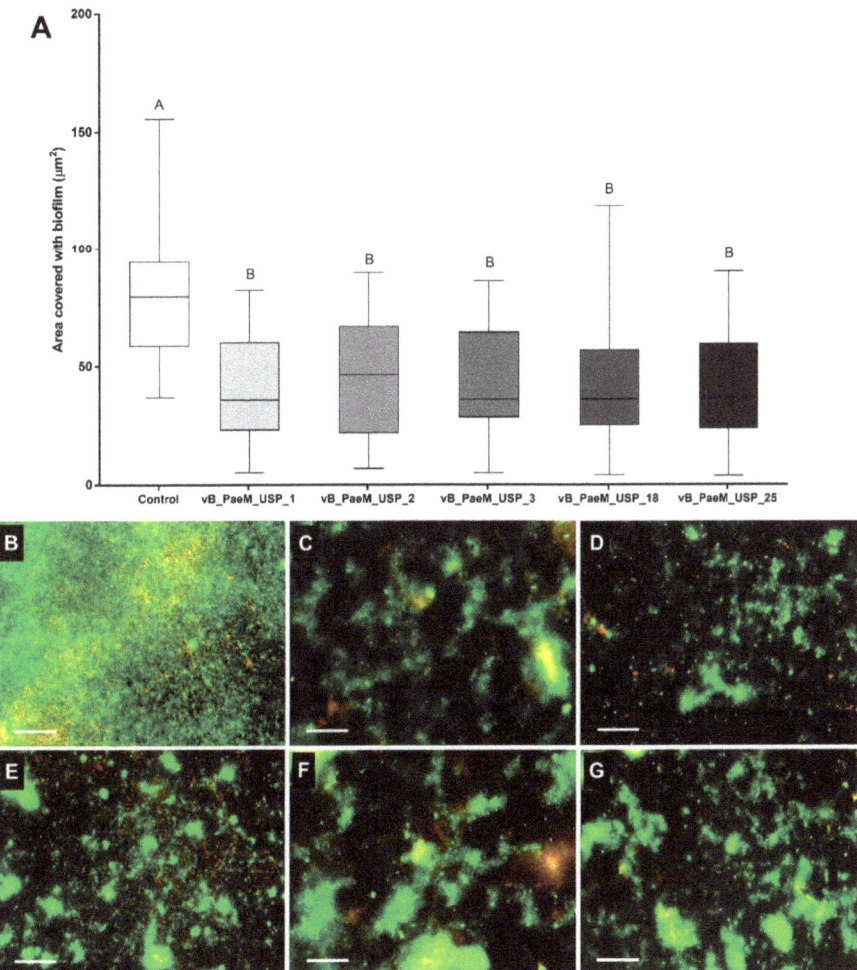

Figure 1. (**A**) Biofilm-covered areas, expressed in μm^2, after phage treatment. Comparisons were conducted among groups by means of multiple comparisons considering strains and bacteriophages in a generalized linear model with Bonferroni correction. ^{AB} Different capital letters indicate statistically significant differences ($p < 0.05$). (**B**–**G**) Representative fluorescent images of *P. aeruginosa* illustrate the control group (**B**) and the action of phages vB_PaeM_USP_1 (**C**), vB_PaeM_USP_2 (**D**), vB_PaeM_USP_3 (**E**), vB_PaeM_USP_18 (**F**), and vB_PaeM_USP_25 (**G**). Scale bar = 50 μm.

2.2. Replication of ET Adsorbed Phage During Biofilm Growth

The phage cocktail that was adsorbed to the ET clearly showed the ability to replicate, since the number of phage particles increased over time. The initial log 3 phage population (0 h) was able to replicate in the presence of the biofilm cells, increasing to log 6 at 24 h and log 8 at 48 h. After 48 up to 168 h, phage concentration remained almost constant without variations among the strains (Figure 2A–C).

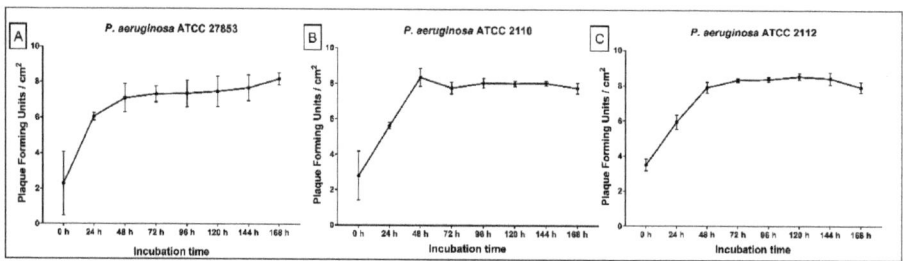

Figure 2. Phage cocktail presence on tube surfaces over 24 to 168 h of dynamic biofilm growth. (**A**) *P. aeruginosa* ATCC 27853; (**B**) *P. aeruginosa* ATCC 2110; (**C**) *P. aeruginosa* ATCC 2112.

2.3. Phage Cocktail Effect on P. aeruginosa Biofilms

The in vivo contamination of an ET was mimicked using a continuous biofilm model system. Biofilm growth rates on non-coated tubes were similar among the three strains. However, on phage-coated tubes, a different growth pattern among the strains was observed (Table S2). This outcome indicated that the cocktail's action was strain dependent. Regarding metabolic activity, phage cocktail coating did not promote substantial changes in the biofilm response. Generally, the absorbance values were lower at early stages and higher in late stages of cultivation time (Figures 3B, 4B and 5B; Table S3).

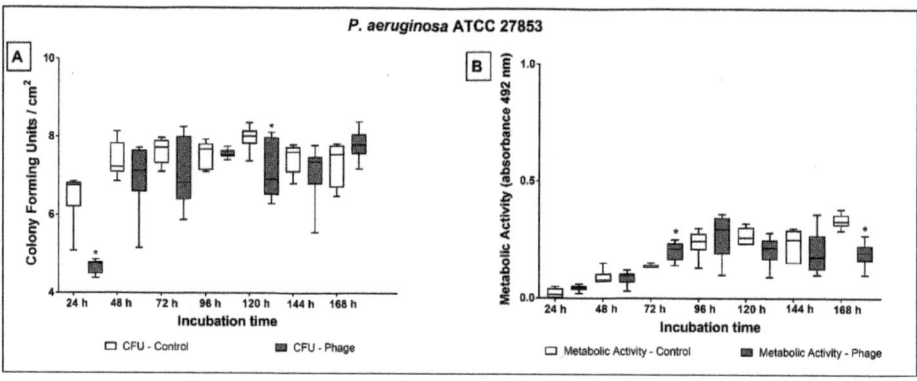

Figure 3. Biofilm growth (**A**) and metabolic activity (**B**) of *P. aeruginosa* ATCC 27853 over 24 to 168 h of dynamic biofilm growth on non-coated and phage cocktail-coated tubes. Comparisons were conducted among groups, at each time point, by means of multiple comparisons considering strains and phage cocktail treatment in a generalized linear model with Bonferroni correction. * indicates statistically significant difference at each time point ($p < 0.05$).

Comparing the CFU values, *P. aeruginosa* ATCC 27853 (Figure 3A) showed a significant reduction of the microbial load on phage cocktail-coated tubes at 24 (1.8 log; $p < 0.001$) and 120 h (0.9 log; $p = 0.035$) of treatment. Even though the CFU values at 48, 72, and 96 h of treatment indicated a slight biofilm reduction on phage cocktail-coated tubes (ranging from 0.1 to 0.6 log), the microbial load did not significantly differ from non-phage coated tubes.

In comparison to control, *P. aeruginosa* ATCC 27853 had higher metabolic activity on phage cocktail-coated tubes at 72 h and lower at 168 h of culture (Figure 3B).

Regarding *P. aeruginosa* ATCC 2110, significant reduction of the microbial load was observed only at 48 h (1 log; $p = 0.004$) of treatment (Figure 4A). The strain exhibited lower metabolic activity on phage cocktail-coated tubes at 72 h of culture in comparison to non-coated tubes (Figure 4B).

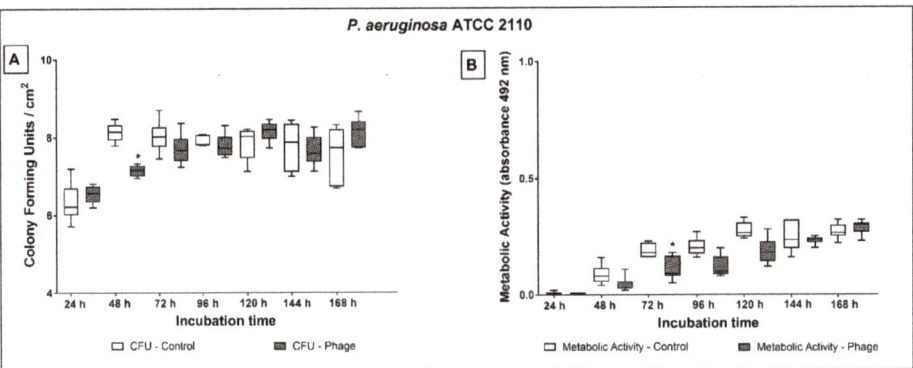

Figure 4. Biofilm growth (**A**) and metabolic activity (**B**) of *P. aeruginosa* ATCC 2110 over 24 to 168 h of dynamic biofilm growth on non-coated and phage cocktail-coated tubes. Comparisons were conducted among groups, at each time point, by means of multiple comparisons considering strains and phage cocktail treatment in a generalized linear model with Bonferroni correction. * indicates statistically significant difference at each time point ($p < 0.05$).

The reduction of *P. aeruginosa* ATCC 2112 on phage cocktail-coated tubes ranged from 1.1 to 1.8 log (Figure 5A) during the entire treatment period ($p \leq 0.001$). Nonetheless, no difference was observed in the evaluation of the metabolic activity (Figure 5B).

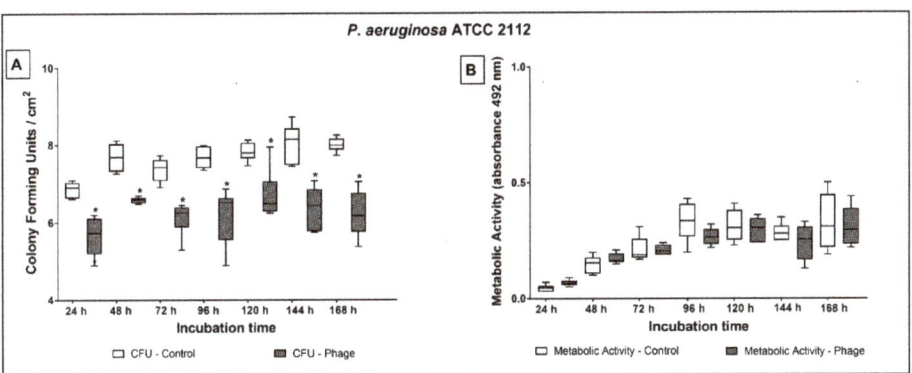

Figure 5. Biofilm growth (**A**) and metabolic activity (**B**) of *P. aeruginosa* ATCC 2112 over 24 to 168 h of dynamic biofilm growth on non-coated and phage cocktail-coated tubes. Comparisons were conducted among groups, at each time point, by means of multiple comparisons considering strains and phage cocktail treatment in a generalized linear model with Bonferroni correction. * indicates statistically significant difference at each time point ($p < 0.05$).

SEM representative biofilm images of *P. aeruginosa* ATCC 2112 for all the cultivation times are shown in Figure 6. The microscopy images of phage cocktail-coated tubes were morphologically distinct from non-phage coated ones. A higher concentration of biofilm cells was noticed covering the tube surface in the control, while tower-like structures could be observed on phage cocktail-coated tubes. In the control tubes, the biofilm grew like a homogeneous layer, while on coated tubes the highest number of cells was observed in the clusters. In addition, on control tubes an extracellular polymeric matrix covered the entire biofilm layer. On phage cocktail-coated tubes, the extracellular polymeric matrix was detected as merely covering the tower-like structures, while in the surrounding areas less matrix and fewer isolated bacteria could be observed during the entire cultivation time.

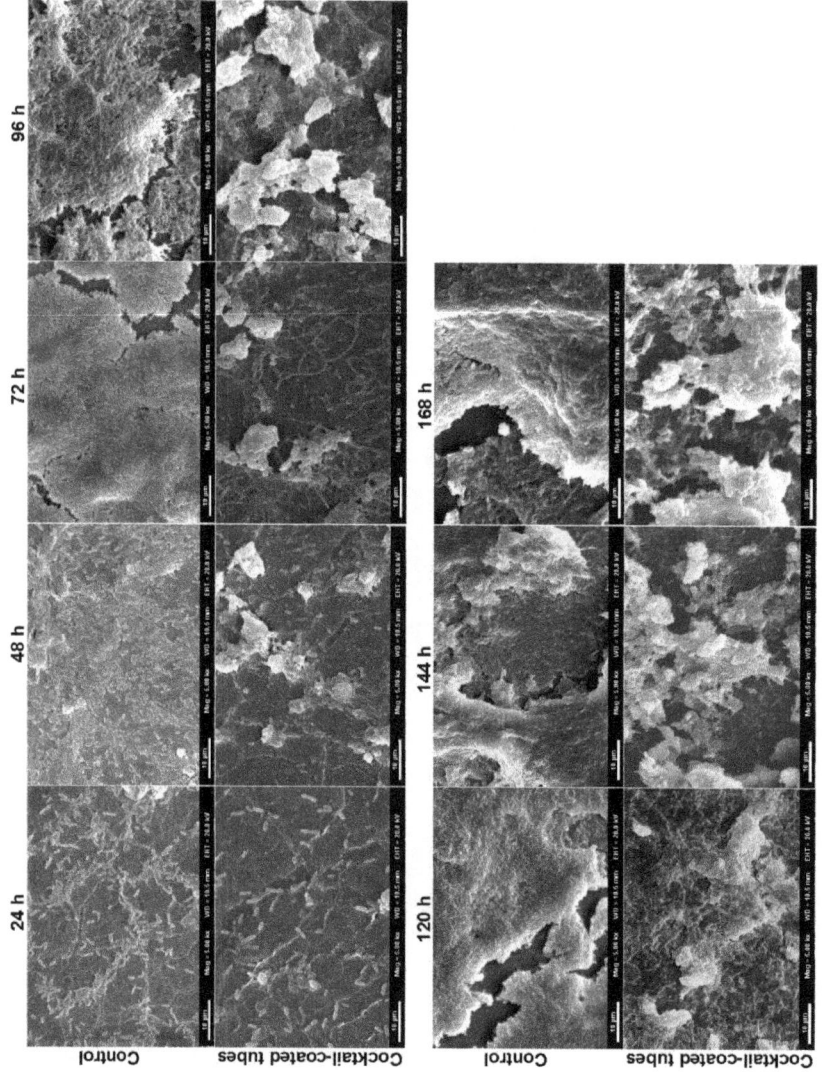

Figure 6. Representative scanning electron micrographs of non-coated (control) and phage cocktail-coated tubes at 24, 48, 72, 96, 120, 144, and 168 h of dynamic biofilm growth. Scale bar = 10 μm.

3. Discussion

In the current study, we assessed whether a phage treatment could efficiently reduce ET-associated biofilm. Firstly, the action of five different phages in a mature biofilm was evaluated. Subsequently, considering the lytic spectrum with multidrug-resistant strains, anti-biofilm screenings, and different efficiency of plating (EOP), two phages were selected as cocktail components and were applied as a strategy to prevent bacterial colonization and biofilm formation. Based on the results, the null hypothesis was rejected, since there were statistical differences for *P. aeruginosa* ET-associated biofilms.

According to biofilm-covered areas, our results demonstrated that phages applied solely exhibited effective anti-biofilm activity against a variety of *P. aeruginosa* strains. Nonetheless, biofilm-covered areas of seven *P. aeruginosa* strains remained unaffected when challenged with phages. Such an observation is in line with another in vitro study that showed varying degrees of biofilm disruption after phage treatment [22] and may be explained by the following reasons: (I) The efficiency of plating of the evaluated phages on five of these strains was considered low according to previously reported data [25]; (II) The antiviral mechanisms developed by the bacteria against phage adsorption, infection, and replication. The bacterial resistance systems have been extensively discussed in the scientific literature [26,27]; (III) Both treatment period and phage dosing might have been insufficient. According to Abedon, elimination of biofilms using phage therapy can require long treatment periods as well as repeated dosing [28]. Here, a single dose and treatment time was evaluated; and (IV) Staining methods and imaging tools have been considered useful for quantitative assessment and spatial structure visualization of biofilm; however, they can also result in misinterpretation of data due to laser penetration, absorption of the dye into the biomass, and auto-fluorescence [29,30]. LIVE/DEAD staining comprises two types of fluorescent stains, which differ in ability to penetrate viable and non-viable bacterial cells [31]. Here, the biofilm-covered areas were calculated according to total image fluorescence. It is known that cell concentration in biofilms can be distributed differently according to their thickness. Our image series may not have precisely recorded the biofilm density, which could in part explain unapparent anti-biofilm effects. Since agar plate counts detect all cultivable cells, the conflicting phage anti-biofilm results, reported by Oliveira et al., could be explained by the method used. The authors demonstrated superior phage anti-biofilm activity, against the same strains, by using colony forming unit counts [25]. Therefore, we consider that additional quantitative methods involving the determination of the number of viable cells by agar plate counts, flow-based cell counting, and assessment of biofilm dry mass or total protein content could lead to efficient determination of the biofilm density.

After describing the phage isolated action, a cocktail composed of vB_PaeM_USP_2 and vB_PaeM_USP_18 was investigated as an additional strategy for biofilm control on the ET surface. We hypothesized that surface coating using multiple phage strains prevents bacterial colonization considering that these two phages have different EOP, distinct lytic spectra with multidrug-resistant strains, and considerable genetic differences that could potentially lead them to bind to different receptors [32].

Efforts have been made to propose methods for phage coating in medical devices [33–35]. For indwelling urological devices, the phage-coating is usually obtained by physical adsorption [33,36] and hydrogel conjugation [34,37,38]. The ETs used in this study were manufactured from reinforced polyvinyl chloride (PVC), and the scientific literature describes neither phage immobilization on PVC surfaces nor on other devices designed for mechanical ventilation. In this sense, we allowed physical adsorption of 1×10^7 PFU/cm^2 to create an antimicrobial surface. After 24 h, the phage immobilized on the tube surface was 1×10^3 PFU/cm^2. The physical adsorption did not promote a large phage immobilization on the ET surface. We consider that the limited anti-biofilm effect, observed in the cocktail-coated tubes, was possibly due to the reduced phage attachment. It might be expected that by maximizing the density of the phages on the ET surface, an enhanced capacity to control *P. aeruginosa* growth would be reached. Even though the physical adsorption comprises a simple and cost-effective method for phage immobilization, the low coverage seems to be unsuitable for producing a largely anti-biofilm effect. In this sense, different studies have been proposed aiming at the development of functionalized surfaces to immobilize phages efficiently. For instance, Wang, Sauvageau, and Elias exhibited that on the plasma-treated polyhydroxyalkanoate surface, the immobilization of phage T4 was greater than on the non-treated surface [39]. Therefore, investigation of different technologies for attaching phages to PVC surfaces, as well as phages displaying plastic-binding peptides, should be performed to ensure a high phage concentration on the ET surface.

Although an initial high phage titer was not immobilized on the tube surface, in the presence of bacterial strains an increasing concentration was observed after 48 h of treatment, which confirmed the phages' ability to replicate and compensate for the initial low dose [40]. Additionally, the 1×10^3 PFU/cm^2 was able to produce differences of bacterial colonization. According to mean differences at each specific time point, *P. aeruginosa* ATCC 27853 and *P. aeruginosa* ATCC 2112 showed evident reduction of biofilm growth on phage cocktail-coated tubes in the early stages of biofilm formation. This result can be related to the biofilm formation stage and the amount of extracellular exopolysaccharide matrix. The scientific literature has shown that inefficiency in phage penetration in mature biofilms is an important factor affecting the tolerance to phages [28]. The initial reduction in biofilm growth could be correlated both to the exponential increase of phage titer and thinner extracellular matrix layer. After 48 h, the constant titer of phages supports the idea that the thicker extracellular matrix could have hindered phage adsorption. On the other hand, a similar pattern was not observed for *P. aeruginosa* ATCC 2112, which exhibited a reduction of biofilm growth during the entire cultivation time. This distinct response can be associated with the metabolic activity of *P. aeruginosa* ATCC 2112. In comparison to *P. aeruginosa* ATCC 27853 and *P. aeruginosa* ATCC 2110, XTT assay revealed high absorbance values for *P. aeruginosa* ATCC 2112. As phages require metabolically active hosts to replicate [41], the cocktail could have more effectively infected this strain. In general, the lowest metabolic activity was observed for *P. aeruginosa* ATCC 2110, which exhibited reduction in biofilm growth only at 48 h. Taken together, these findings suggest that *P. aeruginosa* ATCC 2110 exhibits antiviral mechanisms that result in a phage-insensitive phenotype. Blocking of phage receptors, production of competitive inhibitors, prevention of bacteriophage DNA entry, slicing of bacteriophage nucleic acids, CRISPR/cas system activation, and abortive infection mechanisms are well-known bacterial resistance systems against phage infection [26,27].

The synthetic sputum medium used promotes the formation of *P. aeruginosa* aggregates with sizes similar to those observed in human cystic fibrosis lung tissue [42]. Here, however, coated and non-coated ETs had differences regarding distribution of aggregates. We suggest two different reasons to explain the formation of *P. aeruginosa* aggregates. First, on coated tubes, the formation of large bacterial aggregates, observed in SEM images, seemed to be a protection mechanism against phage invasion as it became more evident in the mature biofilms when phages reached the highest titer. Second, we speculate that this phenomenon may be caused not by the overgrowth of bacteria in some regions but by the lysis of cells by the phage cocktail causing holes on the biofilm. Structures similar to those observed here were also reported by Henriksen et al., who classified them as a defense strategy against phage infection [43]. According to the authors, the continuous phage exposure affected the biofilm growth by stimulating the formation of a highly organized and spatially heterogeneous structure.

Our results did not provide evidence regarding the different phage infection behavior of antibiotic sensitive and resistant strains. Phages have the demonstrated ability to infect both sensitive and multidrug-resistant *P. aeruginosa*. Loc-Carrillo and Abedon pointed out that resistance mechanisms against antibiotics do not affect phage infection [23]. Our results corroborate the author's statement and indicate that phage therapy could be applied as an auxiliary method to treat infections caused by resistant bacteria. Moreover, recombinant phage-encoded enzymes could be applied directly to the tube surface as an alternative to direct phage usage.

The relevance of the present study highlights the urgent need to investigate new therapeutic strategies to control *P. aeruginosa* biofilms on the ET surface. The intubation period through an ET for ≥ 8 days represents a risk factor for VAP occurrences [4]. Here, we demonstrated that phage therapy can reduce bacterial bioburden on the ET surface and therefore might contribute to reducing VAP episodes. Nonetheless, in view of the discrepant titers applied to both strategies in the study, biofilm treatment and biofilm prevention, we were unable to determine whether the phages would be more efficient in the treatment or prophylaxis of *P. aeruginosa* biofilms. Indeed, challenges and limitations of phage therapy are evident, and the scientific literature has reported that the therapeutic or prophylactic use of phages is dependent on the application area. For instance, in the food industry, prophylactic phage administration represents a promising sustainable solution to control pathogenic bacteria and reduce the massive use of antibiotics. In this field, phages are mainly used during food production, sanitization, and preservation [44]. For both animal and human infection treatment, the therapeutic use of phages and phage-encoded enzymes, alone or in combination with antibiotics, has aroused a growing interest in their potential use against multidrug-resistant bacteria, and different routes of administration and dosage effect have been suggested [45]. In order to reduce biofilm growth on implantable medical devices, we consider that immobilization of phages or phage-encoded products, as preventive agents, might decrease colonization more effectively than using them for biofilm removal. Thus, some issues remain and should be addressed in future studies. Experimental ventilator-associated pneumonia models and preclinical assessment would be useful to clarify if the biofilm removal/inhibition promoted by phages could prevent or reduce the severity of the VAP.

4. Materials and Methods

4.1. Bacterial Strains, Growth Conditions, and Bacteriophages

All bacterial strains used in this study are listed in Table 1. Bacteria were thawed and routinely grown in tryptic soy broth (TSB; BD Difco, Sparks, MN, USA) at 37 °C with agitation. After achieving the exponential growth phase, the culture was centrifuged (4200× g, 5 min) and washed twice in phosphate buffered saline (PBS), pH 7.4. The bacteria inoculum was prepared considering its optical density (OD$_{625 \text{ nm}}$) measured in a spectrophotometer (Thermo Scientific, Waltham, MA, USA).

Table 1. Bacterial strains used in the study.

Isolates	Source	Antibiotic Resistance *	Reference
*P. aeruginosa*_Mi_1 [†]	Blood	S	[25]
*P. aeruginosa*_Mi_2 [†]	Sputum	S	[25]
*P. aeruginosa*_Mi_6 [†]	Urine	S	[25]
*P. aeruginosa*_Mi_7 [†]	Sputum	S	[25]
*P. aeruginosa*_Ba_164 [†]	Prosthetic biofilm	S	[25]
*P. aeruginosa*_Ba_168 [†]	Prosthetic biofilm	S	[25]
*P. aeruginosa*_Ba_169 [†]	Prosthetic biofilm	S	[25]
*P. aeruginosa*_Trac_20 [†]	Tracheal secretion	S	[25]
*P. aeruginosa*_Trac_23 [†]	Tracheal secretion	S	[25]
*P. aeruginosa*_Ren_1 [†]	Saliva	S	[25]
*P. aeruginosa*_ATCC 27853 [‡]	Blood	S	[25]
*P. aeruginosa*_ATCC 2108 [‡]	Sputum	AMK, CFZ, CTX, GEN, IMP, TGC	[25]
*P. aeruginosa*_ATCC 2110 [‡]	Sputum	AMP, CFZ, CTX, FOX, NIT, TGC, SXT	[25]
*P. aeruginosa*_ATCC 2112 [‡]	Sputum	AMC, AMP, CFZ, CPD, CRO, CTX, CXM, FOX, NIT, SXT, TET, TGC,	[25]
*P. aeruginosa*_ATCC 2113 [‡]	Sputum	AMP, AMC, CFZ, CTX, NIT, SAM, SXT	[25]

[†] Human Exposome and Infectious Diseases Network collection. [‡] American Type Culture Collection. * S: Susceptible to all antimicrobial agents tested; AMC: amoxicillin-clavulanic acid; AMK: amikacin; AMP: ampicillin; CFZ: cefazolin; CPD: cefpodoxime; CRO: ceftriaxone; CTX: cefotaxime; CXM: cefuroxime; FOX: cefoxitin; GEN: gentamicin; IMP: imipenem; NIT: nitrofurantoin; SAM: ampicillin-sulbactam; SXT: trimethoprim-sulfamethoxazole; TET: tetracycline; TGC: tigecycline.

Five bacteriophages were used in this study: vB_PaeM_USP_1, vB_PaeM_USP_2, vB_PaeM_USP_3, vB_PaeM_USP_18, and vB_PaeM_USP_25. The isolation, characterization, and assessment of the lytic spectrum of the bacteriophages was described previously by Oliveira et al. [25].

4.2. Screening Phages for Anti-Biofilm Activity

The anti-biofilm activity of the bacteriophages was utilized against 10 clinical isolates and five strains from the American Type Culture Collection (ATCC; Table 1). Two hundred microliters of TSB containing standardized bacteria suspension (10^7 colony forming units per milliliter—CFU/mL) was cultured (37 °C, 75 rpm) in black 96-well plates with a flat glass bottom (Corning, New York, NY, USA). After 24 h, half of the culture medium was removed, and the biofilm was supplied with freshly prepared culture medium, then plates were incubated for another 24 h. The culture medium was then discarded, and 200 µL of sterile TSB supplemented with 10^8 plaque forming units per milliliter (PFU/mL) of bacteriophages were added to each well (6×10^5 PFU/mm^2). Culture medium without bacteriophages was used as a control. The plates were incubated for 24 h at 37 °C and 75 rpm.

To evaluate the anti-biofilm activity of the bacteriophages, the culture medium was discarded, and the wells were rinsed with 200 µL of PBS. The biofilm was stained for 15 min, protected from light, with LIVE/DEAD™ Biofilm Viability Kit (Molecular Probes, California, CA, USA) according to the manufacturer's protocol. Afterwards, the plates were scanned, and images were randomly collected (considering peripheral and central regions) with an Operetta CLS High-Content imaging system (PerkinElmer Waltham, MA, USA) at 40× magnification with 15 fields of view/well. The biofilm-covered areas (µm^2) were then analyzed using Harmony High Content Imaging and Analysis Software (PerkinElmer, Version 4.8, MA, USA). The assay was conducted in triplicate.

4.3. Phage Cocktail Pretreatment of Endotracheal Tube Surfaces

Under sterile conditions, the two ends of the ET (8.5 mm diameter, 300 mm length; Rüsh, Meridian, MS, USA) were removed to allow its connection to the tubing of the dynamic biofilm system. A phage cocktail containing 4×10^7 (PFU/mL) of vB_PaeM_USP_2 and vB_PaeM_USP_18 was prepared in elution buffer (SM) (1 M Tris HCl pH 7.5, Sigma-Aldrich, Saint Louis, MO, USA; 8 mM MgSO$_4$, Sigma-Aldrich; 100 mM NaCl, Dinâmica, Indaiatuba, SP, Brazil; 0.002% (*w/v*) gelatin, Dinâmica). Seventeen milliliters of the suspension was added to the inner part of the tube. Then, the extremities were sealed, and the device was maintained under static conditions for 24 h at room temperature. This step was employed to allow phage adsorption to the ET surface. Afterwards, the suspension was discarded, and the tube was rinsed with SM buffer in order to remove unbound phages [33]. Two fragments of 1 cm^2 were removed from the tube to assess the presence of bacteriophages, and the flow system was mounted under sterile conditions, as demonstrated in Figure 7.

4.4. Developing Biofilms on Endotracheal Tube Pretreated with the Phage Cocktail

Three *P. aeruginosa* strains (ATCC 27853, ATCC 2110, and ATCC 2112) were selected for this assay. The strains ATCC 2110 (resistant to ampicillin, cefazolin, cefotaxime, cefoxitin, nitrofurantoin, trimethoprim-sulfamethoxazole, and tetracycline) and ATCC 2112 (resistant to amoxicillin-clavulanic acid, ampicillin, cefazolin, cefpodoxime, ceftriaxone, cefotaxime, cefuroxime, cefoxitin, nitrofurantoin, trimethoprim-sulfamethoxazole tetracycline, and tigecycline) were chosen due to their multidrug-resistant characteristics. The strain ATCC 27853 was selected due to the absence of antibiotic resistance. Each strain was evaluated solely in triplicate.

To simulate in vivo conditions, SCFM2 artificial sputum medium (4 g DNA salmon sperm, GoldBio, St Louis, MO, USA; 5 g swine stomach mucin, Sigma-Aldrich; 5 g casamino acids, Difco; 5.9 mg diethylenetriamine pentaacetic acid, Sigma-Aldrich; 5 g NaCl, Dynamic; 2.2 g KCl, Dynamic; 5 mL egg yolk emulsion; and 1000 mL distilled water, pH = 6.9) that mimics a cystic fibrosis model was employed [42]. After connecting to the flow system, phage cocktail-coated and non-coated tubes were supplied with a continuous flow of SCFM2 culture medium inoculated with 1×10^5 CFU/mL of *P. aeruginosa* strains for 24 h. After 24 up to 168 h, the system was supplied with sterile SCFM2 culture medium without recirculation [33].

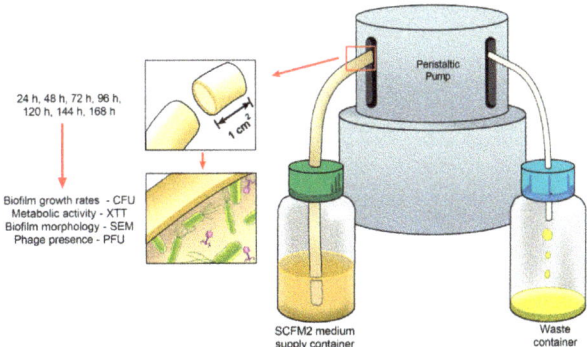

Figure 7. Schematic representation of the dynamic biofilm system showing that biofilm growth was monitored over 24 up to 168 h for colony forming units, metabolic activity, and biofilm morphology. Phage titer was also assessed during the entire cultivation time.

4.5. Analysis of the Phage Cocktail Effect on P. aeruginosa Biofilms

The phage cocktail's ability to prevent ET colonization was determined by means of biofilm growth rates (CFU/cm^2), metabolic activity of the biofilm (XTT), and scanning electron microscopy (SEM) at 24, 48, 72, 96, 120, 144, and 168 h under dynamic conditions. Therefore, at each time point, two fragments of 1 cm^2 of each tube (n = 3) were removed for CFU counts (n = 6) and XTT assessment (n = 6). For biofilm morphology evaluation (SEM), one representative fragment was processed. The CFU and XTT methodology were performed as described previously by Oliveira et al. [25].

For CFU quantification, each fragment was transferred to a tube containing 10 mL of phosphate buffered saline (PBS). The tubes were vortexed for 60 s, sonicated (200 W, 40 kHz; Altsonic, Clean 9CA, Ribeirão Preto, SP, Brazil) for 20 min and vortexed again for 2 min to ensure detachment of all aggregated biofilm. Ten-fold dilution aliquots were seeded in tryptic soy agar (BD Difco) and incubated at 37 °C for 24 h. The number of colonies was registered and expressed as $\log_{10}$CFU/cm^2.

For the evaluation of metabolic activity, the strains were transferred to 24-well plates containing: 948 µL PBS supplemented with 100 mM glucose (Sigma-Aldrich), 240 µL XTT 1 mg/mL (Sigma-Aldrich), and 12 µL 0.4 mM menadione (Sigma-Aldrich). The plates were incubated, protected from light at 37 °C for 2 h, and the OD$_{492\,\text{nm}}$ of the resulting solution was measured in triplicate. The mean of the readings was calculated subtracting the background absorbance.

For SEM analysis, the fragments were fixed with 2.5% glutaraldehyde (v/v) for 24 h and then dehydrated in a graded ethanol series (30%, 50%, 70%, 90%, and 100% (v/v)). After chemical drying using hexamethyldisilazane (Sigma-Aldrich), the specimens were mounted on an aluminum specimen holder and gold coated. The surface morphology of the biofilms was examined at a magnification of 3000× under high vacuum with a scanning electron microscope (EVO 10, CARL ZEISS, Jena, Germany).

4.6. Replication of ET Adsorbed Phage During Biofilm Growth

The replication (infection ability) of phages from the cocktail that were adsorbed on the ET surface was confirmed, at all the time points (from 0 to 168 h), by double-layer-agar plating (tryptic soy agar soft (0.8% agar)—TSAS; BD Difco) [46]. In brief, the suspension employed for CFU quantification was centrifuged and diluted in SM buffer (10^0–10^{-6}). Ten microliters were dropped onto a TSAS medium, with *P. aeruginosa* lawns, and incubated at 37 °C for 24 h. After the incubation period, the phage titer (PFU/mL) was determined by the number of phage plaques observable on the TSAS.

4.7. Statistical Analysis

The adherence of the data to normal distribution (Shapiro–Wilk test) and homogeneous variance (Levene test) was tested. The data set did not exhibit normal distribution and were analyzed by multiple comparisons considering strains and bacteriophages, at specific time points, in a generalized linear model with Bonferroni correction. Comparisons among time points were not conducted in view of significantly phenotypic changes in biofilm growth. The statistical tests were performed through the IBM SPSS Statistics 25.0 software (IBM Corp Armonk, NY, USA). The significance level was set to 0.05.

5. Conclusions

This study is the first step toward enhancing our understanding of biofilm growth in phage-coated ETs. The observed reduction depicts a favorable result but is not enough, suggesting that phages may be used not as an alternative but as a complementary strategy to control biofilms on ET, which can be improved with a better immobilization method. Since this low number of adherent phages caused significant changes in treatment, even better results are expected with an increased immobilization method. Furthermore, special attention should be paid to the potential development of phage resistance mechanisms, since over time phage treatment favors phage-insensitive phenotype development.

Supplementary Materials: The following are available online at https://www.mdpi.com/2079-6382/10/1/78/s1, Table S1: Biofilm-covered areas (μm^2) of *Pseudomonas aeruginosa* strains after 24 h in the presence of five different bacteriophages. Table S2: Colony forming units ($\log_{10}CFU/cm^2$) of different *Pseudomonas aeruginosa* strains after 24, 48, 72, 96, 120, 144, and 168 h of culture in continuous flow, on the surface of endotracheal tubes, in the presence and absence of bacteriophage cocktail. Table S3: Metabolic activity (absorbance at 492 nm) of different *Pseudomonas aeruginosa* strains after 24, 48, 72, 96, 120, 144, and 168 h of culture in continuous flow, on the surface of endotracheal tubes, in the presence and absence of bacteriophage cocktail.

Author Contributions: Conceptualization, V.C.O. and E.W.; data curation, C.H.S.-L., H.F.O.P. and D.A.; formal analysis, A.P.M. and P.R.S.H.; funding acquisition, E.W.; investigation, V.C.O.; methodology, V.C.O. and A.P.M.; project administration, E.W.; supervision, E.W.; validation, L.D.R.M. and S.B.S.; visualization, L.D.R.M. and S.B.S.; writing—original draft, V.C.O.; writing—review and editing, E.W., C.H.S.-L., H.F.O.P., L.D.R.M. and S.B.S. All authors have read and agreed to the published version of the manuscript.

Funding: This work was supported by the São Paulo Research Foundation (FAPESP) under the grants 2018/09757-0, 2019/13271-9 and 2020/03405-5, as well as the National Council for Scientific and Technological Development (CNPq) under the grant 405622/2018-0.

Conflicts of Interest: The authors declare no conflict of interest.

References

1. Francois, B.; Laterre, P.-F.; Luyt, C.-E.; Chastre, J. The challenge of ventilator-associated pneumonia diagnosis in COVID-19 patients. *Crit. Care* **2020**, *24*, 289. [CrossRef] [PubMed]
2. Fernández-Barat, L.; Torres, A. Biofilms in ventilator-associated pneumonia. *Futur. Microbiol.* **2016**, *11*, 1599–1610. [CrossRef] [PubMed]
3. Diaconu, O.; Siriopol, I.; Poloșanu, L.I.; Grigoraș, I. Endotracheal Tube Biofilm and its Impact on the Pathogenesis of Ventilator-Associated Pneumonia. *J. Crit. Care Med.* **2018**, *4*, 50–55. [CrossRef] [PubMed]
4. De Souza, P.R.; De Andrade, D.; Cabral, D.B.; Watanabe, E. Endotracheal tube biofilm and ventilator-associated pneumonia with mechanical ventilation. *Microsc. Res. Tech.* **2014**, *77*, 305–312. [CrossRef] [PubMed]
5. Danin, P.-É.; Girou, E.; Legrand, P.; Louis, B.; Fodil, R.; Christov, C.; Devaquet, J.; Isabey, D.; Brochard, L. Description and Microbiology of Endotracheal Tube Biofilm in Mechanically Ventilated Subjects. *Respir. Care* **2014**, *60*, 21–29. [CrossRef] [PubMed]

6. Bassi, G.L.; Fernandez-Barat, L.; Saucedo, L.; Giunta, V.; Martí, J.D.; Ranzani, O.T.; Xiol, E.A.; Rigol, M.; Roca, I.; Muñoz, L.; et al. Endotracheal tube biofilm translocation in the lateral Trendelenburg position. *Crit. Care* **2015**, *19*, 12–59. [CrossRef] [PubMed]
7. Coppadoro, A.; Bellani, G.; Bronco, A.; Lucchini, A.; Bramati, S.; Zambelli, V.; Marcolin, R.; Pesenti, A. The use of a novel cleaning closed suction system reduces the volume of secretions within the endotracheal tube as assessed by micro-computed tomography: A randomized clinical trial. *Ann. Intensiv. Care* **2015**, *5*, 1–8. [CrossRef]
8. Berra, L.; Coppadoro, A.; Bittner, E.A.; Kolobow, T.; Laquerriere, P.; Pohlmann, J.R.; Bramati, S.; Moss, J.; Pesenti, A. A clinical assessment of the Mucus Shaver: A device to keep the endotracheal tube free from secretions. *Crit. Care Med.* **2012**, *40*, 119–124. [CrossRef]
9. Berra, L.; De Marchi, L.; Yu, Z.-X.; Laquerriere, P.; Baccarelli, A.; Kolobow, T. Endotracheal Tubes Coated with Antiseptics Decrease Bacterial Colonization of the Ventilator Circuits, Lungs, and Endotracheal Tube. *Anesthesiology* **2004**, *100*, 1446–1456. [CrossRef]
10. Kollef, M.H.; Afessa, B.; Anzueto, A.; Veremakis, C.; Kerr, K.M.; Margolis, B.D.; Craven, D.E.; Roberts, P.R.; Arroliga, A.C.; Hubmayr, R.D.; et al. Silver-Coated Endotracheal Tubes and Incidence of Ventilator-Associated Pneumonia: The NASCENT randomized trial. *JAMA* **2008**, *300*, 805–813. [CrossRef]
11. Tokmaji, G.; Vermeulen, H.; Müller, M.C.A.; Kwakman, P.H.S.; Schultz, M.J.; Zaat, S.A.J. Silver-coated endotracheal tubes for prevention of ventilator-associated pneumonia in critically ill patients. *Cochrane Database Syst. Rev.* **2015**, *8*, CD009201. [CrossRef] [PubMed]
12. Ozcelik, B.; Pasic, P.; Sangwan, P.; Be, C.L.; Glattauer, V.; Thissen, H.; Boulos, R.A. Evaluation of the Novel Antimicrobial BCP3 in a Coating for Endotracheal Tubes. *ACS Omega* **2020**, *5*, 10288–10296. [CrossRef] [PubMed]
13. Adair, C.; Gorman, S.P.; Byers, L.; Jones, D.; Feron, B.; Crowe, M.; Webb, H.; McCarthy, G.; Milligan, K. Eradication of endotracheal tube biofilm by nebulised gentamicin. *Intensiv. Care Med.* **2002**, *28*, 426–431. [CrossRef] [PubMed]
14. Guillon, A.; Fouquenet, D.; Morello, E.; Henry, C.O.; Georgeault, S.; Si-Tahar, M.; Hervé, V. Treatment ofPseudomonas aeruginosaBiofilm Present in Endotracheal Tubes by Poly-L-Lysine. *Antimicrob. Agents Chemother.* **2018**, *62*, 00564-18. [CrossRef] [PubMed]
15. Ibis, F.; Ercan, U.K. Inactivation of biofilms in endotracheal tube by cold atmospheric plasma treatment for control and prevention of ventilator-associated pneumonia. *Plasma Process. Polym.* **2020**, *17*, e2000065. [CrossRef]
16. Vandecandelaere, I.; Matthijs, N.; Van Nieuwerburgh, F.; Deforce, D.; Vosters, P.; De Bus, L.; Nelis, H.J.; Depuydt, P.; Coenye, T. Assessment of Microbial Diversity in Biofilms Recovered from Endotracheal Tubes Using Culture Dependent and Independent Approaches. *PLoS ONE* **2012**, *7*, e38401. [CrossRef] [PubMed]
17. Bardes, J.M.; Waters, C.; Motlagh, H.; Wilson, A. The prevalence of oral flora in the biofilm microbiota of the endotracheal tube. *Am. Surg.* **2016**, *82*, 403–406. [CrossRef]
18. Boucher, H.W.; Talbot, G.H.; Bradley, J.S.; Edwards, J.E.; Gilbert, D.; Rice, L.B.; Scheld, M.; Spellberg, B.; Bartlett, J. Bad Bugs, No Drugs: No ESKAPE! An Update from the Infectious Diseases Society of America. *Clin. Infect. Dis.* **2009**, *48*, 1–12. [CrossRef]
19. Moradali, M.F.; Ghods, S.; Rehm, B.H. Pseudomonas aeruginosa Lifestyle: A Paradigm for Adaptation, Survival, and Persistence. *Front. Cell. Infect. Microbiol.* **2017**, *7*, 39. [CrossRef]
20. Otterbeck, A.; Hanslin, K.; Lantz, E.L.; Larsson, A.; Stålberg, J.; Lipcsey, M. Inhalation of specific anti-Pseudomonas aeruginosa IgY antibodies transiently decreases P. aeruginosa colonization of the airway in mechanically ventilated piglets. *Intensiv. Care Med. Exp.* **2019**, *7*, 21. [CrossRef]
21. Dexter, A.M.; Scott, J.B. Airway Management and Ventilator-Associated Events. *Respir. Care* **2019**, *64*, 986–993. [CrossRef] [PubMed]
22. Forti, F.; Roach, D.R.; Cafora, M.; Pasini, M.E.; Horner, D.S.; Fiscarelli, E.V.; Rossitto, M.; Cariani, L.; Briani, F.; Debarbieux, L.; et al. Design of a Broad-Range Bacteriophage Cocktail That ReducesPseudomonas aeruginosaBiofilms and Treats Acute Infections in Two Animal Models. *Antimicrob. Agents Chemother.* **2018**, *62*, 02573-17. [CrossRef] [PubMed]
23. Loc-Carrillo, C.; Abedon, S.T. Pros and cons of phage therapy. *Bacteriophage* **2011**, *1*, 111–114. [CrossRef] [PubMed]
24. Aleshkin, A.V.; Ershova, O.N.; Volozhantsev, N.V.; Svetoch, E.A.; Popova, A.V.; Rubalskii, E.O.; Borzilov, A.I.; Aleshkin, V.A.; Afanas'Ev, S.S.; Karaulov, A.V.; et al. Phagebiotics in treatment and prophylaxis of healthcare-associated infections. *Bacteriophage* **2016**, *6*, e1251379. [CrossRef] [PubMed]
25. Oliveira, V.C.; Bim, F.L.; Monteiro, R.M.; Macedo, A.P.; Santos, E.S.; Silva-Lovato, C.H.; Paranhos, H.F.O.; Melo, L.D.R.; Santos, S.B.; Watanabe, E. Identification and Characterization of New Bacteriophages to Control Multidrug-Resistant Pseudomonas aeruginosa Biofilm on Endotracheal Tubes. *Front. Microbiol.* **2020**, *11*, 580779. [CrossRef]
26. Labrie, S.J.; Samson, J.E.; Moineau, S. Bacteriophage resistance mechanisms. *Nat. Rev. Genet.* **2010**, *8*, 317–327. [CrossRef] [PubMed]
27. Seed, K.D. Battling Phages: How Bacteria Defend against Viral Attack. *PLOS Pathog.* **2015**, *11*, e1004847. [CrossRef]
28. Abedon, S.T. Bacteriophage exploitation of bacterial biofilms: Phage preference for less mature targets? *FEMS Microbiol. Lett.* **2016**, *363*, fnv246. [CrossRef]
29. Azeredo, J.; Azevedo, N.F.; Briandet, R.; Cerca, N.; Coenye, T.; Costa, A.R.; Desvaux, M.; Di Bonaventura, G.; Hébraud, M.; Jaglic, Z.; et al. Critical review on biofilm methods. *Crit. Rev. Microbiol.* **2017**, *43*, 313–351. [CrossRef]

30. Magana, M.; Sereti, C.; Ioannidis, A.; Mitchell, C.A.; Ball, A.R.; Magiorkinis, E.; Chatzipanagiotou, M.S.; Hamblin, M.R.; Hadjifrangiskou, M.; Tegos, G.P. Options and Limitations in Clinical Investigation of Bacterial Biofilms. *Clin. Microbiol. Rev.* **2018**, *31*, e00084-16. [CrossRef]
31. Chan, B.K.; Abedon, S.T.; Loc-Carrillo, C. Phage cocktails and the future of phage therapy. *Futur. Microbiol.* **2013**, *8*, 769–783. [CrossRef] [PubMed]
32. Cademartiri, R.; Anany, H.; Gross, I.; Bhayani, R.; Griffiths, M.; Brook, M.A. Immobilization of bacteriophages on modified silica particles. *Biomaterials* **2010**, *31*, 1904–1910. [CrossRef]
33. Melo, L.D.R.; Veiga, P.; Cerca, N.; Kropinski, A.M.; Almeida, C.; Azeredo, J.; Sillankorva, S. Development of a Phage Cocktail to Control Proteus mirabilis Catheter-associated Urinary Tract Infections. *Front. Microbiol.* **2016**, *7*, 1024. [CrossRef]
34. Milo, S.; Hathaway, H.; Nzakizwanayo, J.; Alves, D.R.; Esteban, P.P.; Jones, B.V.; Jenkins, A.T.A. Prevention of encrustation and blockage of urinary catheters by Proteus mirabilis via pH-triggered release of bacteriophage. *J. Mater. Chem. B* **2017**, *5*, 5403–5411. [CrossRef] [PubMed]
35. Leppänen, M.; Maasilta, I.J.; Sundberg, L.-R. Antibacterial Efficiency of Surface-Immobilized Flavobacterium-Infecting Bacteriophage. *ACS Appl. Bio Mater.* **2019**, *2*, 4720–4727. [CrossRef]
36. Hosseinidoust, Z.; Van De Ven, T.G.M.; Tufenkji, N. Bacterial Capture Efficiency and Antimicrobial Activity of Phage-Functionalized Model Surfaces. *Langmuir* **2011**, *27*, 5472–5480. [CrossRef]
37. Fu, W.; Forster, T.; Mayer, O.; Curtin, J.J.; Lehman, S.M.; Donlan, R.M. Bacteriophage Cocktail for the Prevention of Biofilm Formation by Pseudomonas aeruginosa on Catheters in an In Vitro Model System. *Antimicrob. Agents Chemother.* **2009**, *54*, 397–404. [CrossRef] [PubMed]
38. Lehman, S.M.; Donlan, R. Bacteriophage-Mediated Control of a Two-Species Biofilm Formed by Microorganisms Causing Catheter-Associated Urinary Tract Infections in anIn VitroUrinary Catheter Model. *Antimicrob. Agents Chemother.* **2014**, *59*, 1127–1137. [CrossRef]
39. Wang, C.; Sauvageau, D.; Elias, A.L. Immobilization of Active Bacteriophages on Polyhydroxyalkanoate Surfaces. *ACS Appl. Mater. Interfaces* **2016**, *8*, 1128–1138. [CrossRef]
40. Nilsson, A.S. Pharmacological limitations of phage therapy. *Upsala J. Med Sci.* **2019**, *124*, 218–227. [CrossRef]
41. Pearl, S.; Gabay, C.; Kishony, R.; Oppenheim, A.; Balaban, N.Q. Nongenetic Individuality in the Host–Phage Interaction. *PLoS Biol.* **2008**, *6*, e120. [CrossRef] [PubMed]
42. Darch, S.E.; Kragh, K.N.; Abbott, E.A.; Bjarnsholt, T.; Bull, J.J.; Whiteley, M. Phage Inhibit Pathogen Dissemination by Targeting Bacterial Migrants in a Chronic Infection Model. *mBio* **2017**, *8*, e00240-17. [CrossRef] [PubMed]
43. Henriksen, K.; Rørbo, N.; Rybtke, M.L.; Martinet, M.G.; Tolker-Nielsen, T.; Høiby, N.; Middelboe, M.; Ciofu, O.P. aeruginosa flow-cell biofilms are enhanced by repeated phage treatments but can be eradicated by phage–ciprofloxacin combination. *Pathog. Dis.* **2019**, *77*, ftz011. [CrossRef] [PubMed]
44. Połaska, M.; Sokołowska, B. Bacteriophages—a new hope or a huge problem in the food industry. *AIMS Microbiol.* **2019**, *5*, 324–346. [CrossRef]
45. Melo, L.D.R.; Oliveira, H.; Pires, D.; Dąbrowska, K.; Azeredo, J. Phage therapy efficacy: A review of the last 10 years of preclinical studies. *Crit. Rev. Microbiol.* **2020**, *46*, 78–99. [CrossRef]
46. Sambrook, J.; Russell, D.W. *Molecular Cloning: A Laboratory Manual*; Cold Spring Harbor Laboratory Press: New York, NY, USA, 2001.

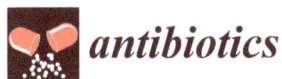

Article

Phytochemical Composition and In Vitro Biological Activity of *Iris* spp. (Iridaceae): A New Source of Bioactive Constituents for the Inhibition of Oral Bacterial Biofilms

Lan Hoang [1], František Beneš [2], Marie Fenclová [2], Olga Kronusová [1,3], Viviana Švarcová [1], Kateřina Řehořová [1], Eva Baldassarre Švecová [4], Miroslav Vosátka [4], Jana Hajšlová [2], Petr Kaštánek [3], Jitka Viktorová [1,*] and Tomáš Ruml [1]

1. Department of Biochemistry and Microbiology UCT Prague, Faculty of Food and Biochemical Technology, Technická 3, 166 28 Prague, Czech Republic; hoangl@vscht.cz (L.H.); kronusova@ecofuel.cz (O.K.); fuchsovv@vscht.cz (V.Š.); rehorova@vscht.cz (K.Ř.); rumlt@vscht.cz (T.R.)
2. Department of Food Analysis and Nutrition UCT Prague, Faculty of Food and Biochemical Technology, Technická 3, 166 28 Prague, Czech Republic; benesfr@vscht.cz (F.B.); fenclovm@vscht.cz (M.F.); hajslovj@vscht.cz (J.H.)
3. EcoFuel Laboratories Ltd., Ocelářská 9, 190 00 Praha, Czech Republic; kastanek@ecofuel.cz
4. Institute of Botany of the Czech Academy of Sciences, Zámek 1, 252 43 Průhonice, Czech Republic; eva.svecova@ibot.cas.cz (E.B.Š.); miroslav.vosatka@ibot.cas.cz (M.V.)
* Correspondence: prokesoj@vscht.cz

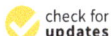

Received: 16 June 2020; Accepted: 8 July 2020; Published: 11 July 2020

Abstract: The inhibition and eradication of oral biofilms is increasingly focused on the use of plant extracts as mouthwashes and toothpastes adjuvants. Here, we report on the chemical composition and the antibiofilm activity of 15 methanolic extracts of *Iris* species against both mono-(*Pseudomonas aeruginosa*, *Staphylococcus aureus*) and multi-species oral biofilms (*Streptococcus gordonii*, *Veillonella parvula*, *Fusobacterium nucleatum* subsp. *nucleatum*, and *Actinomyces naeslundii*). The phytochemical profiles of *Iris pallida* s.l., *Iris versicolor* L., *Iris lactea* Pall., *Iris carthaliniae* Fomin, and *Iris germanica* were determined by ultra-high performance liquid chromatography-high-resolution tandem mass spectroscopy (UHPLC-HRMS/MS) analysis, and a total of 180 compounds were identified among *Iris* species with (iso)flavonoid dominancy. *I. pallida*, *I. versicolor*, and *I. germanica* inhibited both the quorum sensing and adhesion during biofilm formation in a concentration-dependent manner. However, the extracts were less active against maturated biofilms. Of the five tested species, *Iris pallida* s.l. was the most effective at both inhibiting biofilm formation and disrupting existing biofilms, and the leaf extract exhibited the strongest inhibitory effect compared to the root and rhizome extracts. The cytotoxicity of the extracts was excluded in human fibroblasts. The inhibition of bacterial adhesion significantly correlated with myristic acid content, and quorum sensing inhibition correlated with the 7-β-hydroxystigmast-4-en-3-one content. These findings could be useful for establishing an effective tool for the control of oral biofilms and thus dental diseases.

Keywords: biofilm; dental plaque; quorum sensing; microbial resistance

1. Introduction

Bacterial biofilms, communities of microorganisms in a self-produced extracellular polymeric substance matrix, cause more than 60% of human microbial infections [1]. Changes in gene expression and the activation of numerous extracellular communication pathways during biofilm formation often lead to an increase in pathogenicity and overall virulence activity. Startlingly, the antimicrobial resistance of a biofilm can be up to a thousandfold higher than that of free planktonic biota [2].

Quorum sensing (QS) is known as a cell–cell communication pathway that initiates and regulates various physiological activities such as biofilm formation, bioluminescence, and virulence production. Both Gram-positive and Gram-negative bacteria use QS for communication, but they produce distinct signal molecules (autoinducers): N-acyl homoserine lacton (AHL) molecules (autoinducer-1, AI-1) are mainly used by Gram-negative bacteria, while Gram-positive bacteria predominantly use modified oligopeptides (autoinducer peptides, AIP or QS peptides). Another type of signal molecules is autoinducer-2 (AI-2), which are derived from boron-furan and found in both Gram-negative and Gram-positive bacteria. In addition, there is also a fourth class of miscellaneous QS molecules. These QS molecules are not only responsible for inter-kingdom communication, but are possibly also involved in the direct or indirect cross-talk between microorganisms and their environment. Thus, the idea of using antimicrobials, which interfere with the microorganism's QS mechanism, has been a novel antipathogenic method for inhibiting biofilm formation with minimal side effects that is also non-toxic to the host [3].

An oral biofilm contains hundreds of different oral bacteria that may cause serious diseases within the oral cavity. Furthermore, the virulence in response to drastic changes in the biofilm microenvironment can be spread systemically and may induce significant infections in other organs [4]. The presence of *Staphylococcus aureus* in a supra- and subgingival biofilm can induce periodontitis [5], while *Pseudomonas aeruginosa* from a subgingival biofilm may be responsible for a more aggressive form of periodontitis [6]. Dental plaque, consisting of both Gram-positive and Gram-negative bacteria such as *Streptococcus gordonii* and *Fusobacterium nucleatum*, is able to adhere to tooth surfaces, proliferate, and produce lactic acid, causing the demineralization of dental enamel and dentine.

Limitations of conventional antibiotic therapy as well as increasing drug resistance have led to the urgent need for alternative approaches to deal with oral biofilm-related infections. In this context, the use of biologically active plant extracts as antibiotic adjuvants has been of great interest over the last few decades for exhibiting broad biological activities [7]. E.g., various extracts of *Vitis vinifera* have been shown to eradicate oral microorganisms via various mechanisms, including enzyme inhibition, cell wall disruption, and QS inhibition [8,9]. Other studies revealed a high antimicrobial efficacy of *Coffea canephora* [10,11], green tea [12], and *Chesneya nubigena (D. Don) Ali* [13]. Despite these pioneering works and promising results, the antimicrobial potential of a wide range of plants remains to be explored.

Iris spp. is the largest genus of the Iridaceae family and is one of the most important genera of flowering plants, with a rich diversity growing in the territories of Eurasia and North America. The species of this genus have been used in traditional medicine. Due to its rich diversity, the genus *Iris* represents a reservoir of valuable species not only for cultivation purposes, but also as a source of biologically active substances. A broad range of secondary metabolites isolated from *Iris* spp. have exhibited numerous biological activities such as antibacterial, antioxidant, anti-inflammatory, anti-cancer, and immuno-modulatory [14–22]. However, a literature review revealed that there is very limited information about the anti-biofilm activity of *Iris* plants, especially against oral biofilms.

Here, we report on the phytochemical composition and the *in vitro* effect of extracts from five *Iris* spp. on the adherence and disruption of oral microbial biofilms. Moreover, their mechanisms of action against the virulence factors of oral bacteria are described. Given that these bacteria express distinct QS autoinducers that play important roles in the development of virulence factors, we also investigated the effect of *Iris* spp. on the QS communication pathway and provide an additional theoretical basis for its application.

2. Materials and Methods

2.1. Plant Materials and Preparation of Extracts

The different tissues of *Iris* plants (leaves, roots, rhizomes) used in this study were collected from the field collection in the Botanical garden of the Institute of Botany, Czech Republic (July 2018).

Taxonomic identification of the plant materials was confirmed by Dr. Z. Caspers, a herbarium specialist from the Botanical garden.

The plant materials were washed in distilled water and cut into small pieces. After cleaning, the parts were air-dried at room temperature for four days to remove the residual moisture and ground into a fine powder using a laboratory mill. To produce methanol extracts, 1 g of fine plant powder was macerated with 15 mL of 80% methanol at room temperature for 15 h. After that, the extracts (66.7 mg/mL) were filtered using filter paper and stored at −20 °C before their use.

2.2. Phytochemical Analysis: Ultra-High-Performance Liquid Chromatography Coupled with High-Resolution Tandem Mass Spectrometry (UHPLC–HRMS/MS)

For the purpose of phytochemical profiling, an internal database of secondary metabolites reported in *Iris* spp. plants was created based on a scientific literature search [23]. Then, those predicted compounds were screened in a targeted manner in the crude extracts using UHPLC-HRMS/MS analysis, as previously described by [24] with some modifications. Chromatographic separation was achieved using a 150 × 2.1 mm i.d., 1.7 µm Acquity UPLC® BEH C_{18} column (Waters, Milford, MA, USA) in a chromatographic Agilent 1290 Infinity LC System (Agilent Technologies, Santa Clara, CA, USA). The mobile phases consisted of water/acetonitrile (95:5, v/v) (**A**) and 2-propanol/acetonitrile/water (75:20:5, v/v/v) (**B**), both containing ammonium acetate (5 mM) and acetic acid (0.1%). The gradient was as follows: 0–0.5 min, flow 0.3 mL/min, 100% **A**; 0.5–4 min, flow 0.3 mL/min, 100–35% **A**; 4–8 min, flow 0.2 mL/min, 35–22.5% **A**; 8–13 min, flow 0.2 mL/min, 22.5–0% **A**; 13–18 min, flow 0.35 mL/min, 0% **A**. Then, the column was equilibrated for 2 min under the initial conditions. The injection volume was 1.0 µL, and the column temperature was maintained at 60 °C.

The Agilent 6560 quadrupole–time of flight mass spectrometer (Q-TOF) (Agilent Technologies, Santa Clara, CA, USA) was operated in Q-TOF Auto MS/MS acquisition mode. The specific parameters for the mass spectrometer were as follows: electrospray ionization both in positive and negative polarity (separate injections of the samples); drying gas flow rate 12 L/min; drying gas temperature 280 °C; sheath gas flow rate 12 L/min; sheath gas temperature 350 °C; nozzle voltage 400 V; capillary voltage 3500 V; nebulizer 40 psig. In the Auto MS/MS mode, the following parameters were used: mass range 100–1000 m/z (both in MS and MS/MS); acquisition rate 3 spectra/s (MS) and 12 spectra/s (MS/MS); collision energy 20 eV. The predicted compounds of *Iris* spp. were detected and tentatively identified based on the exact masses (*m/z*) of their precursor ions, their isotopic patterns and where possible, the agreement of recorded MS/MS spectra with online mass spectral libraries (such as 'METLIN', 'mzCloud'), or the scientific literature. For some of the detected compounds, several chromatographic peaks meeting the HRMS criteria were observed, probably indicating the presence of structural isomers.

2.3. Antimicrobial Activity

The antimicrobial activity of the extracts was tested against eight pathogenic microorganisms: *Pseudomonas aeruginosa* (CCM, 3955), *Staphylococcus aureus* (ATCC, 25923), *Salmonella enterica* (CCM, 4420), *Candida albicans* (DBM, 2186), *Streptococcus gordonii* (DSMZ, 6777), *Veillonella parvula* (DSMZ, 2008), *Fusobacterium nucleatum* subsp. *nucleatum* (DSMZ, 15643), and *Actinomyces naeslundii* (DSMZ, 43013). The selected strains were according to the EUCAST (European Committee on Antimicrobial Susceptibility Testing) antibiotic-sensitive, which was verified by cefotaxime and penicillin sensitivity. IC_{50} of penicillin [mg/L] was as follows: 0.0059 ± 0.0001 for *S. aureus*; IC_{50} of cefotaxime [mg/L] was as follows: 0.55 ± 0.05 for *P. aeruginosa*, 0.95 ± 0.05 for *C. albicans*, 0.058 ± 0.003 for *S. gordonii*, 0.0047 ± 0.0004 for *V. parvula*, and 0.017 ± 0.0004 for *F. nucleatum* and 0.022 ± 0.001 for *A. naeslundii*.

Susceptibility tests of the target microorganisms, both Gram-positive and Gram-negative bacterial strains, and yeast, were carried out using the standard broth microdilution method, in 96-well plates as described previously [25]. The tested bacteria and yeasts were grown overnight in Brain Heart Infusion Broth (BHI, Sigma-Aldrich, St. Louis, MO, USA) and Malt extract broth (ME broth, Oxoid,

Hampshire, UK), respectively. Resulting suspensions were adjusted to a turbidity of 0.5 McFarland. The extracts were 100× diluted with the suspensions and then binary diluted with the same suspension. These diluted extracts were added to 96-well plates providing concentrations of the extracts ranging from 0.7 up to 666.7 mg/L. All experiments were conducted with a maximum of 1% (v/v) methanol in solution. The suspension of microorganisms without the tested compounds served as a positive control. Bacterial and yeast cultures were incubated for 24 h at 120 rpm and 37 and 28 °C, respectively, and the absorbance was recorded at 500 nm using the SpectraMax i3x Multi-Mode Detection Platform (Molecular Devices, San Jos Tibco Software Inc., San Jose, CA, USA).

2.4. Anti-Biofilm Activity

The activity of the *Iris* extracts on mono- and multi-species bacterial biofilms was tested using *Staphylococcus aureus* (ATCC, 25923), *Pseudomonas aeruginosa* (CCM, 3955), and dental plaque, which consisted of four oral bacterial strains: *Streptococcus gordonii* (DSMZ, 6777), *Veillonella parvula* (DSMZ, 2008), *Fusobacterium nucleatum* subsp. nucleatum (DSMZ, 15643), and *Actinomyces naeslundii* (DSMZ, 43013). *S. aureus* and *P. aeruginosa* were incubated in BHI broth medium at 37 °C aerobically, while all the dental plaque strains were propagated anaerobically using an anaerobic jar (model HP0031A, Thermo Fisher Scientific, MA, USA). An anaerobic atmosphere of 80% N_2, 10% CO_2, and 10% H_2 was obtained with an Oxoid™ AnaeroGen™ 3.5L Sachet with Thermo Scientific™ Resazurin Anaerobic Indicator BR0055 (Thermo Fisher Scientific, MA USA).

For single-species biofilms, the method described by [26] was used. For the mixed biofilm, overnight cultures adjusted to 0.5 McFarland turbidity of all species: *S. gordonii, V. parvula, F. nucleatum,* and *A. naeslundii* were mixed in the same ratio (1:1:1:1, v/v). After that, 100 µL was split into each well and incubated for 48 h. For testing the anti-adhesion activity, a resazurin assay was employed to evaluate the viability of attached cells immediately after 24 h of incubation in the presence of the tested extracts at 37 °C and washing with Phosphate Buffered Saline (PBS) three times (pH 7.4). In the eradication of mature biofilms, the medium was discarded after the adherence incubation period of all strains, and fresh BHI broth medium was replaced every 24 h for 7 days of incubation under anaerobic conditions in order to allow biofilm maturation. After that, the extracts were added in a concentration range of 0.7–666.7 mg/L and incubated for another 24 h. After the final washing of the biofilm, the viability was determined by resazurin assay [27]. The resazurin (Sigma-Aldrich) in PBS (0.03 mg/L) was incubated with the cells for 2 hours at 37 °C avoiding light exposure. The production of resorufin was quantified by measuring fluorescence (560/590 nm, ex./em.) using the SpectraMax i3x Multi-Mode Detection Platform (Molecular Devices, USA). The viability of cells was calculated relative to the viability of cells in the absence of the tested samples.

2.5. Anti-Quorum Sensing Activity

The production of bioluminescence by two commercial (The American Type Culture Collection, ATCC) strains of *Vibrio campbellii*—BAA1118 and BAA1119 in the presence or absence of tested extracts was determined for the evaluation of anti-QS according to the previous protocol [26]. Autoinducer Bioassay (AB-A) medium, consisting of NaCl (17.5 g/L), $MgSO_4$ (12.3 g/L), casamino acids (2 g/L), 10 mM potassium phosphate (pH 7.0), 1 mM L-arginine, and glycerol (10 mL/L) was used for inoculating these two strains and all anti-QS experiments. The 0.2 McFarland overnight culture in AB-A medium was split into each well with the binary dilution of *Iris* extracts (0.7 mg/L–666.7 mg/L). At first, the viability of *V. campbellii* was checked by resazurin assay for setting up the experiment at non-toxic concentrations of the tested samples. IC_{10} was chosen for the anti-QS assay. The extracts were applied at the IC_{10} concentration and further binary diluted with the cell suspension. Then, luminescence was recorded for 16 h with a measurement step of 20 min using a microplate reader set up at 30 °C; integration time of 10,000 ms; and shaking for 60 s prior to measurement. After the measurements, the QS IC_{50} was calculated based on the sum of luminescence recorded by a microplate reader (SpectraMax i3 Multi-Mode Detection Platform, Molecular Devices, UK).

2.6. Cytotoxicity Assay

The extracts were evaluated for their *in vitro* cytotoxicity using human fibroblasts (MRC-5, Sigma-Aldrich, USA) obtained from ATCC (USA). The cell line was grown in Eagle's Minimum Essential Medium (EMEM) culture medium containing 10% fetal bovine serum (FBS) and 1% antibiotic mixture (penicillin, 100 IU/mL and streptomycin, 100 g/mL) at 37 °C in a 5% CO_2 humidified incubator. The cells were counted with a Cellometer Auto T4 (Nexcelom Bioscience, Lawrence, MA), seeded (1×10^5 cells/mL) in a 96-well plate and incubated for 24 h. Then, the cell culture medium was discarded from each well, and the tested extracts were added to assess the effect on cytotoxicity. After 72 h of incubation, a standard resazurin assay [28] was performed to determine the cell viability. The results were expressed as a percentage of viable cells compared to the control (taken as 100%).

2.7. Data Processing and Statistical Analysis

Unless otherwise stated, results are presented as an average of triplicates with the appropriate standard error of the mean (SEM). The relative activity was evaluated as a percentage according to the formula:

$$RA\ (\%) = 100 \frac{(\text{slope of sample} - \text{average slope of PC})}{(\text{average slope of NC} - \text{average slope of PC})}.$$

Values of IC_{50} were determined using an online tool freely provided by AAT Bioquest – IC_{50} Calculator.

The results were subjected to one-way analysis of variance (ANOVA) followed by Duncan's post hoc test ($p < 0.05$) to show significant differences between the means of treated and untreated groups as identified in each assay. Statistica software version 12 (Tibco Software Inc., Tulse, OK, USA) was employed in the ANOVA analysis.

The correlation coefficients were calculated using the automatic function "CORREL" in Microsoft®Office Excel according to [24]. The following variables were used as the matrix: (I) IC_{50} for specific biological activity and (II) the peak areas of compounds detected and tentatively identified by targeted UHPLC–HRMS/MS screening. The significance of the correlation coefficient was evaluated using a comparison of coefficients and the critical values ($\alpha = 0.05$), which were determined using the degrees of freedom (df = n−2).

3. Results

3.1. Phytochemical Analysis of Plant Extracts

The profile of phytochemicals detected using the UHPLC-HRMS/MS method in a methanol extract of leaves, roots, and rhizomes from 5 different species of *Iris* spp. is presented in Tables 1 and A1. As seen in Table 1, more than 50 compounds were found in each extract, with (iso)flavonoids predominating. The highest number of (iso)flavonoids was detected in *I. pallida* leaves and roots, which consisted of 35 and 38 (iso)flavonoids, respectively, while less than half of them were detected in the rhizomes of this species. The lowest deviation in the composition was observed for steroids and fatty acids; in contrast, quinones and flavonoids exhibited variation in their presence within the species. A total of 180 individual compounds were detected and tentatively identified in the samples as a result of the screening analysis. In the extracts, 25 compounds were detected in only 1 sample, while 33 compounds were present in more than half of the extracts. The compound's name, molecular formula, experimentally obtained neutral exact mass, retention time (t_R, min), and presence in 3 different parts of five *Iris* spp. are summarized in Table A1.

3.2. Antimicrobial Activity

For the determination of antimicrobial activity of the *Iris* extracts, both Gram-positive (*S. aureus*, *B. cereus*, *S. gordonii*, *V. parvula*, *A. naeslundii*) and Gram-negative (*P. aeruginosa*, *S. enterica*, *F. nucleatum*) bacteria and yeast (*C. albicans*) were tested. However, no antibacterial or antifungal activity was observed, even at the highest tested concentration of 666.7 mg/L (data not shown). Therefore, this concentration was chosen as the sub-minimum inhibitory concentration (sub-MIC) and used in further experiments.

Table 1. Major chemical constituents present in assessed *Iris* extracts of leaves (L), roots (R), and rhizomes (Rh).

Species	Number of Detected Compounds (Tentative Identity)							
	(Iso)flavonoids	Phenols	Fatty Acids	Terpenoids	Steroids	Xanthones	Quinones	All
I. pallida (L)	35	5	8	14	4	5	2	73
I. pallida (R)	38	7	6	13	3	8	-	75
I. pallida (Rh)	15	11	6	8	3	9	-	52
I. versicolor (L)	8	7	7	20	3	13	-	58
I. versicolor (R)	11	10	7	17	4	9	-	58
I. versicolor (Rh)	5	10	7	22	3	10	-	57
I. lactea (L)	10	9	7	13	3	7	3	52
I. lactea (R)	12	11	5	10	4	7	1	50
I. lactea (Rh)	37	6	7	12	4	7	-	73
I. carthaliniae (L)	11	8	6	12	4	5	1	47
I. carthaliniae (R)	23	8	4	13	5	4	-	57
I. carthaliniae (Rh)	31	7	7	12	4	2	-	63
I. germanica (L)	19	5	9	17	4	6	3	63
I. germanica (R)	46	5	8	15	3	8	-	85
I. germanica (Rh)	43	7	5	10	4	9	-	78

L—leaves; R—roots; Rh—rhizomes.

3.3. Anti-Biofilm Activity

The sub-MIC of *Iris* methanol extracts significantly inhibited the adhesion of Gram-positive (*S. aureus*) and Gram-negative (*P. aeruginosa*) bacteria as well as the dental plaque multispecies biofilm in a concentration-dependent manner (Table 2, Supplementary Table S2). Specifically, activity suppressing biofilm formation was observed more in leaf, root, and rhizome extracts (*I. pallida*, *I. versicolor*), with weaker activity in extracts from leaves and rhizomes (*I. germanica*) and roots (*I. lactea*). Furthermore, the IC_{50} for the multi-species biofilm was significantly higher than those for the mono-species one. Compared to mono-species biofilms, higher concentrations were required to prevent the formation of the multi-species biofilm. Out of all five species, only all the extracts of *I. pallida* and *I. versicolor* reduced multi-species cell adhesion by more than 50%.

Table 2. Concentration of *Iris* spp. extract halving respective activity: (1) adhesion of bacteria forming biofilm and (2) mature biofilm.

Species	Anti-Adhesion IC_{50} [mg/L]			Antibiofilm IC_{50} [mg/L]		
	S. aureus	*P. aeruginosa*	Dental Plaque	*S. aureus*	*P. aeruginosa*	Dental Plaque
I. pallida (L)	139.4 ± 2.0	88.5 ± 1.6	163.5 ± 6.5	406.3 ± 20.4	287.0 ± 10.3	>666.7
I. pallida (R)	177.2 ± 13.0	122.7 ± 4.0	326.9 ± 13.5	>666.7	447.6 ± 45.9	>666.7
I. pallida (Rh)	334.5 ± 8.1	297.2 ± 23.1	556.6 ± 48.3	>666.7	628.2 ± 13.9	>666.7
I. versicolor (L)	169.0 ± 6.1	132.2 ± 14.8	357.0 ± 13.0	>666.7	497.2 ± 22.2	>666.7
I. versicolor (R)	161.0 ± 5.5	177.0 ± 4.3	315.3 ± 38.6	549.6 ± 8.3	526.1 ± 15.9	>666.7
I. versicolor (Rh)	98.5 ± 9.5	112.4 ± 5.2	201.6 ± 12.4	615.6 ± 28.9	500.4 ± 16.4	>666.7
I. lactea (L)	>666.7	>666.7	>666.7	>666.7	>666.7	>666.7
I. lactea (R)	255.3 ± 26.0	393.4 ± 17.0	542.8 ± 46.3	>666.7	>666.7	>666.7
I. lactea (Rh)	370.5 ± 22.6	>666.7	>666.7	>666.7	>666.7	>666.7
I. carthaliniae (L)	494.5 ± 69.1	512.8 ± 14.6	>666.7	>666.7	>666.7	>666.7
I. carthaliniae (R)	427.8 ± 19.1	>666.7	>666.7	>666.7	>666.7	>666.7
I. carthaliniae (Rh)	>666.7	>666.7	>666.7	>666.7	>666.7	>666.7
I. germanica (L)	178.1 ± 23.2	267.5 ± 8.6	357.4 ± 16.3	>666.7	513.0 ± 56.1	>666.7
I. germanica (R)	334.6 ± 8.4	>666.7	>666.7	>666.7	>666.7	>666.7
I. germanica (Rh)	258.1 ± 10.0	630.7 ± 19.0	542.0 ± 23.6	>666.7	>666.7	>666.7

L—leaves; R—roots; Rh—rhizomes; Data are presented as the average of 3 repetitions with SEM. For the statistical analysis, see the Supplementary Supplementary Table S2.

In general, the methanol extracts of *I. pallida* and *I. versicolor* exhibited strong eradication effects on all tested biofilms in both stages: cell adhesion and disruption of a maturated biofilm, with a higher activity against Gram-negative bacteria (*P. aeruginosa*, roots, rhizomes). The leaf extract of *I. pallida* demonstrated the strongest inhibitory effect, as it disrupted the mature *P. aeruginosa* biofilm with the IC$_{50}$ 0.29 ± 0.01 g/L followed by *I. versicolor* root and rhizome extracts. Of the other three extracts, only the leaf extract of *I. germanica* disrupted the matured biofilm observed for *P. aeruginosa*. This activity was not observed in other extracts. Furthermore, none of the *Iris* extracts at the highest tested concentration were able to significantly eradicate the multispecies biofilm of *S. gordonii, V. parvula, F. nucleatum*, and *A. naeslundii* (Figure 1, Supplementary Table S1).

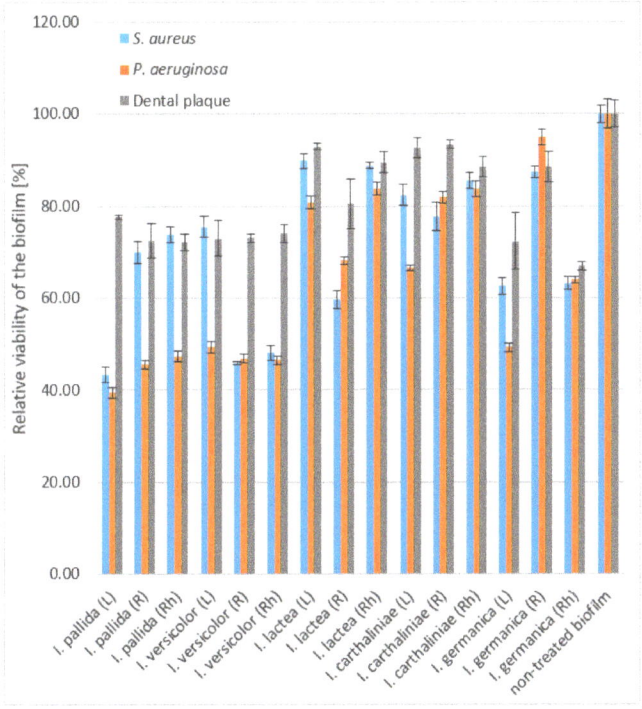

Figure 1. Disruption of mature biofilm by methanol extracts of Iris spp. at concentration of 666.7 mg/L. Data are presented as average of 3 repetitions with SEM. For the statistical analysis, see Supplementary Table S1.

3.4. Cell-To-Cell Communication Inhibition Assay in V. campbellii

In this study, we investigated the QS inhibitory potential of 15 *Iris* methanolic extracts against the QS-dependent phenotypic production of luminescence in mutant sensor strains of *V. campbellii* responding either only to (1) AI-1 autoinducer (BAA1118) or (2) AI-2 autoinducer (BAA1119). To avoid false positive results in the QS inhibition experiment, the concentration of 666.67 mg/L was determined as non-toxic to the tested strains. Thus, the reduced bioluminescence production resulted from an inhibition of cell–cell communication rather than an inhibition of cell growth. In general, only 6 extracts exhibited an inhibition of homoserine lactones-mediated luminescence production in *V. campbellii* BAA1118, responding to autoinducer 1 (AI-1), while AI-2-mediated communication was only inhibited by three extracts (Table 3, Supplementary Table S3). *I. lactea* and *I. carthaliniae* had no effect on QS at all. The *I. pallida* leaf extract inhibited communication based on both AI-1 and AI-2 systems similarly to the root and rhizome extracts of *I. versicolor*. Although they inhibited the cell-to-cell communication system based on boron compounds (AI-2) implemented by many Gram-negative and Gram-positive bacteria, their activities were significantly higher against AI-1. An inhibition of intercellular bacterial communication based on the AI-1 autoinducer was observed in *I. pallida* (leaves, roots), *I. versicolor* (all tissues), and *I. germanica* (leaves). No anti-QS activity was found in other extracts.

Table 3. Concentration of *Iris* spp. extract halving quorum sensing of *Vibrio campbellii*.

	V. campbellii BAA1118	V. campbellii BAA1119
species	QS IC$_{50}$ [mg/L]	QS IC$_{50}$ [mg/L]
I. pallida (L)	533.8 ± 3.2	605.0 ± 3.0
I. pallida (R)	560.6 ± 10.4	>666.7
I. pallida (Rh)	>666.7	>666.7
I. versicolor (L)	543.4 ± 59.5	>666.7
I. versicolor (R)	542.0 ± 1.8	644.0 ± 10.0
I. versicolor (Rh)	638.5 ± 16.2	597.2 ± 33.2
I. lactea (L)	>666.7	>666.7
I. lactea (R)	>666.7	>666.7
I. lactea (Rh)	>666.7	>666.7
I. carthaliniae (L)	>666.7	>666.7
I. carthaliniae (R)	>666.7	>666.7
I. carthaliniae (Rh)	>666.7	>666.7
I. germanica (L)	297.1 ± 10.3	>666.7
I. germanica (R)	>666.7	>666.7
I. germanica (Rh)	>666.7	>666.7
Erythromycin	20.7 ± 1.0	2.6 ± 0.1

L—leaves; R—roots; Rh—rhizomes. Data presented as average of 3 repetitions with SEM. For the statistical analysis, see Supplementary Table S2.

3.5. In Vitro Cytotoxicity

It is necessary to determine the possible toxic effects of antimicrobial agents on human cells to confirm the safety of antimicrobial agents at their effective concentrations intended for application within the oral cavity. The cytotoxic effect of 15 samples on the human fibroblastic cell lines was evaluated by resazurin assay after 72 h of exposure. As shown in Table 4, no toxicity was observed for fibroblasts (MRC cell line) at the highest tested concentration (670 mg/L), except for the rhizome extracts from *I. versicolor* and *I. carthaliniae*.

Table 4. Concentration of *Iris* spp. extract halving viability of fibroblasts (MRC) cell line.

Iris Part	IC$_{50}$ [mg/L]
I. pallida (L)	>666.7
I. pallida (R)	>666.7
I. pallida (Rh)	>666.7
I. versicolor (L)	>666.7
I. versicolor (R)	>666.7
I. versicolor (Rh)	96.0 ± 6.7
I. lacteal (L)	>666.7
I. lacteal (R)	>666.7
I. lacteal (Rh)	>666.7
I. carthaliniae (L)	>666.7
I. carthaliniae (R)	>666.7
I. carthaliniae (Rh)	317.3 ± 40.0
I. germanica (L)	>666.7
I. germanica (R)	>666.7
I. germanica (Rh)	>666.7
Doxorubicin	0.4 ± 0.007

L—leaves; R—roots; Rh—rhizomes. Data are presented as an average of 3 repetitions with SEM.

3.6. Correlation of Biological Activities and Extract Composition

To determine the relationship between the biological activity response in the particular test examined and the amount of the compounds present in the samples, the correlation of the biological activity results with the HRMS/MS responses of detected compounds in each extract was calculated. When plotting the results for all 15 of the extracts, the correlation coefficient (R^2) was determined and assessed. The ability of the extracts to inhibit dental plaque adhesion significantly correlated with the content of myristic acid and germanaism B. Three compounds from different chemical groups: 7-β-hydroxystigmast-4-en-3-one(steroid), amorphene/α-muurolene/β-gurjuenene/γ-elemene (terpenoid), and isomangiferin/mangiferin/nigricanside (xanthone) inhibited the bacterial extracellular communication of *V. campbellii* BAA1118 (see Table 5).

Table 5. Correlation coefficients (R^2) of dependence of biological activity of 15 *Iris* extracts on HRMS/MS responses of compounds detected and tentatively identified by targeted UHPLC–HRMS/MS screening. Note: only substances for which the correlation was significant are presented.

Compound	Inhibition of Dental Biofilm Adhesion			Inhibition of BA1118 Communication		
	df	R_{crit}	R^2	df	R_{crit}	R^2
Myristic acid	7	0.666	0.753			
Germanaism B	1	0.997	0.999			
7-β-hydroxystigmast-4-en-3-one				4	0.811	0.933
Amorphene/α-muurolene/β-gurjuenene/γ-elemene				3	0.878	0.932
Isomangiferin/Mangiferin/Nigricanside				4	0.811	0.827

4. Discussion

Oral diseases, such as dental caries and periodontitis, are mostly linked with microbial biofilms growing in the form of supragingival and subgingival plaque. The development of oral biofilms has led to their persistence with conventional antimicrobial therapies. In view of the growing need for a new remedy for oral infection treatment, naturally occurring molecules found in the plant kingdom may become important candidates for the development of new bacterial biofilm inhibitors. This study assessed the ability of 15 methanol extracts of five different *Iris* plant species to modulate mono- and multi-species oral biofilms. Moreover, in this study, the extracts were further analyzed for potential phytochemical components using UHPLC-HRMS/MS-targeted screening, and some of the detected compounds may associate with the activity observed against the tested bacterial biofilms.

To the best of our knowledge, this is the first report on the phytochemical compounds in methanol extracts of the aforementioned plant species characterized by the UHPLC-HRMS/MS technique. The chemical profile of our *Iris* extracts is similar to what has been previously reported. In many *Iris* species, (iso)flavonoids exist as the main class of polyphenolics as published by [29] and in this study, where more than 90 compounds of this group were identified. Iristectorigenin A, irisflorentin, iriskumaon, and irilone were previously observed in *I. germanica* and *I. pallida* extracts [30], while Rahman et al. (2002, 2003) demonstrated the presence of tectorigenin, irisolidone, irigenin S, iridin, 5-hydroxy-4'-methoxy-6,7-methylenedioxyisoflavone, irilone 4'-O-β-d-glucopyranoside, irifloside, nigricin, and germanasim B in *I. germanica* rhizomes [31,32]. 4'-O-methylapigenin 6-C-hexoside, 4'-O-methylapigenin 8-C-hexoside, already identified in rhizomes of *I. pseudopumila* [33], were also tentatively confirmed in *I. germanica*. On the other hand, the identified terpenoid compounds in our extracts were quite different from those found in the same plant from other sources reported previously. To date, 21-desoxyiridogermanal, 21-desoxyiridogermanal, 26-hydroxyridal, spirocyclic hemiacetal, and 17ε, 26-dihydroxyiridal were not present in any of all five investigated *Iris* spp., while they were isolated and identified in other *Iris* spp. [34,35]. From these data, it appears that there is a species-specific variability in the phytochemical composition of *Iris* extracts.

The formation of bacterial biofilms plays a crucial role in the virulence of oral pathogenic strains and has become one of the major factors in the increasing emergence of antibiotic resistance. In this study, 15 methanolic extracts of *Iris* spp. were tested for their ability to inhibit planktonic cell adhesion to the surface and eradicate maturated biofilms. The obtained results for both monoand multi-species oral biofilms highlight a dramatic reduction in bacterial biofilm formation on a polystyrene surface by extracts from *I. pallida*, *I. versicolor*, even at concentrations far below the MIC. The anti-adhesion activity of these extracts was observed in a concentration-dependent manner for both Gram-positive and Gram-negative bacteria during the initial stages of biofilm development. Furthermore, the application of higher concentrations was required to eliminate half of the bacterial cells attached in the form of a multi-species biofilm compared to the mono-species ones. The result of biofilm eradication demonstrated a reduced biomass of mature biofilm on the polystyrene surface by oral bacterial strains when treated with different concentrations of methanolic extracts of *I. pallida* and *I. versicolor*. The extract from *I. pallida* leaves exhibited the strongest anti-biofilm activity at an IC_{50} of 0.29 ± 0.01 g/L for disrupting a mature *P. aeruginosa* biofilm. The evaluated extracts contain a wide range of secondary metabolites which have been thoroughly investigated for their potential to modulate bacterial activities, including planktonic cell adherence, virulence, and differentiation. Quercetin, a flavonoid also detected in the studied *Iris* extracts, has been previously tested for its inhibition of biofilm development containing oral bacteria, *P. aeruginosa*, *S. aureus* strains, and clinically isolated MRSA strains [36–39]. Interestingly, flavonoids exhibited strong sortase inhibitory activity, which is an enzyme that is responsible for modulating the attachment ability of cells to host tissue and the production of surface protein virulence factors to the peptidoglycan cell wall layer of Gram-positive bacteria such as *Streptococcus mutans* and *Streptococcus pneumoniae* [38,40]. The inhibitory effect on the *S. aureus* sortase A activity of the dryocrassin ABBA flavonoid has been studied [41], and similar activity was also observed with the application of isovitexin at an IC_{50} of 28.98 mg/L [42]. Therefore, it is conceivable that the anti-biofilm potential of the extracts may be related to the ability of their phytochemical components to inactivate bacterial adhesins and enzymes altering the cell membrane, cell–substratum interactions, adherence phase, and biofilm maturation. Although the mechanism behind biofilm modulation is still unclear, the observed effects could result from a combination of multiple factors attributed to several mechanisms, such as interference cell–cell communication pathways such as the quorum sensing system [43].

The production of bioluminescence in *V. campellii* is positively regulated by a typical QS system responding to different autoinducers (AIs)-specifically, *N*-acyl homoserine lactones (AI-1) in Gram-negative bacteria, oligopeptides in Gram-positive bacteria, and a furanosyl borate diester or autoinducer-2 (AI-2) in both Gram-negative and Gram-positive bacteria [44]. As the bacterial QS-deficient mutant exhibits critical deficiencies in colonization and virulence, the modulation of QS systems can be considered an attractive approach to bacterial infection control [45]. Hence, the anti-QS potential of the *Iris* extracts used in our study was tested in terms of their ability to inhibit signal-based cell–cell communication. This activity was explored by using the standard strain of *V. campbellii* BAA1118 and BAA1119 responding to AI-1 and AI-2 autoinducer, respectively, as a biological model. The extracts from *I. lactea* and *I. carthaliniae* did not exhibit anti-QS activity at all, while the leaf extract from *I. pallida* significantly inhibited the bioluminescence production in both AI-1 and AI-2 systems similarly to the *I. versicolor* root and rhizome extracts. Despite the fact that the underlying mechanism of the extracts is not fully understood, our results suggest the involvement of the inhibition of AHL or interference with the cell–cell communication system in the anti-biofilm activity of the tested extracts.

In this work, we found that the *Iris* spp. methanol extracts, excluding the rhizome extracts from *I. versicolor* and *I. carthaliniae*, were not toxic to human fibroblast cells (MRC), suggesting that these extracts could be safely used as a therapeutic agent.

Furthermore, a strong relationship between the biological activity of *Iris* extracts and their phytochemical compounds was confirmed using correlation analysis (Table 5). The ability of myristic acid to prevent the adherence of *Escherichia coli* planktonic cells suggested a potential of *Iris* extracts to inhibit biofilm formation [46], while based on the literature data, there have been no published studies to date that report on the anti-biofilm activity of germanaism. Myristic acid was shown to be a QS inhibitor, and it significantly inhibited the production of four extracellular virulence factors in the *P. aeruginosa* biofilm [47]. Prasath et al. reported the antibiofilm and antivirulence ability of myristic acid against *C. albicans* at a 125 mg/L concentration. The myristic acid-mediated regulation of the composition of lipid rafts may modulate the biofilm formation [48]. Our research also revealed that compounds of three different chemical classes: terpenoids, xanthones and steroids, inhibited QS in *V. campbellii* BAA1118.

Duckworth (2009) published a report about the sufficient effect of a two-minute use of mouthwash [49]. Therefore, the effectiveness of the substances within this short period on the modulation of both mono- and multi-species oral biofilms needs to be further evaluated, as well as the effectiveness of repeated exposures.

5. Conclusions

Natural products represent potential control agents to be used in therapeutic dental treatments. Here, we report on the phytochemical profile and the inhibitory effect on the growth and biofilm formation of mono- and multi-species oral biofilms of phytochemical-rich methanol extracts derived from selected *Iris* species, emphasizing their potency to modulate the virulence properties of dental plaque while maintaining oral health. Based on the highly heterogeneous data and the risk of bias, caution is required when interpreting the presented evidence. The *in vitro* mono- and multi-species biofilms used in our study clearly do not reflect the complex polymicrobial and environmental interactions present in the oral cavity. However, we found the extracts from *I. pallida* and *I. versicolor* in particular to both modulate biofilm formation with a higher effect on Gram-negative bacteria (*P. aeruginosa*), and also interfere with QS phenotype behaviors without affecting the growth of targeting bacteria as well as the human fibroblast cell lines (MRC). Therefore, it appears that *Iris* spp. is a potential candidate as an ecological caries-preventive agent that does not cause antibiotic tolerance and could be valuable in the field of dentistry and pharmacology for the production of oral care products. Further studies of controlled clinical trials with longer observation periods are required to identify multiple mechanisms of action, and efficacious and safe doses of the extracts.

Supplementary Materials: The following are available online at http://www.mdpi.com/2079-6382/9/7/403/s1, Table S1: Disruption of mature biofilm: one-way analysis of variance (ANOVA) followed by Duncan's post hoc test ($p < 0.05$) to show significant differences between methanol extracts of *Iris* spp. at concentration of 666.7 mg/L, Table S2: Concentration of Iris spp. extract halving respective activity: (1) adhesion of bacteria forming biofilm and (2) mature biofilm: one-way analysis of variance (ANOVA) followed by Duncan's post hoc test ($p, <, 005$) showing significant differences between methanol extracts of *Iris* spp. at concentration of 666.7 mg/L, Table S3: Concentration of *Iris* spp. extract halving quorum sensing of *Vibrio campbellii*: one-way analysis of variance (ANOVA) followed by Duncan's post hoc test ($p < 0.05$) showing significant differences between methanol extracts of Iris spp. at concentration of 666.7 mg/L.

Author Contributions: Conceptualization, M.V., J.V., P.K. and T.R.; methodology, E.B.Š., M.V., J.V., F.B., K.Ř., M.F., V.Š., L.H. and T.R.; software, J.V. and M.F.; validation, J.V., M.F., K.Ř. and L.H.; formal analysis, J.V., F.B., M.F. and T.R.; investigation, O.K., J.H. and T.R.; resources, J.H. and T.R.; data curation, J.V., M.F. and L.H.; writing—original draft preparation, L.H., J.V., T.R.; writing—review and editing, J.V., T.R., M.F., F.B. and J.H.; visualization, J.V. and L.H.; supervision, T.R. and J.H.; project administration, P.K., T.R. and J.H.; funding acquisition, P.K., T.R. and J.H. All authors have read and agreed to the published version of the manuscript.

Funding: This research was funded by the Technology Agency of the Czech Republic—National Center of Competence BIOCIRTECH (No. TN010000048) and by the Czech National Program of Sustainability NPU I (LO) (MSMT-43760/2015). It was also supported by the long-term research development project of the Czech Academy of Sciences (RVO 67985939).

Conflicts of Interest: The authors declare no conflict of interest. The funders had no role in the design of the study; in the collection, analyses, or interpretation of data; in the writing of the manuscript, or in the decision to publish the results.

Appendix A

Table A1. Overview of phytochemicals detected and tentatively identified in *Iris* spp. by ultra-high performance liquid chromatography-high-resolution tandem mass spectroscopy (UHPLC–HRMS/MS).

No.	Compound Name	Molecular Formula	Neutral Mass *	t_R (min)	I. pallida.			I. versicolor			I. lactea			I. carthaliniae			I. germanica		
					L	R	Rh	L	R	Rh	L	R	Rh	L	R	Rh	L	Rh	R
Xanthones																			
1	Isomangiferin/Mangiferin/Nigricanside	$C_{19}H_{18}O_{11}$	422.0844	1.03	−	−	−	−	−	+	−	−	−	−	−	−	−	+	+
2	Iriflophenone	$C_{13}H_{10}O_5$	246.0523	2.08	−	−	+	+	+	+	+	+	−	+	+	−	−	−	−
3	Iriflophenone 2-O-hexoside/Iriflophenone 4-O-hexoside	$C_{19}H_{20}O_{10}$	408.1039	2.5	−	−	+	+	+	+	+	+	−	+	+	−	−	−	−
4	Iriflophenone	$C_{13}H_{10}O_5$	246.0521	2.69	−	−	+	+	+	+	+	+	−	+	+	−	−	−	−
5	Iriflophenone	$C_{13}H_{10}O_5$	246.0529	2.87	+	+	+	+	+	+	−	+	−	+	+	−	+	+	+
6	Iriflophenone 2-O-hexoside/Iriflophenone 4-O-hexoside	$C_{19}H_{20}O_{10}$	408.1053	2.88	+	+	+	+	+	+	+	+	+	+	+	−	+	+	+
7	Isomangiferin/Mangiferin/Nigricanside	$C_{19}H_{18}O_{11}$	422.0845	2.96	+	+	+	+	+	+	+	+	+	+	+	−	+	+	+
8	4-O-methyliriflophenone	$C_{14}H_{12}O_5$	260.0685	3.09	+	−	−	−	−	−	−	−	−	−	−	−	−	+	−
9	7-O-methylisomangiferin/7-O-methylmangiferin	$C_{20}H_{20}O_{11}$	436.0995	3.24	−	+	−	−	−	−	−	−	−	−	−	−	+	+	−
10	Iriflophenone	$C_{13}H_{10}O_5$	246.0525	3.37	−	+	+	+	+	+	+	−	−	−	−	−	−	+	−
11	Isomangiferin/Mangiferin/Nigricanside	$C_{19}H_{18}O_{11}$	422.0844	3.39	−	−	−	−	−	−	−	−	−	−	−	+	−	+	+
12	Bellidifolin	$C_{14}H_{10}O_6$	274.047	3.45	−	−	−	−	−	−	−	−	−	−	−	−	−	+	+
13	4-O-methyliriflophenone	$C_{14}H_{12}O_5$	260.0685	3.61	+	−	−	+	+	+	+	+	+	+	+	−	+	+	+
14	Bellidifolin	$C_{14}H_{10}O_6$	274.047	3.62	−	−	−	−	−	+	+	+	−	−	−	−	−	+	+
15	7-O-methylisomangiferin/7-O-methylmangiferin	$C_{20}H_{20}O_{11}$	436.0998	3.64	+	−	−	+	+	+	+	+	+	+	+	+	+	+	+
16	4-O-methyliriflophenone	$C_{14}H_{12}O_5$	260.0674	3.91	+	+	+	+	+	+	+	+	+	+	+	−	+	+	+
17	Isomangiferin/Mangiferin/Nigricanside	$C_{19}H_{18}O_{11}$	422.0836	6.52	+	−	−	−	+	−	+	−	−	−	−	−	−	+	−
18	Bellidifolin	$C_{14}H_{10}O_6$	274.047	4.21	+	−	+	+	+	+	+	+	+	+	+	−	+	+	+
Phenols																			
19	Vanillic acid	$C_8H_8O_4$	168.042	1.68	+	+	+	+	+	+	+	+	+	+	+	+	+	+	+
20	trans-Cinnamic acid	$C_9H_8O_2$	148.0526	2.06	+	+	+	+	+	+	+	+	−	+	+	+	+	+	+
21	Salicylic acid/p-hydroxybenzoic acid	$C_7H_6O_3$	138.0319	2.08	+	−	−	+	+	+	+	+	−	+	+	+	−	+	−
22	Protocatechuic acid	$C_7H_6O_4$	154.0263	2.17	+	+	+	+	+	+	+	+	−	+	+	+	+	+	+
23	Ferulic acid	$C_{10}H_{10}O_4$	194.0574	2.61	+	+	+	−	−	−	−	−	+	−	−	−	+	−	−
24	Salicylic acid/p-hydroxybenzoic acid	$C_7H_6O_3$	138.0319	2.69	−	−	+	+	+	+	+	+	−	+	+	−	−	−	−
25	3-Hydroxy-5-acetophenone/3-Hydroxy-5-methoxyacetonphenoone/Apocynin	$C_9H_{10}O_3$	166.0625	2.91	−	−	−	+	+	+	+	+	+	+	+	+	−	−	−
26	Salicylic acid/p-hydroxybenzoic acid	$C_7H_6O_3$	138.0316	2.96	−	−	−	+	+	+	+	+	+	+	+	+	−	−	−
27	Caffeic acid	$C_9H_8O_4$	180.042	2.96	+	−	+	+	−	−	−	−	−	+	+	−	+	+	−
28	Vanillic acid	$C_8H_8O_4$	168.0419	2.98	+	+	+	+	+	+	+	+	+	+	+	+	−	+	−
29	Vanillic acid	$C_8H_8O_4$	168.0419	3.5	−	−	+	−	+	−	+	+	−	−	−	−	−	−	−
30	Vanillic acid	$C_8H_8O_4$	168.0419	3.75	+	+	+	+	+	+	+	+	−	+	+	−	−	+	+

Table A1. Cont.

No.	Compound Name	Molecular Formula	Neutral Mass *	t_R (min)	I. pallida L	I. pallida R	I. pallida Rh	I. versicolor L	I. versicolor R	I. versicolor Rh	I. lactea L	I. lactea R	I. lactea Rh	I. carthaliniae L	I. carthaliniae R	I. carthaliniae Rh	I. germanica L	I. germanica Rh	I. germanica R
Flavonoids and isoflavonoids																			
31	4',7-di-O-methyldihydroquercetin-5,3,3'-trihydroxy-7,4'-dimethoxyflavanone	$C_{17}H_{16}O_7$	332.0911	1.09	-	-	-	-	-	-	-	-	-	-	-	-	-	-	-
32	Luteolin 7-O-(2''-p-umaroyl) rhamnoside	$C_{30}H_{26}O_{12}$	578.1409	2.71	-	-	-	+	+	+	+	+	-	-	+	-	-	-	-
33	Swertiajaponin/Tectoridin	$C_{22}H_{22}O_{11}$	462.116	2.85	-	-	-	-	-	-	+	+	-	+	+	+	-	-	-
34	Apigenin 8-C-(2''-hexosyl) hexoside/Kaempferol 7-O-(6''-rhamnosyl) hexoside	$C_{27}H_{30}O_{15}$	594.1577	2.85	+	-	-	+	-	-	+	-	-	-	-	+	+	-	-
35	Isorhamnetin 3-O-(2''-hamnosyl) hexoside/Isorhamnetin 3-O-(6''-rhamnosyl)	$C_{28}H_{32}O_{16}$	624.169	2.85	-	-	-	-	-	-	-	-	-	-	-	+	-	-	-
36	hexoside/Tectorigenin-7-O-glucosyl-4'-O-glucoside Luteolin 7-O-(2''-p-oumaroyl)rhamnoside	$C_{30}H_{26}O_{12}$	578.1413	2.88	-	-	-	-	-	-	-	-	-	+	+	-	-	-	-
37	Iristectorigenin A 7-O-hexuronide/Irisdichotin A/Iristectorin B	$C_{23}H_{24}O_{12}$	492.1255	2.9	-	-	-	-	-	-	-	-	-	-	-	+	-	-	-
38	Dichotomitin 3'-O-hexoside	$C_{24}H_{24}O_{12}$	520.1204	2.92	-	-	-	+	-	-	-	-	-	-	-	-	-	-	-
39	Tectorigenin-4'-O-diglucoside/Tectorigenin-7-O-diglucoside	$C_{28}H_{32}O_{17}$	640.1639	2.97	-	-	-	-	-	-	-	-	-	-	-	-	-	+	-
40	Iriflophenone 4-O-(6''-acetyl) hexoside	$C_{21}H_{22}O_{11}$	450.1154	3.03	-	-	+	-	-	+	-	+	-	-	-	+	-	-	-
41	Apigenin 8-C-(2''-pentosyl) hexoside/Isoschaftoside/Schaftoside	$C_{26}H_{28}O_{14}$	564.1477	3.05	-	+	-	+	-	-	-	-	-	-	+	-	-	+	+
42	Kaempferol 3-O-galactoside/Isoorientin/Kaempferol 3-O-glucoside/Luteolin 6-C-glucoside/Luteolin 8-C-hexoside	$C_{21}H_{20}O_{11}$	448.1	3.1	+	-	-	-	-	-	+	-	-	+	-	-	+	-	-
43	Swertiajaponin/Tectoridin	$C_{22}H_{22}O_{11}$	462.115	3.14	+	-	-	-	-	-	-	-	-	+	-	-	+	-	-
44	7,4'-dimethoxy-8,3',5'-trihydroxy-6-O-β-D-glucopyranosylisoflavone	$C_{23}H_{24}O_{13}$	508.1207	3.16	+	+	-	-	-	-	-	-	+	-	-	-	-	-	+
45	Iridin	$C_{24}H_{26}O_{13}$	522.1371	3.16	+	-	-	-	-	-	-	-	+	-	-	-	-	-	-
46	Tectorigenin-4'-O-diglucoside/Tectorigenin-7-O-diglucoside	$C_{28}H_{32}O_{17}$	640.1629	3.17	-	-	-	-	-	-	-	-	-	-	+	-	-	-	-
47	Quercetin 3-O-galactoside/Quercetin 3-O-glucoside	$C_{21}H_{20}O_{12}$	464.0946	3.18	+	-	-	-	-	+	-	-	-	-	-	+	-	+	+
48	Apigenin 6-C-hexoside/Apigenin 8-C-glucoside/Isovitexin	$C_{21}H_{20}O_{10}$	432.1055	3.19	-	-	-	-	-	-	-	-	-	-	+	-	-	-	-
49	Apigenin 8-C-(2''-pentosyl) hexoside/Isoschaftoside/Schaftoside Germanaism	$C_{26}H_{28}O_{14}$	564.1475	3.19	-	-	-	-	-	-	-	-	-	-	+	-	-	-	-
50	A/5,4'-Methoxy-6,7-methylenedioxy-isoflavone-3'-O-β-d-glucopyranoside	$C_{24}H_{24}O_{12}$	504.1253	3.2	-	-	-	-	-	-	-	-	-	+	+	+	-	-	-
51	Isorhamnetin 3-O-(2''-hamnosyl) hexoside/Isorhamnetin 3-O-(6''-rhamnosyl) hexoside/Tectorigenin-7-O-glucosyl-4'-O-glucoside	$C_{28}H_{32}O_{16}$	624.1692	3.2	-	-	-	-	-	-	-	-	-	-	+	-	-	+	+
52	Genistein	$C_{15}H_{10}O_5$	270.0521	3.24	-	-	-	-	-	-	-	-	-	+	+	+	+	+	-
53	Swertiajaponin/Tectoridin	$C_{22}H_{22}O_{11}$	462.1159	3.24	-	-	-	-	-	-	-	-	-	+	+	-	+	+	-
54	Iristectoridin B/Iristectorin A/Iristectorin B	$C_{23}H_{24}O_{12}$	492.1268	3.27	-	-	-	-	-	-	-	-	-	-	-	-	-	+	+
55	Apigenin 8-C-(2''-hexosyl) hexoside/Kaempferol 7-O-(6''-rhamnosyl) hexoside	$C_{27}H_{30}O_{15}$	594.1579	3.27	-	-	-	-	-	-	-	-	-	-	+	-	-	+	+

Table A1. Cont.

No.	Compound Name	Molecular Formula	Neutral Mass*	t_R (min)	I. pallida.			I. versicolor			I. lactea			I. carthaliniae			I. germanica		
					L	R	Rh	L	R	Rh	L	R	Rh	L	R	Rh	L	R	Rh
56	Irilin D	C₁₆H₁₂O₇	316.0571	3.29	-	-	+	-	-	-	-	+	-	-	+	-	-	+	-
57	Iristectorigenin B/Iristectorigenin A	C₁₇H₁₄O₇	330.0739	3.29	+	+	+	-	-	-	+	+	+	-	+	+	-	+	+
58	6,3′,4′-trimethoxy-7,8,5′-trihydroxyisoflavone/Irigenin	C₁₈H₁₆O₈	360.0834	3.32	+	+	+	-	-	-	+	+	-	-	+	+	-	+	+
59	Apigenin 6-C-hexoside/Apigenin 8-C-glucoside/Isovitexin	C₂₁H₂₀O₁₀	432.1043	3.32	+	+	+	-	-	-	+	-	+	-	+	-	+	+	+
60	Genistein	C₁₅H₁₀O₅	270.0533	3.33	+	+	+	-	-	-	-	-	+	-	+	-	-	+	+
61	4′,7-di-O-methyldihydroquercetin-5,3,3′-trihydroxy-7,4′-dimethoxyflavanone	C₁₇H₁₆O₇	332.0895	3.35	-	+	-	-	-	-	-	-	-	-	-	-	-	+	+
62	Quercetin 3-O-galactoside/Quercetin 3-O-glucoside	C₂₁H₂₀O₁₂	464.0948	3.35	+	+	+	+	-	-	+	-	-	-	-	-	-	+	+
63	Apigenin 8-C-(2″-pentosyl)hexoside/Isoschaftoside/Schaftoside	C₂₆H₂₈O₁₄	564.1467	3.35	-	-	-	-	-	-	-	+	-	-	+	-	-	+	-
64	Irilin A/Tectorigenin	C₁₆H₁₂O₆	300.0633	3.37	+	+	+	-	-	-	+	-	+	-	+	-	+	+	+
65	4′-O-Methylapigenin 6-C-hexoside/4′-O-Methylapigenin 8-C-hexoside/Swertisin	C₂₂H₂₂O₁₀	446.1214	3.37	-	+	+	-	-	-	-	-	+	-	+	-	-	+	+
66	3′-Hydroxytectoridin/Isorhamnetin 3-O-galactoside/Isorhamnetin 3-O-glucoside	C₂₂H₂₂O₁₂	478.11	3.43	-	-	-	+	-	-	-	-	-	-	-	-	-	-	-
67	Iristectorigenin B/Iristectorigenin A	C₁₇H₁₄O₇	330.0731	3.44	+	+	+	-	-	-	+	+	+	-	+	-	-	+	+
68	Iristectorigenin A 7-O-hexuronide/Irisdichotin A/Iristectoridin B/Iristectorin A/Iristectorin B	C₂₃H₂₄O₁₂	492.1257	3.45	+	-	+	-	-	-	+	-	+	-	-	-	-	+	+
69	Germanaism B	C₂₃H₂₂O₁₁	474.1161	3.47	+	+	+	-	-	-	-	-	+	-	-	-	-	+	+
70	Swertiajaponin/Tectoridin	C₂₂H₂₂O₁₁	462.1155	3.48	+	+	+	-	-	-	+	+	+	-	-	-	-	+	+
71	Apigenin-6,8-di-C-arabinoside	C₂₅H₂₆O₁₃	534.1363	3.48	-	-	-	-	-	-	-	-	-	+	-	-	-	-	-
72	Apigenin 8-C-(2″-hexosyl)hexoside/Kaempferol 7-O-(6″-rhamnosyl)hexoside	C₂₇H₃₀O₁₅	594.1575	3.48	-	-	-	-	-	-	-	-	-	-	-	-	-	-	-
73	6,3′,4′-trimethoxy-7,8,5′-trihydroxyisoflavone/Irigenin	C₁₈H₁₆O₈	360.0839	3.49	+	+	+	-	-	-	+	+	+	-	-	-	-	+	+
74	Irilin D	C₂₄H₂₆O₁₃	522.1378	3.5	+	+	+	-	-	-	+	+	+	-	+	-	-	+	+
75	Irilin A/Tectorigenin	C₁₆H₁₂O₇	316.0583	3.56	-	-	-	-	-	-	-	-	-	-	+	-	-	-	-
76	Irilone	C₁₆H₁₂O₆	300.0634	3.58	-	-	-	-	-	-	-	-	+	-	-	-	-	+	-
77	Irilone 4′-O-hexoside/Irilone	C₁₆H₁₀O₆	298.0478	3.6	+	-	+	-	-	-	-	-	+	-	-	-	-	+	+
78	Irilone 4′-O-hexoside/Irilone	C₂₂H₂₀O₁₁	460.1007	3.6	+	+	+	-	-	-	-	-	+	-	-	-	-	+	+
79	5,3′,4′,5′-tetramethoxy-6,7-methylenedioxyisoflavone	C₂₀H₁₈O₉	402.0943	3.62	-	-	-	-	-	-	-	-	-	-	+	-	-	-	-
80	Swertiajaponin/Tectoridin	C₂₂H₂₂O₁₁	462.1161	3.62	-	-	-	-	-	-	-	-	+	-	+	-	-	-	-
81	Irilone 4′-O-(6″-hexosyl)hexoside/Irilone 4′-O-β-d-glucopyranoside-(2→1)-l-rhamnoside	C₂₈H₃₀O₁₆	622.1529	3.62	+	-	+	-	-	-	-	-	-	-	-	-	-	+	+
82	Germanaism B	C₂₃H₂₂O₁₁	474.1167	3.67	-	-	-	-	-	-	-	-	+	-	-	-	-	+	-
83	Germanaism A/5,4′-Methoxy-6,7-methylenedioxy-isoflavone-3′-O-β-d-glucopyranoside	C₂₄H₂₄O₁₂	504.1251	3.68	+	+	+	-	-	-	+	+	+	-	+	-	-	+	+
84	Apigenin-6,8-di-C-arabinoside	C₂₅H₂₆O₁₃	534.1365	3.68	+	+	+	-	-	-	-	+	-	-	-	-	-	+	+

Table A1. Cont.

No.	Compound Name	Molecular Formula	Neutral Mass *	t_R (min)	I. pallida.			I. versicolor			I. lactea			I. carthaliniae			I. germanica		
					L	R	Rh	L	R	Rh	L	R	Rh	L	R	Rh	L	R	Rh
85	Apigenin 8-C-(2''-pentosyl)hexoside/Isoschaftoside/Schaftoside	$C_{26}H_{28}O_{14}$	564.1444	3.68	+	+	-	-	-	-	-	-	+	-	-	-	-	+	+
86	4'-O-Methylapigenin 6-C-hexoside/4'-O-Methylapigenin 8-C-hexoside/Swertisin	$C_{22}H_{22}O_{10}$	446.12	3.74	-	-	-	-	-	-	-	-	-	-	-	-	-	+	-
87	4',7-di-O-methyldihydroquercetin-5,3,3'-trihydroxy-7,4'-dimethoxyflavanone	$C_{17}H_{16}O_7$	332.0894	3.77	+	+	-	-	-	-	-	-	+	-	-	-	-	+	+
88	Irigenin S	$C_{19}H_{18}O_8$	374.0989	3.78	+	+	-	-	-	-	-	-	+	-	-	-	-	+	-
89	Irilin B/Irisolidone	$C_{17}H_{14}O_6$	314.0782	3.8	+	-	-	-	-	-	-	-	+	-	-	-	-	+	-
90	Embinin	$C_{29}H_{34}O_{14}$	606.1955	3.81	+	-	-	-	-	-	-	-	-	-	-	-	-	-	-
91	4'-methyltectorigenin-7-glucoside/6,4'-dimethoxy-5-hydroxyflavone-7-glucoside/Irisdichotin C/Irisolidone 7-O-hexoside/Irisolidone-7-O-α-d-glucoside	$C_{23}H_{24}O_{11}$	476.1302	3.82	-	-	-	-	-	-	-	-	-	-	-	-	-	+	-
92	Irilone 4'-O-[6''-(3-hydroxy-3-methylglutaryl)] hexoside	$C_{28}H_{28}O_{15}$	604.1424	3.82	-	+	-	-	-	-	-	-	+	-	-	-	-	-	+
93	7-O-Methyltectorigenin 4'-O-(6''-hexosyl) hexoside	$C_{29}H_{34}O_{16}$	638.1854	3.84	-	-	-	-	-	-	-	-	-	-	-	-	-	+	-
94	Irilone A	$C_{16}H_{10}O_6$	298.0476	3.87	+	+	-	-	-	-	-	-	+	-	-	-	+	+	+
95	Irifloside/Irisflogenin-4'-O-[β-d-glucopyranosyl(1→6)]β-d-glucopyranoside]	$C_{23}H_{22}O_{12}$	490.1096	3.87	+	-	-	-	-	-	-	-	-	-	-	-	-	-	-
96	Irilone 4'-O-hexoside/Irilone 4'-O-β-d-glucopyranoside/Irilone B	$C_{22}H_{20}O_{11}$	460.1006	3.89	+	+	-	-	-	-	-	-	+	-	-	-	-	+	+
97	4'-methyltectorigenin-7-glucoside/6,4'-dimethoxy-5-hydroxyflavone-7-glucoside/Irisdichotin C/Irisolidone 7-O-hexoside/Irisolidone-7-O-α-d-glucoside	$C_{23}H_{24}O_{11}$	476.1315	4.02	-	-	+	-	-	-	-	+	-	-	-	-	-	+	-
98	Irilin D	$C_{16}H_{12}O_7$	316.0577	4.07	-	-	+	-	-	-	-	+	+	+	+	+	-	-	-
99	4'-methyltectorigenin-7-glucoside/6,4'-dimethoxy-5-hydroxyflavone-7-glucoside/Irisdichotin C/Irisolidone 7-O-hexoside/Irisolidone-7-O-α-d-glucoside	$C_{23}H_{24}O_{11}$	476.1307	4.13	-	-	-	-	-	-	-	-	-	-	-	-	-	-	-
100	Irilin B/Irisolidone	$C_{17}H_{14}O_6$	314.0783	4.15	+	+	-	-	-	-	-	-	-	-	-	-	-	+	+
101	6,3',4'-trimethoxy-7,8,5'-trihydroxyisoflavone/Irigenin	$C_{18}H_{16}O_8$	360.084	4.15	+	+	+	-	-	-	-	-	+	-	-	-	+	+	+
102	Iristectorigenin B/Iristectorigenin A Irisoid B/Irisoid	$C_{17}H_{14}O_7$	330.0731	4.18	-	+	+	-	+	-	-	+	+	-	-	+	+	+	-
103	C/Iriskashmirianin/4',5-dimethoxy-3-hydroxy-6,7-methylenedioxyisoflavone/Nigricanin	$C_{18}H_{14}O_7$	342.0737	4.25	-	+	-	+	-	-	-	-	-	-	+	-	-	+	+
104	Iristectorigenin B/Iristectorigenin A	$C_{17}H_{14}O_7$	330.0728	4.27	-	-	-	-	-	-	-	-	-	+	-	-	-	-	-
105	Genistein	$C_{15}H_{10}O_5$	270.0531	4.28	+	-	-	-	-	-	-	-	-	-	+	-	-	+	+
106	5-methoxy-4'-hydroxy-6,7-methylenedioxyisoflavone/Dichotomin/Nigricin	$C_{17}H_{12}O_6$	312.0637	4.28	+	+	-	-	-	-	-	-	+	-	+	-	-	-	+
107	Irilin D	$C_{16}H_{12}O_7$	316.0582	4.3	-	-	-	-	-	-	-	-	-	-	+	+	-	-	-
108	Iristectorigenin B/Iristectorigenin A	$C_{17}H_{14}O_7$	330.0733	4.4	-	-	-	+	+	-	-	-	-	-	+	+	+	+	+
109	Irilin A/Tectorigenin	$C_{16}H_{12}O_6$	300.0627	4.53	-	-	+	+	+	-	-	+	+	+	+	+	-	-	-

Table A1. Cont.

No.	Compound Name	Molecular Formula	Neutral Mass *	t_R (min)	I. pallida.			I. versicolor			I. lactea			I. carthaliniae			I. germanica		
					L	R	Rh	L	R	Rh	L	R	Rh	L	R	Rh	L	R	Rh
110	Irisflorentin a/Iriskumaonin methyl ether	$C_{19}H_{16}O_7$	356.0893	4.53	-	-	-	-	-	-	-	-	+	-	-	-	-	-	+
111	Irigenin S	$C_{19}H_{18}O_8$	374.099	4.54	+	+	+	-	-	-	-	-	-	-	-	-	+	+	+
112	Irisflorentin b	$C_{20}H_{18}O_8$	386.1001	4.55	+	+	+	-	-	-	-	-	-	-	-	-	+	+	+
113	Irilin B/Irisolidone	$C_{17}H_{14}O_6$	314.0778	4.57	+	+	+	-	-	-	-	-	-	-	-	-	+	+	+
114	dichotomitin	$C_{18}H_{14}O_6$	358.0694	4.58	+	+	+	-	-	-	-	-	+	-	-	-	-	-	-
115	Irilone A	$C_{16}H_{10}O_6$	298.0468	4.71	-	-	+	-	-	-	-	-	+	+	+	+	+	+	+
116	Irilin B/Irisolidone	$C_{17}H_{14}O_6$	314.079	4.71	-	-	-	+	+	+	-	-	-	+	-	-	-	-	-
117	Irilin B/Irisolidone	$C_{17}H_{14}O_6$	314.0792	4.86	-	-	-	-	-	-	-	-	-	+	+	+	-	-	-
118	Iristectorigenin B/Iristectorigenin A	$C_{17}H_{14}O_7$	330.0732	4.88	-	-	-	-	-	-	-	-	-	+	+	+	-	-	-
119	Irilin B/Irisolidone	$C_{17}H_{14}O_6$	314.078	5.01	-	-	+	+	+	+	+	+	-	-	-	-	+	+	+
120	Irilin B/Irisolidone	$C_{17}H_{14}O_6$	314.0784	5.15	-	-	-	+	+	-	-	-	-	-	-	-	-	-	-
121	Irilin B/Irisolidone	$C_{17}H_{14}O_6$	314.0782	5.41	-	-	-	-	-	-	+	+	+	-	-	-	-	-	-
122	Genistein	$C_{15}H_{10}O_5$	270.0519	5.52	-	-	-	-	-	-	+	+	+	-	-	-	-	+	+
123	Irilone A	$C_{16}H_{10}O_6$	298.0471	5.98	-	-	+	+	+	+	+	+	+	-	-	-	-	+	+
Terpenoids																			
124	Camphor	$C_{10}H_{16}O$	152.1202	3.87	-	+	-	+	+	-	-	-	-	-	-	-	-	-	-
125	22,23-epoxy-21-hydroxyiridal/tritectol A/Iritectol B	$C_{30}H_{50}O_5$	490.3656	5.59	-	+	-	+	+	+	-	-	-	-	+	-	-	+	+
126	22,23-epoxy-10-deoxy-21-hydroxyiridal/ 22,23-epoxyiridal/Isoiridogermanal	$C_{30}H_{50}O_4$	474.3694	6.28	-	-	-	+	+	-	-	+	-	-	-	-	-	+	+
127	α-Dehydroirigermanal	$C_{30}H_{48}O_3$	456.3604	6.29	-	-	-	+	+	+	-	+	-	-	-	-	-	-	-
128	α-Dehydroirigermanal	$C_{30}H_{48}O_3$	456.3606	6.51	+	+	-	+	+	+	-	+	-	-	+	-	-	-	-
129	22,23-epoxy-10-deoxy-21-hydroxyiridal/ 22,23-epoxyiridal/Isoiridogermanal	$C_{30}H_{50}O_4$	474.3692	6.51	+	+	-	+	+	+	+	+	-	+	+	-	+	+	-
130	spirobicyclic triterpenoid	$C_{30}H_{48}O_5$	488.3487	6.54	+	+	-	-	-	-	+	+	-	-	+	-	-	+	-
131	22,23-epoxy-10-deoxy-21-hydroxyiridal/ 22,23-epoxyiridal/Isoiridogermanal	$C_{30}H_{50}O_4$	474.3702	6.65	+	+	-	-	-	-	+	+	-	+	+	-	+	+	-
132	Belamcandal	$C_{32}H_{48}O_6$	528.3444	6.72	+	+	-	+	+	+	+	+	-	+	+	-	+	+	-
133	α-Dehydroirigermanal	$C_{30}H_{48}O_3$	456.3604	6.91	+	+	-	+	+	+	+	+	-	+	+	-	+	+	-
134	22,23-epoxy-10-deoxy-21-hydroxyiridal/ 22,23-epoxyiridal/Isoiridogermanal	$C_{30}H_{50}O_4$	474.3706	6.92	-	-	-	+	+	+	+	+	-	+	+	-	+	+	-
135	Iridotectoral A/Iridotectoral B	$C_{30}H_{46}O_5$	486.3333	6.96	+	+	-	+	+	+	+	+	-	+	+	-	+	+	-
136	Belamcandal	$C_{32}H_{48}O_6$	528.3434	6.98	+	+	-	+	+	+	+	+	-	+	+	-	+	+	-
137	Belamcandal	$C_{32}H_{48}O_6$	528.344	7.27	+	+	-	+	+	+	+	+	-	+	+	-	+	+	-
138	α-Dehydroirigermanal	$C_{30}H_{48}O_3$	456.3601	7.34	+	+	-	+	+	+	+	+	-	+	+	-	+	+	-
139	spirobicyclic triterpenoid	$C_{30}H_{48}O_6$	488.3486	7.51	+	+	-	+	+	+	+	+	-	+	+	-	+	+	-
140	Iridal/α-irigermanal	$C_{30}H_{50}O_4$	458.3739	7.52	-	-	-	-	-	-	+	+	-	+	+	-	-	-	-
141	Iridotectoral A/Iridotectoral B	$C_{30}H_{46}O_5$	486.3332	7.56	+	+	-	+	+	+	+	+	-	+	+	-	+	+	+
142	Iridotectoral A/Iridotectoral B	$C_{30}H_{46}O_5$	486.3336	7.94	-	-	-	-	+	-	-	-	-	+	+	-	-	+	-
143	22,23-epoxy-10-deoxy-21-hydroxyiridal/ 22,23-epoxyiridal/Isoiridogermanal	$C_{30}H_{46}O_5$	474.3696	7.97	+	-	-	-	+	-	+	+	+	-	-	-	-	+	-
144	Amorphene/α-Muurolene/β-Gurjuenene/γ-Elemene	$C_{15}H_{24}$	204.1866	8.57	+	-	-	-	-	-	-	-	+	-	-	-	-	-	+

Table A1. *Cont.*

No.	Compound Name	Molecular Formula	Neutral Mass *	t_R (min)	I. pallida. L	I. pallida. R	I. pallida. Rh	I. versicolor L	I. versicolor R	I. versicolor Rh	I. lactea L	I. lactea R	I. lactea Rh	I. carthaliniae L	I. carthaliniae R	I. carthaliniae Rh	I. germanica L	I. germanica Rh	I. germanica R
145	α-Dehydroirigermanal	$C_{30}H_{48}O_3$	456.36	8.86	-	-	-	-	+	+	-	-	-	-	-	-	-	+	-
146	Amorphene/α-Muurolene/β-Gurjuenene/γ-Elemene	$C_{15}H_{24}$	204.1877	9.26	-	-	-	+	-	+	-	-	-	-	-	-	-	+	-
147	Iridal/α-irigermanal	$C_{30}H_{50}O_3$	458.3756	9.26	+	-	+	+	+	+	+	+	+	+	+	-	+	+	+
148	iriversical	$C_{31}H_{52}O_3$	472.3899	9.75	+	-	-	+	+	+	+	+	+	+	+	+	+	+	+
149	iriversical	$C_{31}H_{52}O_3$	472.3898	10.03	+	-	+	+	+	+	+	+	+	+	+	+	+	+	+
150	Palmitic acid	$C_{16}H_{32}O_2$	256.2397	10.7	-	+	-	+	+	+	+	+	+	+	+	+	+	+	+
151	Iridotectoral A/Iridotectoral B	$C_{30}H_{46}O_5$	486.3347	10.9	+	-	-	+	+	+	+	+	+	+	+	-	+	+	+
152	Aristolone	$C_{15}H_{22}O$	218.1669	11.02	+	-	-	+	-	+	-	-	-	-	-	-	+	+	+
153	α-Dehydroirigermanal	$C_{30}H_{48}O_3$	456.359	11.29	-	+	-	-	+	+	+	+	+	+	+	+	+	+	+
154	α-Dehydroirigermanal	$C_{30}H_{48}O_3$	456.3594	11.49	+	-	+	+	+	+	+	+	+	+	+	+	+	+	+
155	Iridial	$C_{29}H_{48}O_3$	444.3602	12.19	+	+	-	+	-	+	+	-	+	+	-	-	+	-	-
156	iriversical	$C_{31}H_{52}O_3$	472.3921	13.5	-	-	-	-	+	-	-	-	-	-	+	-	-	+	-
157	Irisgermanic C	$C_{28}H_{48}O_3$	432.36	13.55	+	-	-	+	-	+	-	-	-	-	-	-	+	-	-
158	Iridial	$C_{29}H_{48}O_3$	444.3599	13.55	+	-	-	+	-	+	-	-	-	-	+	-	+	+	+
159	22,23-epoxy-10-deoxy-21-hydroxyiridal/ 22,23-epoxyiridal/Isoiridogermanal	$C_{30}H_{50}O_4$	474.3693	13.46	-	+	-	+	+	-	+	-	-	+	-	-	-	+	+
160	Iridal/α-irigermanal	$C_{30}H_{50}O_3$	458.3731	13.62	+	-	+	-	-	-	-	+	-	-	+	-	+	+	+
161	Amorphene/α-Muurolene/β-Gurjuenene/γ-Elemene	$C_{15}H_{24}$	204.19	14.01	-	-	-	-	-	-	-	-	+	-	-	+	-	+	+
Fatty acids																			
162	Myristic acid	$C_{14}H_{28}O_2$	228.2078	4.98	+	-	-	+	-	-	+	-	-	+	-	-	+	-	-
163	Lauric acid	$C_{12}H_{24}O_2$	200.1766	6.23	+	-	+	+	+	-	+	-	-	-	-	-	-	-	-
164	Myristic acid	$C_{14}H_{28}O_2$	228.2079	7.92	+	+	+	+	+	+	+	+	+	+	+	+	-	+	+
165	Lauric acid	$C_{12}H_{24}O_2$	200.1771	8.08	+	-	+	+	-	+	+	+	-	-	+	+	-	+	+
166	Myristic acid	$C_{14}H_{28}O_2$	228.2084	9.36	+	+	+	+	+	+	+	+	+	+	+	+	+	+	+
167	Lauric acid	$C_{12}H_{24}O_2$	200.1769	11.28	+	+	-	+	+	+	+	+	+	+	+	+	+	+	+
168	Stearic acid	$C_{18}H_{36}O_2$	284.2706	11.87	+	-	+	+	-	-	+	-	-	-	-	+	+	+	+
169	Myristic acid	$C_{14}H_{28}O_2$	228.2081	12.13	+	+	-	+	+	+	+	+	+	+	+	-	+	+	+
170	Myristic acid	$C_{14}H_{28}O_2$	228.208	12.38	+	+	+	+	+	+	+	+	+	+	+	-	+	+	+
171	Palmitic acid	$C_{16}H_{32}O_2$	256.2392	13.46	-	+	-	+	-	-	+	-	+	-	+	-	+	+	+
172	Stearic acid	$C_{18}H_{36}O_2$	284.2704	13.76	+	+	+	+	+	+	+	-	+	+	-	+	+	+	+
Steroids																			
173	Stigmasterol	$C_{29}H_{48}O$	412.3688	9.73	-	-	-	-	-	-	+	+	-	+	+	-	-	-	-
174	Stigmasterol-3-O-b-D-glucopyranoside	$C_{35}H_{58}O_6$	574.422	11.91	+	+	-	+	+	+	+	-	+	+	-	+	+	+	+
175	Stigmasterol-3-O-b-D-glucopyranoside	$C_{35}H_{58}O_6$	574.4219	12.32	+	+	-	+	+	+	+	+	+	+	+	+	+	+	+
176	7-β-Hydroxystigmast-4-en-3-one	$C_{29}H_{48}O_2$	428.3655	12.65	+	+	+	+	-	+	+	-	+	+	+	+	+	+	+
177	Stigmasterol	$C_{35}H_{58}O_6$	412.3701	13.48	+	+	+	+	+	+	+	+	+	+	+	+	+	+	+
Quinones																			
178	Irisoquin B	$C_{24}H_{40}O_4$	392.294	8.4	-	-	-	-	-	-	+	-	-	-	-	-	+	-	-
179	Irisoquinone A	$C_{24}H_{38}O_3$	374.282	11.32	+	-	-	+	-	-	+	-	-	-	-	-	+	-	-
180	Pallasone B Dihydroirisiquinone	$C_{24}H_{40}O_3$	376.2976	12.26	+	-	-	+	-	-	-	-	-	-	-	-	+	-	-

t_R (min)—retention time; L—leaves; R—roots; Rh—rhizomes; + standards for detected and - standards for not detected compound. * Experimentally obtained neutral exact mass.

References

1. Lee, D.; Seo, Y.; Khan, M.S.; Hwang, J.; Jo, Y.; Son, J.; Lee, K.; Park, C.; Chavan, S.; Gilad, A.A.; et al. Use of nanoscale materials for the effective prevention and extermination of bacterial biofilms. *Biotechnol. Bioprocess Eng.* **2018**, *23*, 1–10. [CrossRef]
2. Yu, O.Y.; Zhao, I.S.; Mei, M.L.; Lo, E.C.; Chu, C.H. Dental Biofilm and Laboratory Microbial Culture Models for Cariology Research. *Dent. J.* **2017**, *5*, 21. [CrossRef]
3. Basavaraju, M.; Sisnity, V.S.; Palaparthy, R.; Addanki, P.K. Quorum quenching: signal jamming in dental plaque biofilms. *J. Dent. Sci.* **2016**, *11*, 349–352. [CrossRef] [PubMed]
4. Kolenbrander, P.E.; Palmer, R.J.; Periasamy, S.; Jakubovics, N.S. Oral multispecies biofilm development and the key role of cell-cell distance. *Nat. Rev. Microbiol.* **2010**, *8*, 471–480. [CrossRef] [PubMed]
5. Zuanazzi, D.; Souto, R.; Mattos, M.B.A.; Zuanazzi, M.R.; Tura, B.R.; Sansone, C.; Colombo, A.P.V. Prevalence of potential bacterial respiratory pathogens in the oral cavity of hospitalised individuals. *Arch. Oral Biol.* **2010**, *55*, 21–28. [CrossRef]
6. Da Silva-Boghossian, C.M.I.; Do Souto, R.M.; Luiz, R.R.; Colombo, A.P.V. Association of red complex, A. *Actinomycetemcomitans* and non-oral bacteria with periodontal diseases. *Arch. Oral Biol.* **2011**, *56*, 899–906. [CrossRef]
7. Al-Jumaili, A.; Kumar, A.; Bazaka, K.; Jacob, M.V. Plant secondary metabolite-derived polymers: a potential approach to develop antimicrobial films. *Polymers* **2018**, *10*, 515. [CrossRef]
8. Furiga, A.; Roques, C.; Badet, C. Preventive effects of an original combination of grape seed polyphenols with amine fluoride on dental biofilm formation and oxidative damage by oral bacteria. *J. Appl. Microbiol.* **2014**, *116*, 761–771. [CrossRef]
9. Furiga, A.; Lonvaud-Funel, A.; Dorignac, G.; Badet, C. In vitro anti-bacterial and anti-adherence effects of natural polyphenolic compounds on oral bacteria. *J. Appl. Microbiol.* **2008**, *105*, 1470–1476. [CrossRef]
10. Antonio, A.G.; Iorio, N.L.P.; Pierro, V.S.S.; Candreva, M.S.; Farah, A.; Dos Santos, K.R.N.; Maia, L.C. Inhibitory properties of *Coffea canephora* extract against oral bacteria and its effect on demineralisation of deciduous teeth. *Arch. Oral Biol.* **2011**, *56*, 556–564. [CrossRef]
11. Antonio, A.; Iorio, N.P.; Farah, A.; Dos Santos, K.N.; Maia, L. Effect of *Coffea canephora* aqueous extract on microbial counts in ex vivo oral biofilms: a case study. *Planta Med.* **2012**, *78*, 755–760. [CrossRef] [PubMed]
12. Gartenmann, S.J.; Steppacher, S.L.; Von Weydlich, Y.; Heumann, C.; Attin, T.; Schmidlin, P.R. The effect of green tea on plaque and gingival inflammation: a systematic review. *J. Herb. Med.* **2020**, *21*, 100337. [CrossRef]
13. Moon, K.H.; Lee, Y.; Kim, J.N. Effects of foreign plant extracts on cell growth and biofilm formation of *Streptococcus mutans*. *J. Life Sci.* **2019**, *29*, 712–723. [CrossRef]
14. Burcu, B.; Aysel, U.; Nurdan, S. Antimicrobial, antioxidant, antimutagenic activities, and phenolic compounds of *Iris germanica*. *Ind. Crop. Prod.* **2014**, *61*, 526–530. [CrossRef]
15. Fang, R.; Houghton, P.J.; Hylands, P.J. Cytotoxic effects of compounds from *Iris tectorum* on human cancer cell lines. *J. Ethnopharmacol.* **2008**, *118*, 257–263. [CrossRef]
16. Ibrahim, S.R.M.; Mohamed, G.A.; Al-Musayeib, N.M. New constituents from the rhizomes of Egyptian *Iris germanica* L. *Molecules* **2012**, *17*, 2587–2598. [CrossRef]
17. Kostić, A.; Gašić, U.M.; Pešić, M.B.; Stanojević, S.P.; Barać, M.B.; Mačukanović-Jocić, M.P.; Avramov, S.N.; Tešić, Ž.L. Phytochemical analysis and total antioxidant capacity of rhizome, above-ground vegetative parts and flower of three *Iris* species. *Chem. Biodivers.* **2019**, *16*, e1800565. [CrossRef]
18. Moaket, S.; Oguzkan, S.B.; Kilic, I.H.; Selvi, B.; Karagoz, I.D.; Erdem, M.; Erdoğan, N.; Tekin, H.; Ozaslan, M. Biological activity of *Iris sari* Schott ex Baker in Turkey. *J. Biol. Sci.* **2017**, *17*, 136–141. [CrossRef]
19. Mocan, A.; Zengin, G.; Mollica, A.; Uysal, A.; Gunes, E.; Crişan, G.; Aktumsek, A. Biological effects and chemical characterization of *Iris schachtii* Markgr extracts: a new source of bioactive constituents. *Food Chem. Toxicol.* **2018**, *112*, 448–457. [CrossRef]
20. Nadaroğlu, H.; Demir, Y.; Demir, N. Antioxidant and radical scavenging properties of *Iris germanica*. *Pharm. Chem. J.* **2007**, *41*, 409–415. [CrossRef]
21. Singab, A.N.B.; Ayoub, I.M.; El-Shazly, M.; Korinek, M.; Wu, T.Y.; Cheng, Y.B.; Chang, F.R.; Wu, Y.C. Shedding the light on iridaceae: ethnobotany, phytochemistry and biological activity. *Ind. Crop. Prod.* **2016**, *92*, 308–335. [CrossRef]

22. Xie, G.Y.; Qin, X.Y.; Liu, R.; Wang, Q.; Lin, B.B.; Wang, G.K.; Xu, G.K.; Wen, R.; Qin, M.J. New isoflavones with cytotoxic activity from the rhizomes of *Iris germanica* L. *Nat. Prod. Res.* **2013**, *27*, 2173–2177. [CrossRef] [PubMed]
23. Kaššák, P. Secondary metabolites of the chosen genus *Iris* species. *Acta Univ. Agric. Silvic. Mendel. Brun.* **2013**, *60*, 269–280. [CrossRef]
24. Viktorova, J.; Stranska-Zachariasova, M.; Fenclova, M.; Vitek, L.; Hajslova, J.; Kren, V.; Ruml, T. Complex evaluation of antioxidant capacity of milk thistle dietary supplements. *Antioxidants* **2019**, *8*, 317. [CrossRef] [PubMed]
25. Pogačnik, L.; Bergant, T.; Skrt, M.; Ulrih, N.P.; Viktorová, J.; Ruml, T. In Vitro Comparison of the Bioactivities of Japanese and Bohemian Knotweed Ethanol Extracts. *Foods* **2020**, *9*, 544. [CrossRef] [PubMed]
26. Viktorová, J.; Stupák, M.; Řehořová, K.; Dobiasová, S.; Hoang, L.; Hajšlová, J.; Van Thanh, T.; Van Tri, L.; Van Tuan, N.; Ruml, T. Lemon grass essential oil does not modulate cancer cells multidrug resistance by citral—its dominant and strongly antimicrobial compound. *Foods* **2020**, *9*, 585. [CrossRef]
27. Sandberg, M.E.; Schellmann, D.; Brunhofer, G.; Erker, T.; Busygin, I.; Leino, R.; Vuorela, P.M.; Fallarero, A. Pros and cons of using resazurin staining for quantification of viable *Staphylococcus aureus* biofilms in a screening assay. *J. Microbiol. Methods* **2009**, *78*, 104–106. [CrossRef]
28. Tran, V.N.; Viktorova, J.; Augustynkova, K.; Jelenova, N.; Dobiasova, S.; Rehorova, K.; Fenclova, M.; Stranska-Zachariasova, M.; Vitek, L.; Hajslova, J.; et al. In silico and in vitro studies of mycotoxins and their cocktails; Their toxicity and its mitigation by silibinin pre-treatment. *Toxins* **2020**, *12*, 148. [CrossRef]
29. Kukula-Koch, W.; Sieniawska, E.; Widelski, J.; Urjin, O.; Główniak, P.; Skalicka-Woźniak, K. Major secondary metabolites of *Iris* spp. *Phytochem. Rev.* **2015**, *14*, 51–80. [CrossRef]
30. Roger, B.; Jeannot, V.; Fernandez, X.; Cerantola, S.; Chahboun, J. Characterisation and quantification of flavonoids in *Iris germanica* L. and *Iris pallida* Lam. resinoids from Morocco. *Phytochem. Anal.* **2012**, *23*, 450–455. [CrossRef]
31. Nasim, S.; Baig, I.; Jalil, S.; Orhan, I.; Sener, B.; Choudhary, M.I. Anti-inflammatory isoflavonoids from the rhizomes of *Iris germanica*. *J. Ethnopharmacol.* **2003**, *86*, 177–180. [CrossRef]
32. Nasim, S.; Baig, I.; Jalil, S.; Orhan, I.; Sener, B.; Choudhary, M.I. Isoflavonoid glycosides from the rhizomes of *Iris germanica*. *Chem. Pharm. Bull.* **2002**, *50*, 1100–1102. [CrossRef]
33. Rigano, D.; Formisano, C.; Grassia, A.; Grassia, G.; Perrone, A.; Piacente, S.; Vuotto, M.L.; Senatore, F. Antioxidant flavonoids and isoflavonoids from rhizomes of *Iris pseudopumila*. *Planta Med.* **2007**, *73*, 93–96. [CrossRef] [PubMed]
34. Krick, W.; Marner, F.-J.; Jaenicke, L. Isolation and structural determination of a new methylated triterpenoid from rhizomes of *Iris versicolor* L. *Zeitschrift fur Naturforsch C J. Biosci.* **1983**, *38*, 689–692. [CrossRef]
35. Marner, F.J.; Longerich, I. Isolation and structure determination of new iridals from *Iris sibirica* and *Iris versicolor*. *Liebigs Ann. Chem.* **1992**, 269–272. [CrossRef]
36. Ouyang, J.; Sun, F.; Feng, W.; Sun, Y.; Qiu, X.; Xiong, L.; Liu, Y.; Chen, Y. Quercetin is an effective inhibitor of quorum sensing, biofilm formation and virulence factors in *Pseudomonas aeruginosa*. *J. Appl. Microbiol.* **2016**, *120*, 966–974. [CrossRef]
37. Lee, J.H.; Park, J.H.; Cho, H.S.; Joo, S.W.; Cho, M.H.; Lee, J. Anti-biofilm activities of quercetin and tannic acid against *Staphylococcus aureus*. *Biofouling* **2013**, *29*, 491–499. [CrossRef]
38. Wang, J.; Song, M.; Pan, J.; Shen, X.; Liu, W.; Zhang, X.; Li, H.; Deng, X. Quercetin impairs *Streptococcus pneumoniae* biofilm formation by inhibiting sortase A activity. *J. Cell. Mol. Med.* **2018**, *22*, 6228–6237. [CrossRef]
39. Zeng, Y.; Nikitkova, A.; Abdelsalam, H.; Li, J.; Xiao, J. Activity of quercetin and kaemferol against *Streptococcus mutans* biofilm. *Arch. Oral Biol.* **2019**, *98*, 9–16. [CrossRef]
40. Yang, W.Y.; Kim, C.K.; Ahn, C.H.; Kim, H.; Shin, J.; Oh, K.B. Flavonoid glycosides inhibit sortase A and sortase A-mediated aggregation of *Streptococcus mutans*, an oral bacterium responsible for human dental caries. *J. Microbiol. Biotechnol.* **2016**, *26*, 1557–1565. [CrossRef]
41. Zhang, B.; Wang, X.; Wang, L.; Chen, S.; Shi, D.; Wang, H. Molecular mechanism of the flavonoid natural product dryocrassin ABBA against *Staphylococcus aureus* sortase A. *Molecules* **2016**, *21*, 1428. [CrossRef] [PubMed]
42. Mu, D.; Xiang, H.; Dong, H.; Wang, D.; Wang, T. Isovitexin, a potential candidate inhibitor of sortase A of *Staphylococcus aureus* USA300. *J. Microbiol. Biotechnol.* **2018**, *28*, 1426–1432. [CrossRef] [PubMed]

43. Slobodníková, L.; Fialová, S.; Rendeková, K.; Kováč, J.; Mučaji, P. Antibiofilm activity of plant polyphenols. *Molecules* **2016**, *21*, 1717. [CrossRef] [PubMed]
44. Pande, G.S.J.; Natrah, F.M.I.; Sorgeloos, P.; Bossier, P.; Defoirdt, T. The *Vibrio campbellii* quorum sensing signals have a different impact on virulence of the bacterium towards different crustacean hosts. *Vet. Microbiol.* **2013**, *167*, 540–545. [CrossRef] [PubMed]
45. Asfour, H. Anti-quorum sensing natural compounds. *J. Microsc. Ultrastruct.* **2018**, *6*, 1–10. [CrossRef] [PubMed]
46. Gomes, L.C.; Moreira, J.M.; Araújo, J.D.; Mergulhão, F.J. Surface conditioning with *Escherichia coli* cell wall components can reduce biofilm formation by decreasing initial adhesion. *AIMS Microbiol.* **2017**, *3*, 613–628. [CrossRef]
47. Abd-Alla, M.H.; Bashandy, S.R. Production of quorum sensing inhibitors in growing onion bulbs infected with *Pseudomonas aeruginosa* E (HQ324110). *ISRN Microbiol.* **2012**, *2012*, 161890. [CrossRef]
48. Prasath, K.G.; Sethupathy, S.; Pandian, S.K. Proteomic analysis uncovers the modulation of ergosterol, sphingolipid and oxidative stress pathway by myristic acid impeding biofilm and virulence in *Candida albicans*. *J. Proteom.* **2019**, *208*, 103503. [CrossRef]
49. Duckworth, R.M.; Maguire, A.; Omid, N.; Steen, I.N.; McCracken, G.I.; Zohoori, F.V. Effect of rinsing with mouthwashes after brushing with a fluoridated toothpaste on salivary fluoride concentration. *Caries Res.* **2009**, *43*, 391–396. [CrossRef]

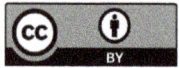

© 2020 by the authors. Licensee MDPI, Basel, Switzerland. This article is an open access article distributed under the terms and conditions of the Creative Commons Attribution (CC BY) license (http://creativecommons.org/licenses/by/4.0/).

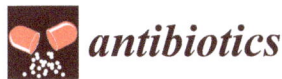

Article

Nanovectorized Microalgal Extracts to Fight *Candida albicans* and *Cutibacterium acnes* Biofilms: Impact of Dual-Species Conditions

Virginie Lemoine [1], Clément Bernard [1], Charlotte Leman-Loubière [2], Barbara Clément-Larosière [3], Marion Girardot [1], Leslie Boudesocque-Delaye [2], Emilie Munnier [4] and Christine Imbert [1,*]

1. Laboratoire Ecologie et Biologie des Interactions, Université de Poitiers, UMR CNRS 7267, 86073 Poitiers, France; lemoinev60@gmail.com (V.L.); clement.bernard@univ-poitiers.fr (C.B.); marion.girardot@univ-poitiers.fr (M.G.)
2. Laboratoire SIMBA EA 7502, Faculté de Pharmacie, Université de Tours, 31 avenue Monge, 37200 Tours, France; charlotte.leman-loubiere@clarins.com (C.L.-L.); leslie.boudesocque@univ-tours.fr (L.B.-D.)
3. Dénitral, Groupe COOPERL, 7 rue des Blossières Maroue BP 60328, 22403 Lamballe, France; barbara.clement-larosiere@cooperl.com
4. Laboratoire Nanomédicaments et Nanosondes EA 6295, Faculté de Pharmacie, Université de Tours, 31 avenue Monge, 37200 Tours, France; emilie.munnier@univ-tours.fr
* Correspondence: christine.imbert@univ-poitiers.fr

Received: 30 April 2020; Accepted: 23 May 2020; Published: 26 May 2020

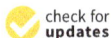

Abstract: Biofilm-related infections are a matter of concern especially because of the poor susceptibility of microorganisms to conventional antimicrobial agents. Innovative approaches are needed. The antibiofilm activity of extracts of cyanobacteria *Arthrospira platensis*, rich in free fatty acids, as well as of extract-loaded copper alginate-based nanocarriers, were studied on single- and dual-species biofilms of *Candida albicans* and *Cutibacterium acnes*. Their ability to inhibit the biofilm formation and to eradicate 24 h old biofilms was investigated. Concentrations of each species were evaluated using flow cytometry. Extracts prevented the growth of *C. acnes* single-species biofilms (inhibition > 75% at 0.2 mg/mL) but failed to inhibit preformed biofilms. Nanovectorised extracts reduced the growth of single-species *C. albicans* biofilms (inhibition > 43% at 0.2 mg/mL) while free extracts were weakly or not active. Nanovectorised extracts also inhibited preformed *C. albicans* biofilms by 55% to 77%, whereas the corresponding free extracts were not active. In conclusion, even if the studied nanocarrier systems displayed promising activity, especially against *C. albicans*, their efficacy against dual-species biofilms was limited. This study highlighted that working in such polymicrobial conditions can give a more objective view of the relevance of antibiofilm strategies by taking into account interspecies interactions that can offer additional protection to microbes.

Keywords: antibiofilm; antimicrobial agent; bacteria; fungi; polymicrobial biofilm; microalga; free fatty acids; encapsulation

---

1. Introduction

Biofilms are involved in numerous diseases, both superficial and systemic, for instance those affecting the oral cavity, skin or related to an implanted medical device. They can be single species, but most often they are polymicrobial and contain both fungi and bacteria. For example, dermal wounds are colonized by aerobic and anaerobic bacterial and fungal species, most of them belonging to resident microbiota of the surrounding skin, oral cavity and gut, or from the external environment [1]. It has been shown that 60% of chronic wounds exhibit a biofilm which is a major factor in delayed wound healing [2–5]. Also, it is considered that *Candida* spp. are among the primary causes of delayed healing and infection in both acute and chronic wounds, especially those of a surgical nature [6,7]. Literature data suggest that *Candida* spp. rarely colonize human skin but can cause infection especially in specific conditions such as immune deficiency, diabetes or after antibiotic use [8,9].

Gram-positive bacteria *Cutibacterium acnes* (formerly *Propionibacterium acnes*) [10] are a main colonizer and inhabitant of the skin [11,12] and a good biofilm former, producing both single species and polymicrobial biofilms [13–16]. Its involvement in chronic skin disease such as acne vulgaris is very well-known and this species is also occasionally involved in non-skin-related infections such as prosthetic joint infections, some of them being related to the formation of a biofilm [17,18]. As for many other microbial species, sessile *C. acnes* cells as well as *Candida albicans* cells have been shown to be more tolerant to conventional antibiotics than their planktonic counterparts [19–21].

Our team recently showed that *C. acnes* and *C. albicans* can form dual-species biofilms, with *C. acnes* adhering to both hyphal and yeast forms of *C. albicans* [15]. The presence of metabolically active *C. albicans* cells enhanced the early growth of *C. acnes* under aerobic conditions, while no influence was observed in anaerobic conditions. We also recently demonstrated that the co-presence of these species in biofilms influenced their sensitivity to micafungin, a major conventional antifungal agent. Actually, *C. acnes* was shown to protect *C. albicans* cells from the effect of micafungin in dual-species biofilms [22]. Along the same lines, Montelongo-Jauregui et al. showed that the resistance of *C. albicans* to amphotericin B and caspofungin, as well as the resistance of *Streptococcus gordonii* to clindamycin were increased due to a dual-species biofilm produced by *C. albicans* and with *Streptococcus gordonii*, compared to single-species conditions [23]. Therefore, a double issue should be thus observed—biofilm lifestyle causes itself a decreased susceptibility to antimicrobial agents and the polymicrobial nature of the biofilm can make this lack of susceptibility even worse.

Biofilms are infectious reservoirs and the most effective way to prevent biofilm-related infections requires the eradication of these complex microbial structures, that is their detachment, their disorganization and the killing of all released microbial cells, with these three events needing to be concomitant. Unfortunately, the available antimicrobial conventional molecules fail to reach this challenging goal.

Free fatty acids (FFAs) are physiological antimicrobial agents occurring on skin, exhibiting a wide antimicrobial spectrum (antibacterial, antifungal, antibiofilm . . .) [24,25]. Microalgae have been well-described as abundant sources of lipids and especially FFAs [26,27]. Those FFAs, especially polyunsaturated (PUFAs), may also represent a potential source of topical drugs against polymicrobial biofilms. Indeed, a previous screening of 29 FFAs based on topical antibacterial activity highlighted that PUFAs were among the most active [25]. *Arthrospira platensis* (formerly *Spirulina platensis*) appeared as a good model among all microalgae as it was the most studied microalgae with a well-known FFA profile.

Due to their lipid nature, FFAs are not able to penetrate the biofilm made of highly hydrophilic exopolysaccharide. Recently, nanosized systems showed their ability to vectorize active molecules in biofilms. Core-shell nanosystems, with a hydrophilic shell and a lipophilic core, seem to be very appropriate vectors for low-polarity active molecules [28,29]. Alginate-based nanocarriers, nanosystems made of a triglyceride core and an alginate gel shell, were shown to be efficient to vectorize FFAs in *C. albicans* biofilm [30]. The reproducibility of the preparation, the stability of the systems and their FDA-approved ingredients constitute key advantages for their use in dermatology. Moreover, they were shown to be stable in dermatological preparations [31].

We previously developed a proof of concept of the potential of *A. platensis* extracts and alginate-based nanocarriers combination as a possible strategy to fight *C. albicans* single-species biofilms. The antibiofilm strategies are all the more innovative and promising in that they are able to act on taxonomically distant and diverse microbial species, because of the polymicrobial nature of most biofilms developing in humans.

Thus, this current study aimed to obtain lipid extracts from Cyanobacteria *A. platensis*, to develop extract-loaded copper alginate-based nanocarriers able to carry a lipid extract and to evaluate the antibiofilm activity of these lipid extracts nanovectorized or free, against both single-species fungal and bacterial biofilms and interkingdom dual-species biofilms.

2. Results

2.1. A. platensis Extraction

A. platensis biomass was extracted using two sustainable solvents—EtOAc and DMC. Resulting extracts were enriched in lipids (Table 1), with a closely related FFA profile. Both extracts contained mainly ω6 PUFA, i.e., linoleic and γ-linolenic acid (more than 60% of total FFAs) (Table 2). Also, lipophilic dyes (chlorophyll and carotenoids) were co-extracted (Table 2), but their content remained low, highlighting again the good selectivity of these solvents towards lipids.

Table 1. *A. platensis* extracts composition (total lipids, chlorophylls, carotenoids).

Extract	EtOAc	DMC
Total lipids (mg of equiv. castor oil/g of extract)	1115.1 ± 87.2	980.3 ± 67.9
Chlorophylls (mg/g of extract)	82.0 ± 8.1	52.6 ± 2.5
Carotenoids (mg/g of extracts)	53.5 ± 8.1	61.0 ± 2.6

Data are shown as mean ± SD; $n = 3$.

Table 2. Free fatty acid (FFA) ratios in *A. platensis* extracts, in relative percentage of total FFA.

	EtOAc	DMC
Saturated		
Myristic acid	nd	nd
Palmitic acid	27.0%	21.9%
Stearic acid	5.1%	5.7%
MUFA		
Myristoleic acid	nd	nd
Palmitoleic acid	nd	nd
Oleic acid	4.8%	4.8%
PUFA		
Linoleic acid	41.1%	42.3%
γ-Linolenic acid	22.0%	25.2%

nd = nondetected; $n = 1$.

2.2. A. platensis Extracts Vectorization

Extract-loaded ANCs were prepared with EtOAc extract and DMC extract. Physicochemical characteristics are shown in Table 3.

Table 3. Physicochemical characteristics of extract-loaded alginate-based nanocarriers.

	Hydrodynamic Diameter (nm) (Mean ± SD, $n = 3$)	Polydispersity Index (Mean ± SD, $n = 3$)	Zeta Potential (mV) (Mean ± SD, $n = 3$)
Empty ANC	249 ± 9	0.129 ± 0.044	−24.5 ± 0.7
EtOAc extract-loaded ANC	236 ± 2	0.147 ± 0.018	−24.2 ± 0.2
DMC-extract loaded ANC	250 ± 1	0.139 ± 0.015	−24.1 ± 0.9

Extract-loaded ANCs show similar size and surface potential as empty ANCs with a pure Labrafac®® WL 1349 core. The polydispersity index lower than 0.2 shows a monodispersity of the suspensions, guaranteeing the reproducibility of the dosage. The negative surface charge of the nanocarriers participates to the colloidal stability of the nanocarriers and should not limit their interaction with the biofilms. Indeed, even if biofilms are generally considered negatively charged and could thus bind more easily to cationic nanoparticles [32], several negatively charged systems displayed antibiofilm efficacy [28,33]. The native ANC suspension shows a concentration in *A. platensis* extract of ~1 mg/mL.

2.3. Ability of A. platensis Extracts to Prevent Biofilm Formation

In single-species conditions, EtOAc extract used at 0.2 mg/mL displayed a significant ($p = 0.0001$) but very limited antibiofilm formation effect against *C. albicans* (24.4% inhibition) (Figure 1A). This extract used at 0.1 mg/mL was not active against *C. albicans*, and DMC extracts (at both 0.1 and 0.2 mg/mL) as well. Both EtOAc and DMC extracts significantly reduced the growth of *C. acnes* biofilms, regardless of the tested concentrations—inhibition ranged between 66.0% and 78.4% (EtOAc extract, $p \leq 0.003$) and between 67.6% and 86.2% (DMC extract, $p \leq 0.0008$) (Figure 1C). However, no real conclusion can be made in the case of EtOAc (0.1 and 0.2 mg/mL) and DMC (0.1 mg/mL) as the error bars are very high.

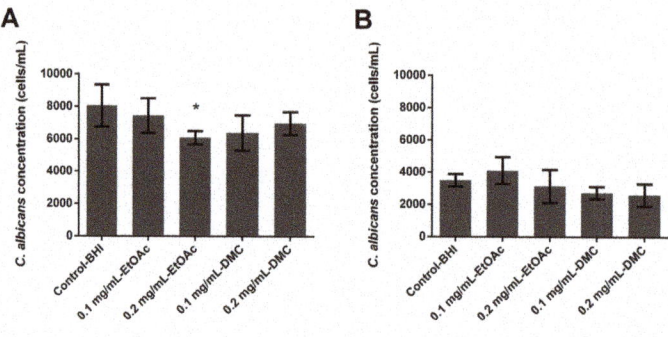

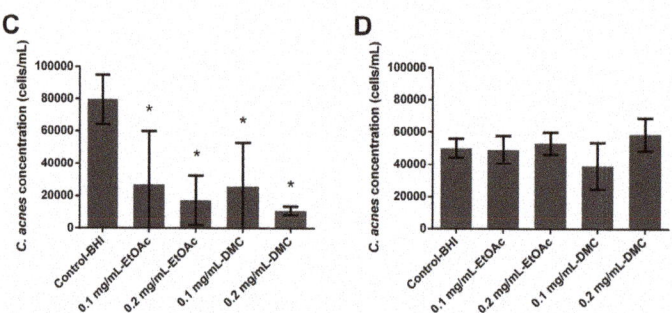

Figure 1. Ability of *Arthrospira fusiformis* extracts to prevent biofilm formation. Single-species biofilms (*C. albicans*) (**A**); *C. albicans* concentration obtained in dual-species biofilms (*C. albicans* + *C. acnes*) (**B**); single-species biofilms (*C. acnes*) (**C**); *C. acnes* concentration obtained in dual-species biofilms (*C. albicans* + *C. acnes*) (**D**). Results are expressed as mean ± SD. * $p < 0.005$: test condition vs. BHI-control (biofilms treated with BHI only).

In dual-species conditions, neither EtOAc nor DMC extract solutions were able to reduce the biofilm formation of *C. albicans* and no reduction was observed in the fungal and bacterial populations.

2.4. Ability of A. platensis Extracts to Eradicate Preformed Biofilms

None of the extracts, whatever the tested concentration, had any effect on *C. albicans* or *C. acnes* preformed single-species or dual-species biofilms. No reduction was observed in the fungal and bacterial populations after a 24 h treatment (Figure 2).

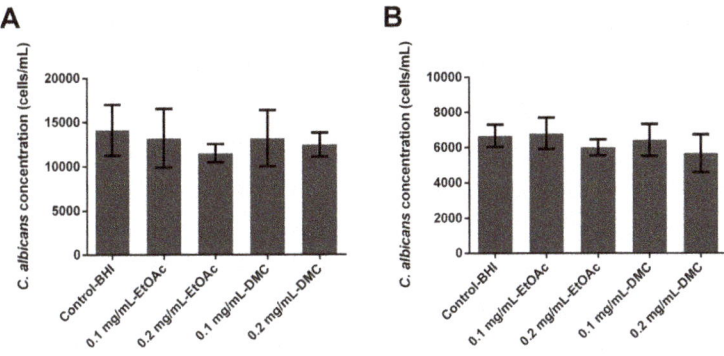

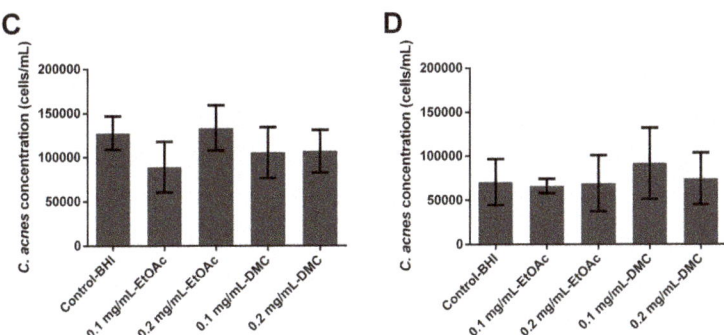

Figure 2. Ability of *Arthrospira fusiformis* extracts to eradicate preformed biofilm. Single-species biofilms (*C. albicans*) (**A**); *C. albicans* concentration obtained in dual-species biofilms (*C. albicans* + *C. acnes*) (**B**); single-species biofilms (*C. acnes*) (**C**); *C. acnes* concentration obtained in dual-species biofilms (*C. albicans* + *C. acnes*) (**D**). Results are expressed as mean ± SD. * $p < 0.005$: test condition vs. BHI-control (biofilms treated with BHI only).

2.5. Ability of A. platensis Extracts Encapsulated in Alginate-Based Nanocarriers to Prevent Biofilm Formation

In single-species conditions, empty nanocarriers inhibited the growth of *C. albicans* biofilms by 51.55% (0.1_emptyNC, $p = 0.001$) or 54.14% (0.2_emptyNC, $p = 0.0002$), while they had no effect on *C. acnes* biofilms (Figure 3A,C). Nanocarriers loaded with extract solutions at 0.2 mg/mL (0.2 mg/mL_EENC) inhibited the growth of *C. albicans* biofilms by 51.35% (EtOAc, $p = 0.0031$) or 43.77% (DMC, $p = 0.0021$) while those loaded with extract solutions at 0.1 mg/mL (0.1 mg/mL_EENC) had no significant influence. Regarding the growth of *C. acnes* biofilms, only nanocarriers loaded with EtOAc extract at 0.2 mg/mL and DMC extract at 0.1 mg/mL demonstrated a weak inhibitory activity of 22.48% ($p = 0.0016$) and 32.74% ($p = 0.0004$), respectively (Figure 3C).

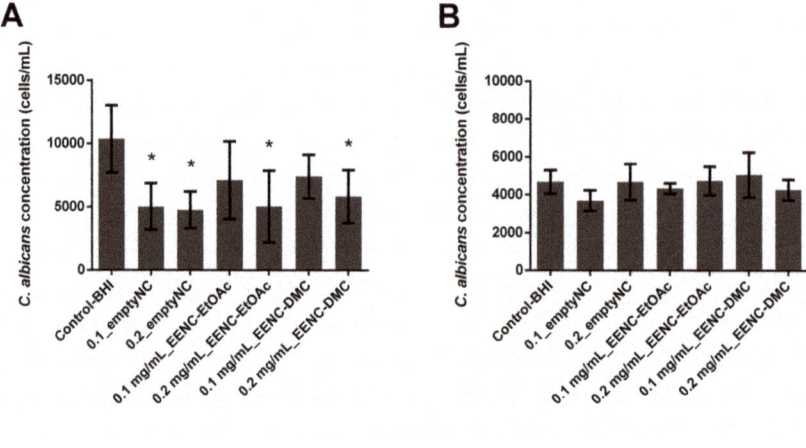

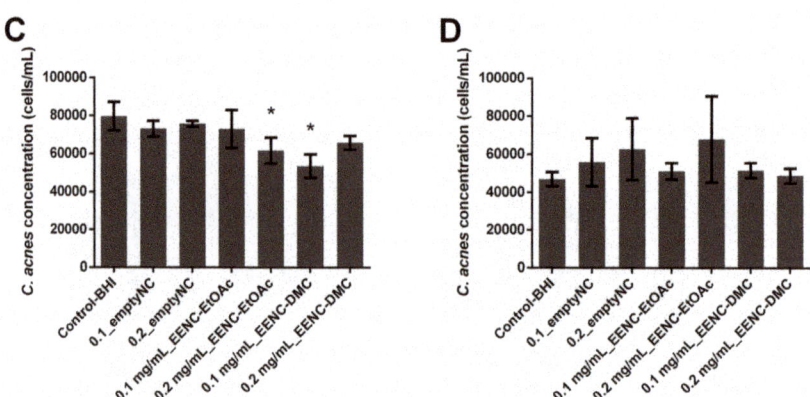

Figure 3. Ability of *Arthrospira fusiformis* extracts encapsulated in alginate nanocarriers to prevent biofilm formation. Single-species biofilms (*C. albicans*) (**A**); *C. albicans* concentration obtained in dual-species biofilms (*C. albicans* + *C. acnes*) (**B**); single-species biofilms (*C. acnes*) (**C**); *C. acnes* concentration obtained in dual species biofilms (*C. albicans* + *C. acnes*) (**D**). Results are expressed as mean ± SD. * $p < 0.005$: test condition vs. BHI-control (biofilms treated with BHI only).

In dual-species conditions, nanocarriers loaded with extract solutions did not limit the growth of either *C. albicans* or *C. acnes* in biofilms. Only empty nanocarriers (0.1_emptyNC, $p = 0.0046$) displayed a weak activity but were not significant ($p > 0.005$) against *C. albicans* growth (21.0%) and no reduction was observed on *C. acnes* population (Figure 3B,D).

2.6. Ability of A. platensis Extracts Encapsulated in Alginate-Based Nanocarriers to Eradicate Preformed Biofilms

In single-species conditions, empty nanocarriers inhibited preformed biofilms of *C. albicans* by 58.7% (0.1_emptyNC, $p < 0.0001$) or 76.69% (0.2_emptyNC, $p < 0.0001$), whereas they had no effect on *C. acnes* biofilms (Figure 4A,B). Whatever the conditions, all nanocarriers loaded with extract solutions inhibited preformed single species *C. albicans* biofilms ($p < 0.0001$) by at least 55%; nanocarriers loaded with EtOAc extracts inhibited biofilms by 76.9% (0.1 mg/mL_EENC-EtOAc) and 62.35% (0.2 mg/mL_EENC-EtOAct) whereas those loaded with DMC extracts induced a 55.69% (0.1 mg/mL_EENC-DMC) and a 77.32% (0.2 mg/mL_EENC-DMC) inhibition. On the contrary, whatever the conditions, both empty and loaded nanocarriers failed to significantly reduce an already formed single-species biofilm of *C. acnes* ($p > 0.005$) (Figure 4C).

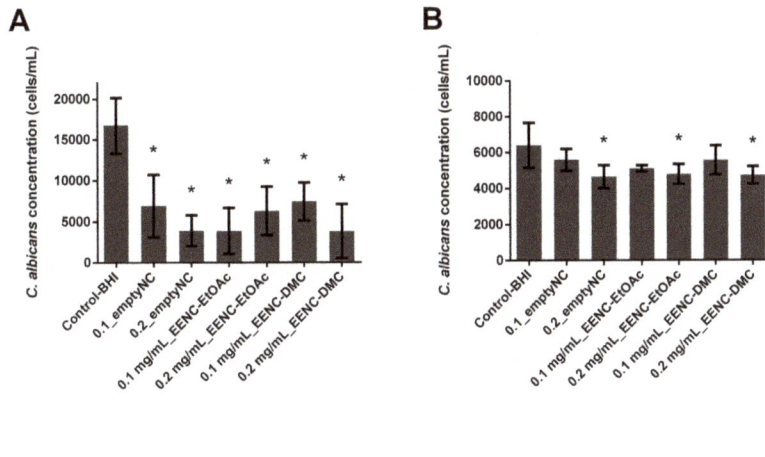

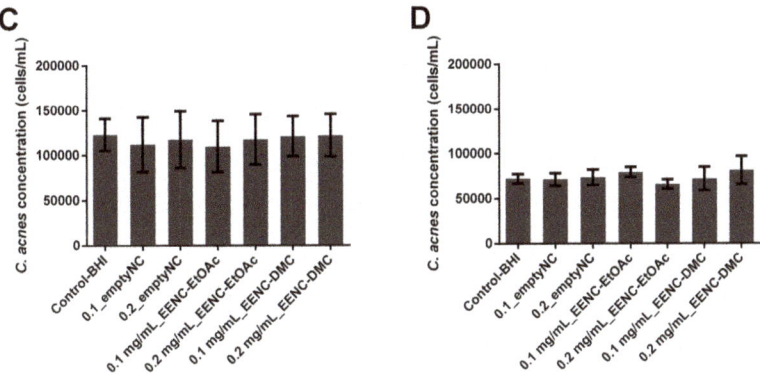

Figure 4. Ability of *Arthrospira fusiformis* extracts encapsulated in alginate nanocarriers to eradicate preformed biofilm. Single-species biofilms (*C. albicans*) (**A**); *C. albicans* concentration obtained in dual-species biofilms (*C. albicans* + *C. acnes*) (**B**); single-species biofilms (*C. acnes*) (**C**); *C. acnes* concentration obtained in dual-species biofilms (*C. albicans* + *C. acnes*) (**D**). Results are expressed as mean ± SD. * $p < 0.005$: test condition vs BHI-control (biofilms treated with BHI only).

In dual-species conditions, empty nanocarriers as well as those loaded with extract solutions induced inhibition always less than 28% of already formed dual-species biofilms, whatever the target population (*C. albicans* or *C. acnes*) (Figure 4B,D). Significant *p*-values demonstrating an inhibition of the *C. albicans* population were only observed in the case of 0.2_emptyNC (inhibition: 27.5%), 0.2 mg/mL_EENC-EtOAc (inhibition: 25.3%) and 0.2 mg/mL_EENC-DMC (inhibition: 26.3%) (Figure 4B).

3. Discussion

The results are in accordance with those previously obtained when studying the activity of EtOAc extract at 0.2 mg/mL on *C. albicans* biofilms [30]. The ability of EtOAct extract at 0.2 mg/mL to inhibit *C. albicans* biofilms growth evidenced by the significant decrease in the number of cells forming treated biofilms (FCM approach) (Figure 1A) agrees with previous results showing that this extract was able to reduce the metabolic activity of *C. albicans* forming treated biofilms (XTT method). However, EtOAc extract at 0.1 mg/mL and DMC extract at 0.1 or 0.2 mg/mL did not manage to decrease yeast concentration in biofilms, although they previously showed antimetabolic activity. The XTT method is a classical method used to quantify fungal biofilms [34–36]. However, this method does not allow a differentiation between bacterial and fungal populations in dual-species biofilms. That is why the FCM approach used for the current study was recently developed [22,37]. A comparative study previously suggested that results provided by colony-forming unit (CFU) counts, XTT reduction or FCM counts were generally comparable and occasional differences could be explained by the specificity and targets of each method [37]. For example, metabolic activity can be reduced without any change in the cell number explaining some divergence in XTT versus CFU or FCM count results. Slight differences between previous and present results could also be at least partially explained by the fact that two different *A. platensis* biomasses were used in these studies, leading to different compositions of extracts. Growth conditions impact the FFA profile as large amounts of ω6-MUFAs and PUFAs were highlighted here, with decreased rates of saturated FFAs, the latter being known to exhibit higher antifungal activity.

By comparing results obtained from growing biofilms (prophylactic activity) and preformed ones (curative activity), we observed that EtOAc extract at 0.2 mg/mL loses its activity once the biofilm is formed (Figures 1A and 2A). Similarly, although all tested extracts significantly limited the growth of single species *C. acnes* biofilms, they were not active anymore once the biofilm was preformed (Figures 1C and 2C). The extracts, whether free or nanovectorized, were not active against dual-species biofilms, growing or already formed as well (Figure 1C,D and Figure 2B,D). Moreover, since single-species *C. albicans* biofilms were prepared aerobically and those involving *C. acnes* anaerobically, a role of the presence of oxygen could not be excluded to explain the different levels of antibiofilm activity that have been observed. In fact, the mechanism of action of the FFA is not completely elucidated. Some studies suggested that their antimicrobial activity would be partly explained by the formation of PUFA peroxidation products [24], which would be favored in an aerobic environment. These oxidized metabolites would act according to a mechanism different from that of native FFAs [24], explaining the residual activity observed on *C. acnes*. As we could expect, these results suggest that preventing the formation of a biofilm is easier than eradicating this biofilm once it is formed.

Different teams demonstrated that biofilms made of more than one species presented reduced susceptibility to antimicrobial treatment compared to single-species biofilms [38,39]. In addition to studying the activity of the extracts and nanocarriers loaded or not by extracts on single-species biofilms, our work assessed the impact of the dual-species nature of the biofilms. Indeed, our results showed that nanocarriers loaded or otherwise with *A. platensis* EtOAc extracts or loaded or not with *A. platensis* DMC extracts as well significantly reduced both already formed and formation of *C. albicans* single-species biofilms, but displayed no or poor activity against *C. albicans* in dual-species biofilms (Figure 3; Figure 4A,B). These results thus suggest that *C. albicans* growing with *C. acnes* in dual-species biofilms is more difficult to inhibit than in single-species ones, which agrees with previous studies on the efficacy of micafungin against *C. albicans* in these two conditions [22]. More generally, results published in recent years suggest that bacteria and fungi from dual-species biofilms such as *C. albicans*–*Staphylococcus* spp. or *C. albicans*–*Streptococcus* spp. often exhibit reduced susceptibilities towards antibiotic or antifungal agents, which is at least partially caused by their synergistic interaction [23,38,40–43]. This study confirmed the activity of the empty nanocarriers against *C. albicans* biofilms which was already observed by Boutin et al. in 2019 [30], suggesting that copper ions could efficiently reach *C. albicans* cells through this single-species biofilm. Cheong et al., 2020 recently confirmed that copper displayed a high antifungal activity against *C. albicans* [44]. Unfortunately, we observed that empty nanocarriers lose their activity at least partially against *C. albicans* as soon as *C. acnes* is present in biofilms, whatever the age of the studied biofilm. Punniyakotti et al. 2020, recently reported the antibiofilm activity of copper nanoparticles studying *Pseudomonas* and *Staphylococcus* species [45]. They hypothesized that Cu^{2+} ions liberated from the nanoparticles would be engrossed by the bacterial cell surface and cause cell damage, affecting biofilm development. These authors suggested that the surface binding capability of copper ions would play a key role in the biofilm inhibition. Although we can hypothesize a similar mechanism to explain the activity against fungi, there is no clear explanation as to why empty nanocarriers failed to inhibit biofilm in the presence of *C. acnes*. Nanocarriers loaded with *A. platensis* extracts failed to significantly prevent the formation of *C. acnes* biofilms whereas *A. platensis* extracts without nanocarriers did it in the range of 66.0% to 86.2%. As empty nanocarriers display no activity either, we can hypothesize that nanocarrier loading would counteract the action of extracts against these bacteria (Figure 1; Figure 3C). Conversely, the encapsulation of *A. platensis* extracts induced up to 51.35% of inhibition against the formation of *C. albicans* single-species biofilms (Figures 1A and 3A). As the empty nanocarriers inhibited *C. albicans* single-species biofilm formation and eradicated biofilms, the activity cannot be totally attributed to the extracts. Unfortunately, this encapsulation did not allow the growth inhibition of dual-species biofilms, whatever the studied species (Figure 1; Figure 3B,D).

Finally, *A. platensis* extracts alone or encapsulated in nanosystems displayed an absence of activity against *C. acnes* preformed biofilms (Figures 2C and 4C) whereas the encapsulation of *A. platensis* extracts gave a promising activity against *C. albicans* preformed single-species biofilms, inducing inhibition up to 77.32% (Figures 2A and 4A). Whatever the microorganism studied, the encapsulation does not lead to the obtention of an efficient and significant inhibition of preformed dual-species biofilms (Figure 2B,D and Figure 4B,D)

Very few authors compared the effect of nanosystems vectorizing antimicrobial agents on mono- or multispecies biofilms [46,47], and even less on biofilms mixing Gram-positive bacteria and fungi. It is now established that the efficacy of nanosystems on biofilms is linked to their capacity for deeply penetrating the matrix [32]. However, the penetration of nanoparticles into biofilms is highly dependent on the surface characteristics of the nanoparticles [46,48]. Our results suggest that ANCs can diffuse through the extracellular polymeric substance (EPS) of *C. albicans* biofilm, but are not able to diffuse in the EPS of *C. acnes* and in that of polymicrobial biofilm matrix as well. Anjum et al. showed that PLGA nanoparticules loaded with xylitol successfully penetrated into the EPS matrix of single-species biofilms of *S. aureus* or *Pseudomonas aeruginosa*, and also of dual-species biofilms [46]. In the study of Anjum et al., penetration was made easier by adding a ligand onto the nanoparticle surface targeting the biofilm matrix. Tan et al. measured the antibiofilm activity of nanoparticles including enzymes targeting the matrix of biofilms composed of *S. aureus* and *C. albicans* [47]. The particles were able to disrupt in a similar manner single-species or dual-species biofilms, but it was observed that adhesion of bacteria to *Candida* hyphae made their surface less accessible to antimicrobial molecules. This obstacle was already described for free antimicrobial molecules in dual-species biofilms of *S. aureus* and *Fusarium falciforme* [49]. This interaction between the microbial species was also observed for *C. acnes* et *C. albicans* [22] and could participate in the loss of activity of ANCs on *C. albicans* in the dual-species biofilm.

In conclusion, our results highlight the interest of *A. platensis* extracts in preventing the formation of *C. acnes* single-species biofilms. They also suggest that even if the nanocarrier developed by our team offers interesting features, especially in the case of *C. albicans*, its activity against dual-species biofilms is much more limited at the concentrations tested. Even if in vitro models represent simplified models, far from real clinical conditions, developing polymicrobial conditions gives a more realistic representation of clinical biofilms that develop in the human body. This study clearly demonstrated the impact of polymicrobial conditions on the antibiofilm efficacy of nanovectorized antimicrobial systems and highlighted the importance of working in such polymicrobial conditions to have a more objective view of the tested molecules or systems.

4. Materials and Methods

4.1. Chemicals

Ethyl acetate (EtOAc), methanol (MeOH), toluene, hexane, formic acid, diethylether, glacial acetic acid, petroleum ether, sulfuric acid 96% (H_2SO_4) and dimethylsulfoxide (DMSO) were purchased from Carlo Erba (Val de Reuil, France). Dimethyl carbonate (DMC), sodium alginate, (±)-α-tocophérol 96% (vitamin E), oleic acid, linoleic acid, palmitic acid, myristic acid, stearic acid, palmitoleic acid, γ-linolenic acid, 2,3-bis-(2-methoxy-4-nitro-5-sulfophenyl)-2H-tetrazolium-5-carboxanilide (XTT), menadione and glucose were purchased from Sigma Aldrich (Saint-Quentin Fallavier, France). Phosphoric acid 85% was purchased from Merck pro analysis (Darmstad, Germany). Labrafac®® WL 1349 was purchased from Gattefossé (Saint-Priest, France). Montane 80®® and Montanox 80®® were purchased from Seppic (Castres, France). Copper nitrate $Cu(NO_3)_2$ was purchased from Fisher Scientific SAS (Illkirch, France). Vanillin, acetic acid trihydrate 99+% were purchased from Acros Organics (Geel, Belgium). Water was purified using a Milli-Q system (Millipore Corporation, Bedford, MA, USA).

4.2. Biomass

Arthrospira platensis was cultivated and harvested by DENITRAL SA (Lamballe, France) and kindly provided by Dr Barbara Clément-Larosière.

4.3. Extraction Protocol and Extracts Analyses

A total of 1 g of biomass was extracted with DMC or EtOAc according to the protocol described by Boutin et al. [30]. The calibration curve was built up using castor oil and results were expressed as mg of equivalent of castor oil in the extract.

Pigments and total lipid rates were obtained using protocol described in Boutin et al. (2019) [30]. FFA profiles were obtained using the LC-ESI-MS protocol adapted from Samburova et al. (2013) [50]. Briefly, LC-ESI-MS analyses were performed on an Acquity H-Class with an SQD detector (Waters, Saint Quentin en Yvelines, France). The system was fitted with a BEH C18 (50 × 2.1 mm; 1.7 μm particle size). The column oven was set at 40 °C. Mobile phases were A Water 0.1% NH_3 aq; B acetonitrile 0.1% NH_3 aq. Flow rate was 0.25 mL/min and the gradient was set as follows—initial solvent B content was 10%, raised to 40% in 2 min, 90% in 23 min and 100% in 1 min and maintained for 9 min. ESI in negative mode was performed with cone voltage set at 50 V and capillary voltage at 2.8 kV.

4.4. Alginate-Based Nanocarriers Preparation and Characterization

Alginate-based nanocarriers (ANCs) were prepared using ultrasound oil-in-water emulsification followed by surface gelation with cupric ions inspired by Nguyen et al. [31] and adapted by Boutin et al. [30]. Briefly, an *A. platensis* lipid extract solution in Labrafac ® WL 1349 (6 mg/mL) was emulsified with a sodium alginate solution in presence of nonionic surfactant, using an ultrasonic probe (Vibra-cell ultrasonic processor, Sonics, Newtown, CT, USA, 20 kHz). The resulting nanoemulsion was mixed under ultrasounds stirring with a solution of copper ions, which complex alginates to form an insoluble copper-alginate gel at the surface of the nanodroplets.

The hydrodynamic diameter and polydispersity index (PdI) of the ANC aqueous suspensions were measured using a dynamic light scattering (DLS) instrument (NanoZS, Malvern Panalytical,

Malvern, UK). Each sample was diluted 1:50 in ultrapure water before measurements. Zeta potential was determined on the same sample with the same instrument. Measurements were made in triplicate at 25 °C.

4.5. Bacterial and Fungal Organisms

C. albicans ATCC® 28367™ and *C. acnes* ATCC® 6919 were used for this study.

Yeasts were cultured on Sabouraud Glucose with Chloramphenicol agar plates aerobically at 37 °C whereas *C. acnes* was cultured on Brain Heart Infusion (BHI) agar plates supplemented with 10% of defibrinated horse blood anaerobically at 37 °C. Before biofilm experiments, *C. albicans* and *C. acnes* were cultured overnight in BHI at 37 °C in aerobic and anaerobic conditions, respectively. Following incubation, cultures were washed with PBS (centrifugation at 2000× g, 10 min) and adjusted to 2×10^7 cells/mL and 2×10^8 cells/mL in fresh BHI for *C. albicans* and *C. acnes* respectively.

4.6. Antibiofim Formation Assay

Single-species *C. albicans*, single-species *C. acnes* and polymicrobial *C. albicans-C. acnes* biofilms were formed in 96-wells flat bottom nontreated polystyrene microplates. In the single-species condition, wells received 100 µL of microbial suspensions. In polymicrobial condition, wells received 50 µL of both microbial suspensions.

Antibiofilm formation activities of lipid extracts previously dissolved in DMSO were tested at two concentrations—0.1 and 0.2 mg/mL. Final DMSO concentrations did not exceed 2% of the overall volume in wells. For extracts included in nanocarriers (NCs), nanosystem tested concentrations were chosen to display extracts at 0.1 and 0.2 mg/mL in ultrapure water—"extract equivalent in nanocarrier" (mg/mL_EENC). Finally, empty nanocarriers were tested as controls and the studied concentrations corresponded to those present in nanocarriers loaded with extracts at 0.1 and 0.2 mg/mL (0.1_emptyNC and 0.2_emptyNC). A total of 100 µL of extract or nanosystem solutions diluted in BHI were then added to the wells. Some wells without extract or nanosystem solution were reserved as a control and received 100 µl of fresh BHI (BHI control). Microplates containing only *C. albicans* were incubated 24 h at 37 °C in aerobic conditions while microplates containing *C. acnes* or both microorganisms were incubated in anaerobic conditions.

After incubation, cell concentrations were determined using a protocol adapted from the work of Kerstens et al., 2015 [51]. Planktonic cells were eliminated (2 rounds of washing with 200 µL of PBS) and sessile cells were scraped off from the microplate bottom using sterile tips. An extensive rinsing of the microplate bottom was performed to detach remaining microorganisms. The obtained suspensions were sonicated for 10 min to break down aggregates (Elmasonic S 30, Elma Electronic, Wetzikon, Switzerland, 37 Hz). This procedure has no effect on both *C. albicans* and *C. acnes* viability according to literature data [18,51].

In these microbial suspensions, cells concentrations were determined using flow cytometry (FCM). For dual-species conditions, FCM allowed us to distinguish the yeast population from that of bacteria according to their respective sizes and morphologies [22]. Measurements were performed on a CytoFLEX (Beckman Coulter, Indianapolis, IN USA) managed by CytExpert 2.0.0.153 software (Beckman Coulter, Indianapolis, IN, USA) and equipped with a blue laser (λ_{ex} = 488 nm) and a 488/8 bandpass filter. The flow rate used was 30 µL·min^{-1}.

4.7. Anti-Preformed Biofilm Assay

Single-species *C. albicans*, single-species *C. acnes* and polymicrobial *C. albicans-C. acnes* biofilms were formed in 96-well flat-bottom nontreated polystyrene microplates. In single-species condition, wells received 100 µL of microbial suspensions. In polymicrobial condition, wells received 50 µL of both microbial suspensions. Final volume was adjusted to 200 µL using fresh BHI in all conditions. Microplates containing only *C. albicans* were incubated 24 h at 37 °C in aerobic conditions whereas microplates containing *C. acnes* or both microorganisms were incubated in anaerobic conditions.

After incubation, supernatants were removed, and biofilms were carefully rinsed twice with 200 µL of PBS. A total of 100 µL of fresh BHI was added to all wells. Then, wells received 100 µL of extract or nanosystem solutions diluted in BHI. Tested conditions were similar to those presented for antibiofilm formation assays. Some wells without extract or nanosystem solution were reserved as a control. A total of 100 µL of fresh BHI was also used in control wells. Microplates containing only *C. albicans* were incubated 24 h at 37 °C in aerobic conditions whereas microplates containing *C. acnes* or both microorganisms were incubated in anaerobic conditions.

After incubation, cell concentrations were determined as described previously for the antibiofilm formation assay.

4.8. Statistical Analysis

Experiments were performed at least in duplicate with four replicates for each condition. Mann–Whitney U test was applied to determine statistical significance of the differences between the groups using GraphPad Prism® version 6.01 (GraphPad Software Inc, San Diego, CA USA). Differences were considered significant if $p < 0.005$.

Author Contributions: Conceptualization, C.I., E.M., M.G. and L.B.-D.; Methodology, C.B., M.G., L.B.-D., E.M. and C.I.; Resources, B.C.L., M.G., L.B.-D., E.M. and C.I.; Investigation, V.L., C.B. and C.L.-L.; Formal analysis, C.B., E.M., L.B. and C.I.; Writing–Original Draft Preparation, C.B., L.B.-D., E.M. and C.I. and S.M.; Writing–Review & Editing, C.B., B.C.-L., M.G., L.B.-D., E.M. and C.I.; Supervision, L.B.-D, E.M. and C.I.; Project administration, L.B.-D., E.M. and C.I. All authors have read and agree to the published version of the manuscript.

Funding: This work was supported by a grant (2018–2019) of the AAP Collaborative Research Action of the universities of Tours and Poitiers; This work was also supported by the 2015–2020 State-Region Planning Contracts (CPER), European Regional Development Fund (FEDER), and intramural funds from the Centre National de la Recherche Scientifique (CNRS) and the University of Poitiers. The authors thanks the ARD Cosmétosciences and the Centre Val de Loire Region for financial support (ARD 2017-00118114).

Acknowledgments: The authors also wish to thank Didier Debail and Garry Holding for revising the English text.

Conflicts of Interest: The authors have nothing to declare.

References

1. Bowler, P.G.; Duerden, B.I.; Armstrong, D.G. Wound microbiology and associated approaches to wound management. *Clin. Microbiol. Rev.* **2001**, *14*, 244–269. [CrossRef] [PubMed]
2. Kalan, L.; Grice, E.A. Fungi in the wound microbiome. *Adv. Wound Care* **2018**, *7*, 247–255. [CrossRef] [PubMed]
3. Johnson, T.R.; Gómez, B.I.; McIntyre, M.K.; Dubick, M.A.; Christy, R.J.; Nicholson, S.E.; Burmeister, D.M. The cutaneous microbiome and wounds: New molecular targets to promote wound healing. *Int. J. Mol. Sci.* **2018**, *19*. [CrossRef] [PubMed]
4. Vindenes, H.; Bjerknes, R. Microbial colonization of large wounds. *Burns* **1995**, *21*, 575–579. [CrossRef]
5. James, G.A.; Swogger, E.; Wolcott, R.; Pulcini, E.D.; Secor, P.; Sestrich, J.; Costerton, J.W.; Stewart, P.S. Biofilms in chronic wounds. *Wound Repair Regen.* **2008**, *16*, 37–44. [CrossRef]
6. Duerden, B.I. Virulence Factors in Anaerobes. *Clin. Infect. Dis.* **1994**, *18*, S253–S259. [CrossRef]
7. Mangram, A.J.; Horan, T.C.; Pearson, M.L.; Silver, L.C.; Jarvis, W.R. Guideline for Prevention of Surgical Site Infection, 1999. Centers for Disease Control and Prevention (CDC) Hospital Infection Control Practices Advisory Committee. *Am. J. Infect. Control* **1999**, *27*, 97–134. [CrossRef]
8. Noble, W.C. Skin microbiology: Coming of age. *J. Med. Microbiol.* **1984**, *17*, 1–12. [CrossRef]
9. Peleg, A.Y.; Hogan, D.A.; Mylonakis, E. Medically important bacterial–fungal interactions. *Nat. Rev. Microbiol.* **2010**, *8*, 340–349. [CrossRef]
10. Scholz, C.F.P.; Kilian, M. The natural history of cutaneous propionibacteria, and reclassification of selected species within the genus *Propionibacterium* to the proposed novel genera *Acidipropionibacterium* gen. Nov., *Cutibacterium* gen. nov. and *Pseudopropionibacterium* gen. nov. *Int. J. Syst. Evol. Microbiol.* **2016**, *66*, 4422–4432. [CrossRef]
11. Grice, E.A.; Segre, J.A. The skin microbiome. *Nat. Rev. Microbiol.* **2011**, *9*, 244–253. [CrossRef] [PubMed]

12. Cogen, A.L.; Nizet, V.; Gallo, R.L. Skin microbiota: A source of disease or defence? *Br. J. Dermatol.* **2008**, *158*, 442–455. [CrossRef] [PubMed]
13. Kuehnast, T.; Cakar, F.; Weinhäupl, T.; Pilz, A.; Selak, S.; Schmidt, M.A.; Rüter, C.; Schild, S. Comparative analyses of biofilm formation among different *Cutibacterium acnes* isolates. *Int. J. Med. Microbiol.* **2018**, *308*, 1027–1035. [CrossRef] [PubMed]
14. Achermann, Y.; Goldstein, E.J.C.; Coenye, T.; Shirtliffa, M.E. *Propionibacterium acnes*: From Commensal to opportunistic biofilm-associated implant pathogen. *Clin. Microbiol. Rev.* **2014**, *27*, 419–440. [CrossRef]
15. Bernard, C.; Lemoine, V.; Hoogenkamp, M.A.; Girardot, M.; Krom, B.P.; Imbert, C. *Candida albicans* enhances initial biofilm growth of *Cutibacterium acnes* under aerobic conditions. *Biofouling* **2019**, *35*, 350–360. [CrossRef]
16. Tyner, H.; Patel, R. Propionibacterium acnes biofilm—A sanctuary for *Staphylococcus aureus*? *Anaerobe* **2016**, *40*, 63–67. [CrossRef]
17. Bojar, R.A.; Holland, K.T. Acne and *Propionibacterium acnes*. *Clin. Dermatol.* **2004**, *22*, 375–379. [CrossRef]
18. Bayston, R.; Ashraf, W.; Barker-Davies, R.; Tucker, E.; Clement, R.; Clayton, J.; Freeman, B.J.C.; Nuradeen, B. Biofilm formation by *Propionibacterium acnes* on biomaterials in vitro and in vivo: Impact on diagnosis and treatment. *J. Biomed. Mater. Res. Part A* **2007**, *81A*, 705–709. [CrossRef]
19. Coenye, T.; Peeters, E.; Nelis, H.J. Biofilm formation by *Propionibacterium acnes* is associated with increased resistance to antimicrobial agents and increased production of putative virulence factors. *Res. Microbiol.* **2007**, *158*, 386–392. [CrossRef]
20. Kuhn, D.M.; George, T.; Chandra, J.; Mukherjee, P.K.; Ghannoum, M.A. Antifungal susceptibility of *Candida* biofilms: Unique efficacy of amphotericin B lipid formulations and echinocandins. *Antimicrob. Agents Chemother.* **2002**, *46*, 1773–1780. [CrossRef]
21. Mukherjee, P.K.; Chandra, J. *Candida* biofilm resistance. *Drug Resist. Updat.* **2004**, *7*, 301–309. [CrossRef] [PubMed]
22. Bernard, C.; Renaudeau, N.; Mollichella, M.L.; Quellard, N.; Girardot, M.; Imbert, C. *Cutibacterium acnes* protects *Candida albicans* from the effect of micafungin in biofilms. *Int. J. Antimicrob. Agents* **2018**, *52*, 942–946. [CrossRef] [PubMed]
23. Montelongo-Jauregui, D.; Srinivasan, A.; Ramasubramanian, A.K.; Lopez-Ribot, J.L. An in vitro model for oral mixed biofilms of *Candida albicans* and *Streptococcus gordonii* in synthetic saliva. *Front. Microbiol.* **2016**, *7*, 1–13. [CrossRef] [PubMed]
24. Desbois, A.P.; Smith, V.J. Antibacterial free fatty acids: Activities, mechanisms of action and biotechnological potential. *Appl. Microbiol. Biotechnol.* **2010**, *85*, 1629–1642. [CrossRef]
25. Ruffell, S.E.; Müller, K.M.; McConkey, B.J. Comparative assessment of microalgal fatty acids as topical antibiotics. *J. Appl. Phycol.* **2016**, *28*, 1695–1704. [CrossRef]
26. D'Alessandro, E.B.; Antoniosi Filho, N.R. Concepts and studies on lipid and pigments of microalgae: A review. *Renew. Sustain. Energy Rev.* **2016**, *58*, 832–841. [CrossRef]
27. Hess, S.K.; Lepetit, B.; Kroth, P.G.; Mecking, S. Production of chemicals from microalgae lipids—Status and perspectives. *Eur. J. Lipid Sci. Technol.* **2018**, *120*, 1700152. [CrossRef]
28. Kłodzińska, S.N.; Wan, F.; Jumaa, H.; Sternberg, C.; Rades, T.; Nielsen, H.M. Utilizing nanoparticles for improving anti-biofilm effects of azithromycin: A head-to-head comparison of modified hyaluronic acid nanogels and coated poly (lactic-co-glycolic acid) nanoparticles. *J. Colloid Interface Sci.* **2019**, *555*, 595–606. [CrossRef]
29. Sánchez, M.C.; Toledano-Osorio, M.; Bueno, J.; Figuero, E.; Toledano, M.; Medina-Castillo, A.L.; Osorio, R.; Herrera, D.; Sanz, M. Antibacterial effects of polymeric PolymP-n Active nanoparticles. An in vitro biofilm study. *Dent. Mater.* **2019**, *35*, 156–168. [CrossRef]
30. Boutin, R.; Munnier, E.; Renaudeau, N.; Girardot, M.; Pinault, M.; Chevalier, S.; Chourpa, I.; Clément-Larosière, B.; Imbert, C.; Boudesocque-Delaye, L. *Spirulina platensis* sustainable lipid extracts in alginate-based nanocarriers: An algal approach against biofilms. *Algal Res.* **2019**, *37*, 160–168. [CrossRef]
31. Nguyen, H.T.P.; Munnier, E.; Souce, M.; Perse, X.; David, S.; Bonnier, F.; Vial, F.; Yvergnaux, F.; Perrier, T.; Cohen-Jonathan, S.; et al. Novel alginate-based nanocarriers as a strategy to include high concentrations of hydrophobic compounds in hydrogels for topical application. *Nanotechnology* **2015**, *26*, 255101. [CrossRef] [PubMed]
32. Fulaz, S.; Vitale, S.; Quinn, L.; Casey, E. Nanoparticle–Biofilm Interactions: The Role of the EPS Matrix. *Trends Microbiol.* **2019**, *27*, 915–926. [CrossRef]

33. Lopes, L.Q.S.; Santos, C.G.; de Almeida Vaucher, R.; Raffin, R.P.; Santos, R.C.V. Nanocapsules with glycerol monolaurate: Effects on *Candida albicans* biofilms. *Microb. Pathog.* **2016**, *97*, 119–124. [CrossRef] [PubMed]
34. Lohse, M.B.; Gulati, M.; Valle Arevalo, A.; Fishburn, A.; Johnson, A.D.; Nobile, C.J. Assessment and optimizations of *Candida albicans* in vitro biofilm assays. *Antimicrob. Agents Chemother.* **2017**, *61*. [CrossRef] [PubMed]
35. Taff, H.T.; Nett, J.E.; Andes, D.R. Comparative analysis of *Candida* biofilm quantitation assays. *Med. Mycol.* **2012**, *50*, 214–218. [CrossRef]
36. Dhale, R.P.; Ghorpade, M.V.; Dharmadhikari, C.A. Comparison of various methods used to detect biofilm production of *Candida* species. *J. Clin. Diagn. Res.* **2014**, *8*, DC18-c20. [CrossRef]
37. Juin, C.; Perrin, F.; Puy, T.; Bernard, C.; Mollichella, M.L.; Girardot, M.; Costa, D.; Guillard, J.; Imbert, C. Anti-biofilm activity of a semi-synthetic molecule obtained from resveratrol against *Candida albicans* biofilm. *Med. Mycol.* **2019**. [CrossRef]
38. Harriott, M.M.; Noverr, M.C. *Candida albicans* and *Staphylococcus aureus* form polymicrobial biofilms: Effects on antimicrobial resistance. *Antimicrob. Agents Chemother.* **2009**, *53*, 3914–3922. [CrossRef]
39. Morales, D.K.; Hogan, D.A. *Candida albicans* interactions with bacteria in the context of human health and disease. *PLoS Pathog.* **2010**, *6*, 1–4. [CrossRef]
40. Harriott, M.M.; Noverr, M.C. Ability of *Candida albicans* mutants to induce *Staphylococcus aureus* vancomycin resistance during polymicrobial biofilm formation. *Antimicrob. Agents Chemother.* **2010**, *54*, 3746–3755. [CrossRef]
41. Kim, D.; Liu, Y.; Benhamou, R.I.; Sanchez, H.; Simon-Soro, A.; Li, Y.; Hwang, G.; Fridman, M.; Andes, D.R.; Koo, H. Bacterial-derived exopolysaccharides enhance antifungal drug tolerance in a cross-kingdom oral biofilm. *ISME J.* **2018**, *12*, 1427–1442. [CrossRef] [PubMed]
42. Bernard, C.; Girardot, M.; Imbert, C. *Candida albicans* interaction with Gram-positive bacteria within interkingdom biofilms. *J. Mycol. Med.* **2019**. [CrossRef]
43. Adam, B.; Baillie, G.S.; Douglas, L.J. Mixed species biofilms of *Candida albicans* and *Staphylococcus epidermidis*. *J. Med. Microbiol.* **2002**, *51*, 344–349. [CrossRef] [PubMed]
44. Cheong, Y.-K.; Arce, M.P.; Benito, A.; Chen, D.; Luengo Crisóstomo, N.; Kerai, L.V.; Rodríguez, G.; Valverde, J.L.; Vadalia, M.; Cerpa-Naranjo, A.; et al. Synergistic Antifungal Study of PEGylated Graphene Oxides and Copper Nanoparticles against *Candida albicans*. *Nanomaterials* **2020**, *10*. [CrossRef] [PubMed]
45. Punniyakotti, P.; Panneerselvam, P.; Perumal, D.; Aruliah, R.; Angaiah, S. Anti-bacterial and anti-biofilm properties of green synthesized copper nanoparticles from *Cardiospermum halicacabum* leaf extract. *Bioprocess Biosyst. Eng.* **2020**, 1–9. [CrossRef]
46. Anjum, A.; Chung, P.Y.; Ng, S.F. PLGA/xylitol nanoparticles enhance antibiofilm activity: Via penetration into biofilm extracellular polymeric substances. *RSC Adv.* **2019**, *9*, 14198–14208. [CrossRef]
47. Tan, Y.; Ma, S.; Leonhard, M.; Moser, D.; Ludwig, R.; Schneider-Stickler, B. Co-immobilization of cellobiose dehydrogenase and deoxyribonuclease I on chitosan nanoparticles against fungal/bacterial polymicrobial biofilms targeting both biofilm matrix and microorganisms. *Mater. Sci. Eng. C* **2020**, *108*, 110499. [CrossRef]
48. Wang, T.; Bai, J.; Jiang, X.; Nienhaus, G.U. Cellular uptake of nanoparticles by membrane penetration: A study combining confocal microscopy with FTIR spectroelectrochemistry. *ACS Nano* **2012**, *6*, 1251–1259. [CrossRef]
49. Bautista-Hernández, L.A.; Gómez-Olivares, J.L.; Buentello-Volante, B.; Dominguez-Lopez, A.; Garfias, Y.; Acosta-García, M.C.; Calvillo-Medina, R.P.; Bautista-de Lucio, V.M. Negative interaction of *Staphylococcus aureus* on *Fusarium falciforme* growth ocular isolates in an in vitro mixed biofilm. *Microb. Pathog.* **2019**, *135*, 103644. [CrossRef]
50. Samburova, V.; Lemos, M.S.; Hiibel, S.; Kent Hoekman, S.; Cushman, J.C.; Zielinska, B. Analysis of triacylglycerols and free fatty acids in algae using ultra-performance liquid chromatography mass spectrometry. *JAOCS J. Am. Oil Chem. Soc.* **2013**, *90*, 53–64. [CrossRef]
51. Kerstens, M.; Boulet, G.; Van kerckhoven, M.; Clais, S.; Lanckacker, E.; Delputte, P.; Maes, L.; Cos, P. A flow cytometric approach to quantify biofilms. *Folia Microbiol.* **2015**, *60*, 335–342. [CrossRef] [PubMed]

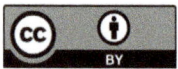

© 2020 by the authors. Licensee MDPI, Basel, Switzerland. This article is an open access article distributed under the terms and conditions of the Creative Commons Attribution (CC BY) license (http://creativecommons.org/licenses/by/4.0/).

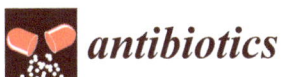

Article

Carbapenem-Resistant *Klebsiella pneumoniae* Clinical Isolates: In Vivo Virulence Assessment in *Galleria mellonella* and Potential Therapeutics by Polycationic Oligoethyleneimine

Dalila Mil-Homens [1], Maria Martins [1], José Barbosa [1], Gabriel Serafim [1], Maria J. Sarmento [2], Rita F. Pires [1], Vitória Rodrigues [3], Vasco D.B. Bonifácio [1,*] and Sandra N. Pinto [1,*]

1. iBB—Institute for Bioengineering and Biosciences, Department of Bioengineering, Instituto Superior Técnico, Universidade de Lisboa, Av. Rovisco Pais, 1049-001 Lisboa, Portugal; dalilamil-homens@tecnico.ulisboa.pt (D.M.-H.); mald.martins@campus.fct.unl.pt (M.M.); josembarbosa@tecnico.ulisboa.pt (J.B.); gabriel.serafim@tecnico.ulisboa.pt (G.S.); ritafpires@tecnico.ulisboa.pt (R.F.P.)
2. J. Heyrovský Institute of Physical Chemistry of the Czech Academy of Sciences, Dolejskova 3, 18223 Prague, Czech Republic; maria.sarmento@jh-inst.cas.cz
3. Secção de Microbiologia, Laboratório SYNLAB-Lisboa, Grupo SYNLAB Portugal, Av. Columbano Bordalo Pinheiro, 75 A, 2° Andar, 1070-061 Lisboa, Portugal; vitoria.rodrigues@synlab.pt
* Correspondence: vasco.bonifacio@tecnico.ulisboa.pt (V.D.B.); sandrapinto@ist.utl.pt (S.N.P.)

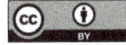

Abstract: *Klebsiella pneumoniae*, one of the most common pathogens found in hospital-acquired infections, is often resistant to multiple antibiotics. In fact, multidrug-resistant (MDR) *K. pneumoniae* producing KPC or OXA-48-like carbapenemases are recognized as a serious global health threat. In this sense, we evaluated the virulence of *K. pneumoniae* KPC(+) or OXA-48(+) aiming at potential antimicrobial therapeutics. *K. pneumoniae* carbapenemase (KPC) and the expanded-spectrum oxacillinase OXA-48 isolates were obtained from patients treated in medical care units in Lisbon, Portugal. The virulence potential of the *K. pneumonia* clinical isolates was tested using the *Galleria mellonella* model. For that, *G. mellonella* larvae were inoculated using patients KPC(+) and OXA-48(+) isolates. Using this in vivo model, the KPC(+) *K. pneumoniae* isolates showed to be, on average, more virulent than OXA-48(+). Virulence was found attenuated when a low bacterial inoculum (one magnitude lower) was tested. In addition, we also report the use of a synthetic polycationic oligomer (L-OEI-h) as a potential antimicrobial agent to fight infectious diseases caused by MDR bacteria. L-OEI-h has a broad-spectrum antibacterial activity and exerts a significantly bactericidal activity within the first 5-30 min treatment, causing lysis of the cytoplasmic membrane. Importantly, the polycationic oligomer showed low toxicity against in vitro models and no visible cytotoxicity (measured by survival and health index) was noted on the in vivo model (*G. mellonella*), thus L-OEI-h is foreseen as a promising polymer therapeutic for the treatment of MDR *K. pneumoniae* infections.

Citation: Mil-Homens, D.; Martins, M.; Barbosa, J.; Serafim, G.; Sarmento, M.J.; Pires, R.F.; Rodrigues, V.; Bonifácio, V.D.; Pinto, S.N. Carbapenem-Resistant *Klebsiella pneumoniae* Clinical Isolates: In Vivo Virulence Assessment in *Galleria mellonella* and Potential Therapeutics by Polycationic Oligoethyleneimine. *Antibiotics* **2021**, *10*, 56. https://doi.org/10.3390/antibiotics10010056

Received: 30 September 2020
Accepted: 6 January 2021
Published: 8 January 2021

Publisher's Note: MDPI stays neutral with regard to jurisdictional claims in published maps and institutional affiliations.

Keywords: *Klebsiella pneumoniae*; KPC and OXA-48-like carbapenemases; *Galleria mellonella* infection model; linear oligoethyleneimine hydrochloride

Copyright: © 2021 by the authors. Licensee MDPI, Basel, Switzerland. This article is an open access article distributed under the terms and conditions of the Creative Commons Attribution (CC BY) license (https://creativecommons.org/licenses/by/4.0/).

1. Introduction

The widespread use of antibiotics in clinics caused an increased frequency of multidrug-resistance bacteria mainly due to bacterial mutations [1]. In particular, the emergence of resistance to last resource antibiotic treatment options (including carbapenems) has contributed to the limitation of effective therapeutics. Recent reports revealed a weak pipeline for novel antibiotics. From all the compounds under development, very few target infections were caused by Gram-negative bacteria [2–4]. This is clinically relevant, as Gram-negative bacteria infections are significantly more lethal compared to those caused by the Gram-positive [3]. Several factors contribute to the scarcity of new antibiotics, market failure being the most relevant. As result of a low return investment, pharmaceutical companies lack incentives for novel antibiotics development. Antibiotics are fast-acting drugs (limiting patient requirements to a small-time window) and the use of novel antibiotics is often reserved since, ultimately, an unpredictable resistance may occur [1,5]. Therefore, the development of novel and efficient antimicrobial agents is of utmost priority.

Klebsiella pneumonia, a pathogen of the *Enterobacteriaceae* family, is resistant to last resource antibiotics and is the source of some of the most complicated hospital-acquired infections [6–8]. Resistance to carbapenem in *K. pneumonia* poses a significant threat to patients in hospitals as this organism can cause life-threatening infections such as pneumonia, bloodstream infections and sepsis [9]. Several factors are associated with the acquisition of *K. pneumonia* KPC(+) and OXA-48(+) bacteria, including prolonged hospitalization, infections caused by medical devices (including contamination of ventilators and catheters) and overuse of antibiotics (e.g., carbapenems). Carbapenems-resistant *K. pneumonia* bacteria are capable of inactivating carbapenems via the production of carbapenemase enzymes. Several carbapenemases have been identified and categorized into classes. The ambler classes A (KPC, plasmid-mediated clavulanic acid-inhibited β-lactamases) and D (OXA-48, expanded-spectrum oxacillinase) categories are considered relevant carbapenemases, being highly resistant to all β-lactam molecules, including carbapenems [10].

To investigate the in vivo relevance of MDR *K. pneumonia* infection, we obtained different KPC(+) and OXA-48(+) isolates and determined their virulence using *Galleria mellonella*, a caterpillar model of infection. The success of MDR *K. pneumonia* infections depends, "among other factors", on the ability of the pathogen to escape the host's defense mechanisms. The larvae of the greater wax moth *G. mellonella* have been successfully employed as a model host to study virulence of human pathogenic agents, including several human pathogens, and to investigate the efficacy of therapeutic drugs [11–14]. *G. mellonella* possess only an innate immune system (that includes melanization, hemolymph, and several antimicrobial peptides). However, this is enough to offer powerful resistance to microbial infections [15]. Additionally, their innate immune system shares a high degree of structural and functional homology with the innate immune systems of mammal's [16]. Thus, evaluation of *G. mellonella* responses to *K. pneumonia* isolates infection can provide indication of the mammalian response to these pathogens.

Very few treatment options are available for patients infected with *K. pneumoniae* producing KPC or OXA-48-like carbapenemases and are often limited to administration of multiple antibiotic therapies and to colistin [17,18]. In the light of this, in this study, we report the use of a polycationic synthetic oligomer, linear oligoethyleneimine hydrochloride (L-OEI-h), as an antimicrobial agent for the treatment of *K. pneumonia* KPC(+) and OXA-48(+) bacterial infections. We have previously reported the synthesis and biocidal activity of L-OEI-h against *Streptococcus aureus* and *Escherichia coli* [19]. Herein, we evaluate L-OEI-h antibacterial activity against MDR bacteria clinical isolates, namely *K. pneumoniae*, and investigate the underlying mechanism of action, which, as found for other polycationic antimicrobial agents, might involve disruption of the cell wall and/or the disintegration of the cytoplasmic membrane [10].

2. Results

2.1. Evaluation of K. pneumoniae Virulance in G. mellonella Infection Model

Ten *K. pneumoniae* isolates (Table S1) with reduced sensitivity to carbapenems were obtained from different clinical specimens. To investigate the virulence of *K. pneumoniae* isolates in vivo, we used the *G. mellonella* infection model (Figure 1). In this case, larvae survival rates were measured by injecting inoculums, incubating at 37 °C and recording the survival rate daily for up to three days. In all experiments, control groups with administration of phosphate-buffered saline (PBS) solution resulted in a 100% survival rate.

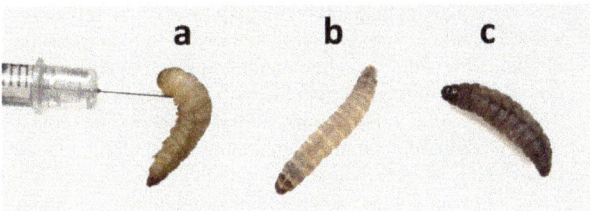

Figure 1. In vivo assays using the *Galleria mellonella* larva model. Inoculation by injection of different bacteria inoculum (**a**), healthy larva (**b**), and dead larva (**c**) as a result of *Klebsiella pneumoniae* infection.

Most larvae were found healthy following infection with 1×10^4 CFU (colony-forming unit) of each isolate per larva (Figure S1), which suggests that at this bacterial density the humoral immunity of the insects is enough to produce an adequate response to the infection. However, the larvae survival was significantly altered upon increase of infection ratio (1×10^5 CFU per larva). As shown in Figure 2, the virulence of isolates varied widely, with some KPC(+) isolates promoting total larvae mortality (e.g., SYN7 KPC clinical isolate). These differences in virulence are in accordance with data reported for patients suffering from *K. pneumoniae* KPC(+) infections [20], confirming the reliability of the *G. mellonella* infection model in reporting pathogenicity differences between all *K. pneumoniae* isolates. This infection model (*G. mellonella* infected with 1×10^5 CFU *K. pneumoniae* per larva) is now well established in our lab, and we believe that will be very helpful in future development of *K. pneumoniae* therapeutics.

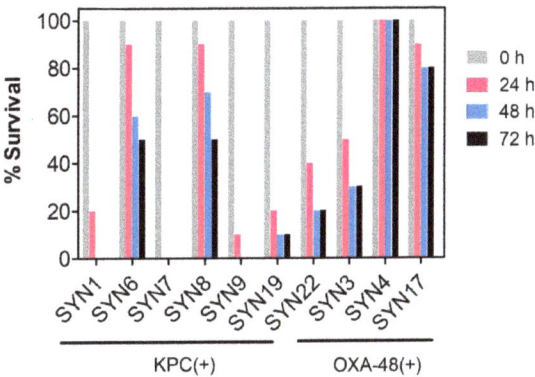

Figure 2. Evaluation of virulence of *Klebsiella pneumoniae* KPC(+) and OXA-48(+) isolates in *Galleria mellonella*. Survival of *G. mellonella* was followed for three days after infection with *K. pneumoniae* KPC(+) and OXA-48(+) with 1×10^5 CFU per larva. Ten larvae were analyzed in each condition and larvae survival was monitored daily. In all cases, no larvae death was observed upon administration of PBS (control). KPC(+) isolates: SYN1, SYN6, SYN7, SYN8, SYN9 SYN19 and SYN22; OXA-48(+) isolates: SYN3, SYN4 and SYN17.

2.2. Antimicrobial Activity of L-OEI-h

The oligomer L-OEI-h was synthesized following our reported protocol [19]. We evaluated the antimicrobial activity of L-OEI-h against *K. pneumoniae* isolates by determination of the minimum inhibitory concentration (MIC) and the minimum bactericidal concentration (MBC). MIC is defined as the lowest drug concentration that prevents visible growth of bacteria. The MBC is the lowest concentration of an antimicrobial agent required to kill $\geq$99.9% bacteria over an extended period (18–24 h). The antimicrobial assays were conducted according with CLSI guidelines in Mueller Hinton broth (MHB), a nutrient rich bacterial growth medium. The obtained results for the different isolates are shown in Table 1. We included other Gram-negative bacteria (*Pseudomonas aeruginosa* PAO and *E. coli* AB1157) and a Gram-positive strain (*S. aureus* MRSA JE2) as control strains. Except for SYN7 KPC, which is also the most virulent isolate, L-OEI-h displayed good antibacterial activity against Gram-negative strains with particular relevance for *P. aeruginosa* PAO and *E. coli* AB1157. The MIC and MBC values were almost identical, which is indicative that the oligomer exerts a bactericidal activity.

Table 1. Antimicrobial activity of linear oligoethyleneimine hydrochloride (L-OEI-h) against *Klebsiella pneumoniae* isolates, control bacterial strains (*P. aeruginosa* PAO, *E. coli* AB1157) and the methicillin-resistant *Staphylococcus* strain *S. aureus* JE2.

Clinical Isolate	MIC (µg/mL)	MBC (µg/mL)
SYN1 KPC	458	458
SYN3 OXA-48	915	>915
SYN4 OXA-48	458	915
SYN6 KPC	915	915
SYN7 KPC	>915	>915
SYN8 KPC	458	458
SYN9 KPC	229	229–458
SYN17 OXA-48	915	915
SYN19 KPC	915	915
SYN22 KPC	915	>915
P. aeruginosa PAO	114	114
E. coli AB1157 *	90	90
S. aureus JE2	>915	>915

* Data acquired in a previous study [13].

We previously demonstrated that L-OEI-h is also able to target some Gram-positive bacteria with low efficiency [19], as demonstrated here for methicillin-resistant *S. aureus* JE2 (MIC > 915 µg/mL).

2.3. Biocompatibility Studies

Some membrane-lytic agents are known to display selectivity towards bacterial membranes, allowing for elevated antibiotic activity and low toxicity to mammalian cells [21]. The differences in composition and lipid arrangement in bacterial and mammalian cell membranes can support the selectivity observed in these antimicrobial agents [21,22]. Here, we evaluated the cytotoxicity of L-OEI-h using in vitro (L929 mouse fibroblasts) and in vivo models (*G. mellonella* larvae) (Figure 3).

The polycationic oligomer compound has very little cytotoxicity against mammalian cell lines, even at the highest dose tested against clinical isolates (915 µg/mL, Figure 3a,b). The larvae were injected with 5 µL of different concentrations of L-OEI-h, and then incubated in Petri dishes at 37 °C and daily scored for survival. Up to a concentration of 915 µg/mL, all larvae were found healthy for a three-day period (Figure 3c). To obtain more differences in larvae health, we also determined the health index scores (Figure 3d), which scores four main parameters: larvae activity, cocoon formation, melanization and survival. The injection of the larvae with L-OEI-h even after 72 h resulted in high health index scores. The higher activity and more cocoon formation are regularly associated to a healthier wax worm [23].

All experiments included a control group injected only with a PBS solution. Overall, our results corroborate the biocompatibility of L-OEI-h.

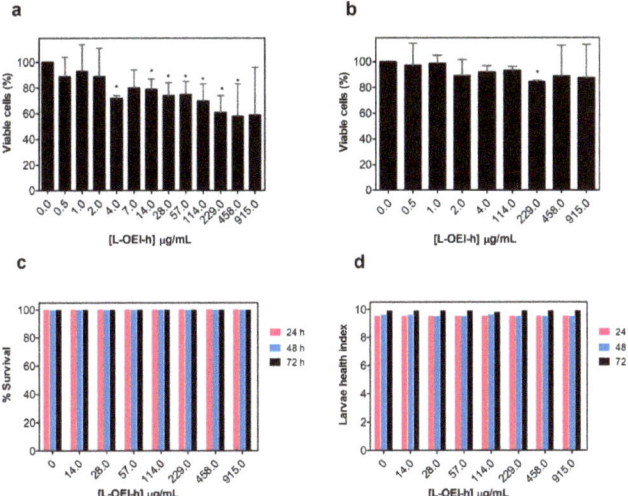

Figure 3. Evaluation of linear oligoethyleneimine hydrochloride (L-OEI-h) toxicity and biocompatibility using in vitro mammalian cells (L929 mouse and A549 human epithelial cells) (**a**,**b**) and in vivo assays (*Galleria mellonella* larvae) (**c**). The health index scores of wax worms injected with L-OEI-h was also evaluated (**d**). Asterisks (*) represent statistical significance in *t*-student tests ($p < 0.05$) compared to the untreated samples.

2.4. Exploring the L-OEI-h Mechanism of Action

Cationic polymers are expected to target the microbial cell surface, via binding to negatively charged components, and to disrupt the cytoplasmic membrane [24]. A fast-killing kinetics is associated with surface membranolytic processes, while slow kinetics is usually associated with activation of intracellular processes [25–28]. In this sense a time-kill assay based on traditional colony count was carried out to discriminate between fast and slow kinetics of antibacterial activity.

Time-kill curves of a selected OXA-48(+) (SYN4 OXA-48) and KPC(+) isolates (SYN8 KPC) were obtained in the presence of two different oligomer concentrations. As shown in Figure 4 and Figure S2, after the addition of L-OEI-h, the number of *K. pneumoniae* viable and culturable colonies decreases significantly in the first 30 min of treatment, with almost complete bacterial removal achieved at 2 h treatment. This observation illustrates a possible fast L-OEI-h bactericidal activity. For other Gram-negative bacteria (e.g., *E. coli* AB1157 [19]), L-OEI-h had a very fast killing effects (within 5 min). In both cases, the verified fast activity is supportive of a surface membranolytic mechanism of action for L-OEI-h.

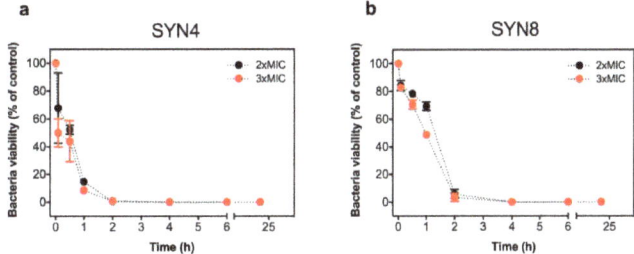

Figure 4. Killing kinetics of *Klebsiella pneumonia* SYN4 OXA-48 (**a**) and SYN8 KPC (**b**) clinical isolates induced by L-OEI-h. The killing kinetics was evaluated with a colony count assay using two different oligomer concentrations, $2 \times$ MIC and $3 \times$ MIC.

The higher antimicrobial activity of L-OEI-h against Gram-negative bacteria (e.g., *E. coli* AB1157 vs. *S. aureus* NCTC8325-4 [19]) may indicate that the presence of lipopolysaccharides (LPS) in the outer leaflet of the outer membrane of Gram-negative may facilitate the initial binding of the compound. Antibacterial cationic polymers are expected to permeabilize bacterial membrane by one of two possible mechanisms: (i) Perpendicular insertion in the membrane followed by pore formation and membrane permeabilization/depolarization, or (ii) accumulation at the membrane surface until a certain threshold concentration is achieved, which leads to membrane disruption and cell lysis.

To further characterize the mechanism of action of L-OEI-h, studies with membrane mimetics were carried out. In these simplified membrane models, size, geometry, and composition can be tailored with great precision.

The effect of L-OEI-h on the membrane was thus, studied using large unilamellar vesicles (LUVs) of controlled lipid composition, serving as mimetics of bacterial and mammalian cell membranes. The bacterial membrane model, with an overall negative charge, was composed of different ratios of phosphatidylcholine (POPC) and phosphatidylglycerol (POPG), while the healthy mammalian plasma membrane model contained only POPC [20]. POPC zwitterionic liposomes are not affected by the addition of L-OEI-h, but higher amount of negatively charged lipids (>20%) led to the formation of large clusters within a few seconds (Figure 5). We hypothesize that the formation of large clusters (>100 nm) is consistent with the binding/accumulation of the polymer in membranes with high negatively charged lipids.

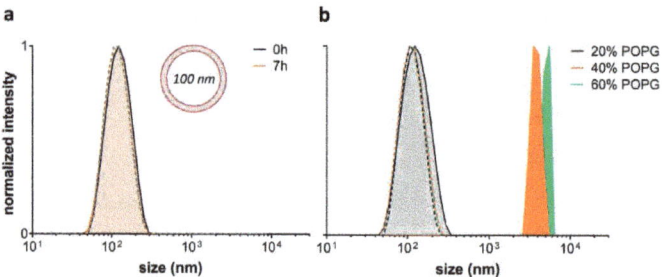

Figure 5. Effect of L-OE-h on model liposomes composed of phosphatidylcholine (POPC) (**a**) and POPC with varying phosphatidylglycerol (POPG) content (**b**). Vesicle sizes were measured by DLS at 25 °C. Dashed lines are the respective controls without polymer.

Upon electrostatic binding of L-OEI-h to anionic lipid vesicles, and after a certain threshold concentration, the oligomer induces vesicle aggregation and/or vesicle fusion, which explains the appearance of a LUV population larger in size (Figure 5b). Vesicle aggregation and fusion are not unusual occurrences, being also observed in the case of cationic peptides addition to anionic vesicles [29]. Ultimately, accumulation of L-OEI-h in the membrane may induce micelle formation or the formation of transient pores, as illustrated for the mechanism of action of some antimicrobial peptides (e.g., [29]). In both cases membrane disintegration is a consequence of these events (Figure 6).

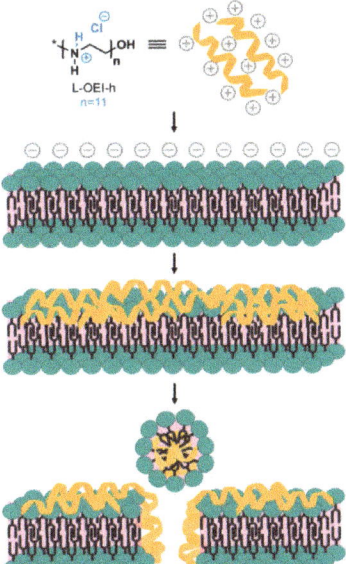

Figure 6. Hypothetical mechanism of action of L-OEI-h (model II) towards bacterial cell membranes. The accumulation of the polycationic oligomer at the membrane surface, due to electrostatic interactions, results in an oligomer threshold concentration capable of cell disruption and lysis.

3. Discussion

Bacterial infections are becoming a major human health problem. Resistance towards antibiotics is becoming increasingly common, including to the ones only reserved for the treatment of severe infections. The World Health Organization has recently included *Klebsiella* in the critical list of microorganisms for which new therapeutics are urgently needed [30]. In the light of this demand, in this study we examine the sensitivity of *G. mellonella* to *K. pneumoniae* isolates that are resistant to last resources antibiotics and focused our attention towards a polycationic oligomer [19], a synthetic mimic of host defense peptides (HDPs), as a novel treatment for MDR *K. pneumonia* infections.

HDPs are a class of innate immunity components expressed by all multicellular organisms [31]. It is believed that their function is, in part, to kill invasive cells without prejudice to the host and without presenting itself as a stress agent for the development of resistance traits [31]. The discovery of HDPs was accompanied by the development of disinfectant polymers, which in the late 1990s led to HDP-mimicking polymers [32]. Although antimicrobial peptides (AMPs)/HDPs are an excellent alternative to conventional antibiotics, cheap and scalable bioprocessing is not yet available [33]. Additionally, AMPs are poorly stable in vivo due to protease liability.

In this way, HDP-mimicking polymers are considered a more cost-effective and stable alternative to HDP/AMP [31]. The relationship between structure and activity of HDP-mimetic polymers relies on two main design principles: (i) Hydrophobic/hydrophilic component ratio and (ii) presence of a structured cationic group. It was demonstrated that a poly(methacrylate) random copolymer with 40% methyl side chains (hydrophobic segment) and 60% aminoethyl side chains (hydrophilic segment) show potent antibacterial activity and low hemolytic activity [34].

The effect of primary amine groups, instead of traditional quaternary ammonium salt (QAS), was already investigated [35]. For the same type of polymer, primary amines outperformed in comparison with tertiary or quaternary amines in terms of antimicrobial activity and toxicity. Following this study, it was found that primary ammonium groups can form a stronger complex with phospholipid headgroups when compared to QAS analogues [36].

Additionally, the effect of amine groups density is quite relevant since increasing the amine density by monomer unit enhances the polymers efficacy and decreases hemolysis in great extent [37].

The synthetic polymer polyethyleneimine (PEI), due to its intrinsic features, is regarded as a good alternative to fight antibiotic resistant organisms. The abundance of reactive amine groups in the backbone allows post-modifications to display both hydrophobicity and a positive charge density, primary requirements for a good antimicrobial activity [38]. In previous studies, we found that L-OEI-h, a PEI analogue, is a very effective biocidal oligomer [19], whose activity may be attributed to high positive charge density (hydrochloride salt, quaternary nitrogen atoms), if compared with commercial L-PEI (non-quaternary nitrogen atoms) [39] (see Figure 7). As we and others demonstrated, a higher positive charge density leads to higher antimicrobial efficacy [40].

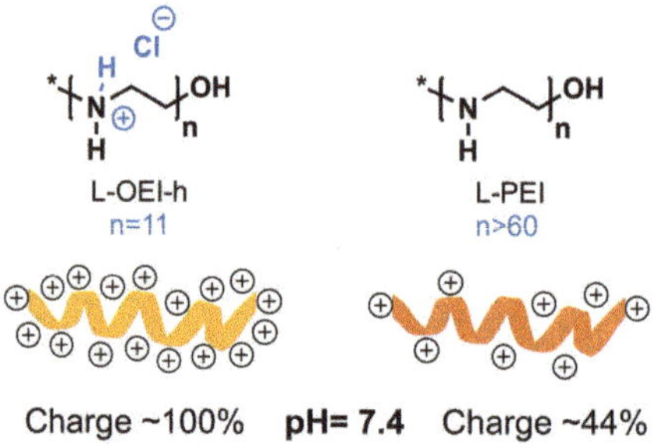

Figure 7. Comparison of positive charge density between linear oligoethyleneimine hydrochloride (L-OEI-h) and linear polyethyleneimine (L-PEI) at physiological pH.

In this work, we evaluated the antimicrobial activity of L-OEI-h against a variety of *K. pneumonia* strains. The antimicrobial efficiency is attributed to favorable electrostatic interactions between the polycationic oligomer (having *ca.* +11 formal net charge, one positive charge per monomer unit) and the anionic bacterial membrane. This interaction can induce a very fast-bactericidal activity, as demonstrated by us [19]. Such a fast mode of action strongly suggests that membranolytic processes are responsible for antimicrobial activity. Through direct permeabilization of the lipidic membrane, instead of action on a specific cellular target, the probability of bacteria to develop resistance to this treatment is extremely low.

For *K. pneumoniae* clinical isolates, the bactericidal activity of the oligomer does not occur earlier than 30 min, in contrast with what we and others verified for other membrane disruption agents, whereby membrane permeabilization and/or lysis happened within 5 min [19,41,42]. It is likely that, for *K. pneumoniae* clinical isolates, L-OEI-h cannot diffuse so efficiently (or diffuses slowly) through the bacterial cell wall to reach the plasma membrane. This could be associated with the fact that the capsule (composed of extracellular polysaccharides) of *K. pneumoniae* is more "robust" than what was verified for other gram-negative bacteria, and, in this sense, constitutes an efficient barrier against several antimicrobial agents [43,44] including HDPs. Despite this, L-OEI-h was able to efficiently kill several *K. pneumoniae* clinical isolates (Table 1, Figure 4 and Figure S2).

Importantly, the L-OEI-h antimicrobial action against some *K. pneumoniae* clinical isolates such as SYN4 OXA-48 and SYN9 KPC (a highly virulent clinical isolate) is verified under a possible therapeutic window, since L-OEI-h induces low cytotoxicity against in vitro mammalian cell lines (<80% cell viability [45] within statistical error) and, more importantly, no visible cytotoxicity was detected against the in vivo model (*G. mellonella*). As shown here, low toxicity in these models is likely associated with reduced interaction with the plasma membrane of eukaryotic cells. Liposomes with a lipid composition mimicking the outer leaflet of eukaryotic plasma membranes were not affected by the presence of L-OEI-h (Figure 5a). On the other hand, liposomes rich in phosphatidylglycerol, mimicking bacterial membrane lipid composition, showed dramatic aggregation upon interaction with this compound. Large unilamellar vesicles (LUVs) were used in these studies as their size is more amenable to DLS resolution. Other membrane models, such as multilamellar vesicles (MLVs), due to their multi-layered character, prevent polymer interactions with the internal bilayers (that could mask possible effects occurring only in the outer membrane), while small unilamellar vesicles (SUV)'s small size results in membranes with excessive curvature that do not mimic bacterial membranes. On the other hand, very large vesicles such as giant unilamellar vesicles (GUVs) have a less controlled lipid concentration/size and thus frequently show significant vesicle heterogeneity within the same sample.

Although we obtained promising data for some *K. pneumoniae* isolates, we verified that in some cases MIC and MBC values were still high (if compared with the results obtained for the Gram-negative control strains). The polymer design and the polymer-membrane interactions are crucial issues for bacterial infection eradication. In a recent study, linear and branched PEI polymers were found to have very similar MIC values, while ε-polycaprolactone showed superior broad-spectrum antimicrobial properties over L-PEI [46]. Hence, in future work we will consider the use of a coarse-grain (CG) molecular dynamics model of L-OEI-h to better understand its interactions with bacterial and mammalian membranes. This study will allow the identification of key oligomer-membrane interactions which could lead to enhanced polymer antimicrobials.

4. Materials and Methods

4.1. Synthesis of Linear Oligoethyleneimine Hydrochloride (L-OEI-h)

The preparation of L-OEI-h was made in two steps following our previous protocol. First, linear 2-ethyl(2-oligooxazoline) (OEtOx) was synthesized by cationic ring-opening polymerization (CROP) in supercritical carbon dioxide, a green polymerization methodology [47]. The living OEtOx polymer was terminated with water and isolated as a brownish sticky oil. Next, OEtOx was hydrolyzed overnight using a HCl 5M solution. After this period, the precipitated solid was filtered and washed with acetone to obtain L-OEI-h as an off-white solid in quantitative yield. After vacuum drying, L-OEI-h is ready to use [19].

4.2. Clinical Isolates Collection and Identification

The KPC and OXA-48-positive carbapenems-resistant *K. pneumoniae* clinical isolates were collected from patients treated in medical care units (Lisbon, Portugal). All strains were identified with matrix-assisted laser desorption/ionization time-of-flight (MALDI-TOF) spectrometry [48,49] using the VITEK MS system (bioMérieux). Briefly, inoculation loops were used to select and smear the isolates onto the sample spots/target slide. Then 1 µL VITEK mass spectrometry α-cyano-4-hydroxycinnamic acid (MS-CHCA) matrix was applied over the sample and air dried (1–2 min). The target slide was loaded into the VITEK MS system to acquire the mass spectra of whole bacterial cell protein (which is mainly composed of ribosomal proteins). Then, the mass spectra acquired for each sample were compared to the mass spectra contained in the database.

In addition, the following antimicrobials were included in the microorganism's characterization: β-lactams (ceftazidime, cefepime, cefuroxime/axetil, amoxicillin/clavulanate, ticarcillin/clavulanate and piperacillin/tazobactam), carbapenems (meropenem, ertapenem), aminoglycosides (gentamicin, amikacin), nitrofurantoin fluoroquinolones (ciprofloxacin), polymyxin (colistin), fosfomycin, trimethoprim/sulfamethoxazole. The production of carbapenemases in these strains is evidenced through the antibiotic resistance profile and the type of carbapenemase (OXA-48-like, KPC, NDM or VIM) was identified through an immunochromatographic method (RESIST-4 O.K.N.V., Coris). CASFM-EUCAST 2016-defined breakpoints for *Enterobacteriaceae* were used to interpret susceptibility data for *K. pneumoniae* (http://www.sfm-microbiologie.org).

From pure culture on MacConkey agar plates, all identified *K. pneumoniae* isolates were transferred to 1.5 mL Eppendorf tubes contain Luria–Bertani (LB) broth with 20%

(v/v) glycerol and were maintained at $-80\ °C$ for long-term storage. For the antimicrobial activity studies, bacterial cultures were inoculated in Mueller-Hinton broth (MHB) (Difco), at 37 °C. Tryptic soy agar (TSA) agar plates (bioMérieux, Marcy l'Etoile, France) were used to subculture *K. pneumoniae* isolates, *P. aeruginosa* PAO and *E. coli* AB1157. *S. aureus* MRSA JE2 was streaked on Columbia agar +5% sheep blood plates (COS, bioMérieux, Marcy l'Etoile, Auvergne-Rhône-Alpes, France) and grown overnight at 37 °C. *P. aeruginosa* PAO, *E. coli* AB1157 and *S. aureus* JE2 were used as reference strains. The antimicrobial activity of L-OEI-h against *E. coli* AB1157 was previously investigated by us [19].

4.3. Galleria mellonella Infection Model

G. mellonella wax moth larvae were reared in our lab at 25 °C in the dark, from egg to last-instar larvae, on a natural diet (beeswax and pollen grains). Worms of the final-instar larval stage, weighing 250 ± 25 mg, were selected for the experiments. The *G. mellonella* survival experiment was adapted from previous studies with small changes [11,14]. Briefly, all *K. pneumoniae* isolates were grown overnight in TSA plates. Then, the assay was carried out by preparing two distinct inoculums of 2×10^6 and 2×10^7 CFU/mL in PBS. Using a hypodermic microsyringe, the larvae were injected with 5 µL of each bacterial suspension via the hindmost left proleg, previously surface sanitized with 70% (v/v) alcohol. Different groups were used (n = 10 each)—larvae injected with PBS to monitor the killing due to injection trauma (control) and larvae injected with *K. pneumoniae* isolates. After inoculation, larvae were kept in Petri dishes and maintained in the dark at 37 °C for 72 h. The larval survival was assessed daily during that period, and caterpillars were considered dead based on the lack of mobility in response to touch. Each larva was also scored daily to the *G. mellonella* health index, which scores four main parameters: Larvae activity, cocoon formation, melanization and survival, as described in [23].

All experiments were performed using a minimum of two independent experiments.

4.4. Antimicrobial Activity

4.4.1. Minimum Inhibitory Concentration (MIC) Determination

To determine the MIC values, the bacterial suspension was initially adjusted to a concentration of 1×10^6 CFU/mL in MHB (according to CLSI guidelines) [50]. On a 96-well plate (Orange Scientific, Braine-l'Alleud, Belgium), two-fold serial dilution (in MHB) of L-OEI-h was then added to each well that contained the bacterial inoculums (dilution 1:1). Final bacteria inoculum in each well were diluted to 5×10^5 CFU/mL. The 96-well tissue culture plates were incubated for 18–20 h at 37 °C. All experiments were performed using a minimum of three independent experiments performed with three technical replicates each.

4.4.2. Minimum Bactericidal Concentration (MBC) Determination

The MBC values were determined by the traditional colony count assay [51]. At the end of the MIC assay, 20 µL samples from each well (corresponding to $\frac{1}{2}$ MIC, MIC, $2 \times$ MIC, $3 \times$ MIC of L-OEI-h) were transferred to a new 96-well plate and successively diluted (10-fold) in MHB. Then, each dilution was sub-cultured in TSA plates. After incubation at 37 °C for 24 h, the resultant viable colonies were counted. All experiments were performed using a minimum of three independent experiments performed with three technical replicates each.

4.4.3. In Vitro Time-Kill Curves

Time-kill curves of L-OEI-h were determined according to literature [52,53]. Briefly, a final inoculum of 1×10^6 to 1×10^7 CFU/mL was exposed to distinct doses of L-OEI-h and incubated at 37 °C. Aliquots at specified time points were taken; 10-fold dilutions of each well were prepared and plated onto a TSA plate for CFU enumeration. TSA plates were incubated for 24 h at 37 °C and bacterial colonies were counted. Viable cells (CFU/mL) are reported here as percentage of the control (bacterial suspension without

L-OEI-h exposition). From the number of bacterial colonies obtained, viable bacteria (in CFU/mL) are reported as percentage of the control. All experiments were performed using two independent experiments with three technical replicates each.

4.5. Biocompatibility Assays

4.5.1. MTT Viability Assay

L-929 and A549 cell lines were cultured in T-75 cell culture flasks (Filter caps) using Dulbecco's modified Eagle's medium (DMEM, Catalog number 41966-029) supplemented with 10% fetal bovine serum (Thermo Fisher Scientific, Catalog number 10500-064, heat inactivated) and 1% penicillin-streptomycin (Thermo Fisher Scientific, catalogue number 15140-122) and maintained in a humidified atmosphere with 5% CO_2 at 37 °C. All cell culture lines were maintained with routinely subcultures (using TrypLE Express without phenol red, GIBCO™, for chemical detaching). Mammalian cell lines were counted with a hemocytometer.

The MTT assay was used to detect changes on metabolic activity of mammalian cells [54]. Briefly, the L-929 and A549 cell lines were seeded in 96-well flat-bottomed polystyrene plates with a density of 1×10^4 cells/well and left to adhere overnight in a CO_2 incubator (5%) at 37 °C. After 24 h, the cell medium was discarded and replaced with fresh medium containing different concentrations of L-OEI-h. Cells were then incubated for a period of 24 h at 37 °C in a humidified 5% CO_2 incubator. After this incubation period, the medium was discarded and 20 μL of MTT (5 mg/mL) were added to each well together with 100 μL of fresh DMEM and incubated at 37 °C for 3.5 h. The formazan crystals formed in the wells were dissolved using 150 μL of MTT solvent (4 mM of HCl, 0.1% of Nondet P-40 in isopropanol). The formation of formazan was monitored by measuring the absorbance at 590 nm in a microplate reader (BMG Labtech, Polar Star Optima). Cell viability was determined relatively to the untreated sample after correcting the data with the negative control.

All experiments were performed using a minimum of two independent experiments with three technical replicates each.

4.5.2. *Galleria mellonella* Toxicity Assay

The L-OEI-h toxicity was also evaluated in the larvae infection in vivo model. The *G. mellonella* killing assays were based on the above descriptions with small modifications. L-OEI-h doses were prepared and injected into the larvae hindmost left proleg. The larvae survival was assessed daily during a period of 72 h. A control group was also included in the assay. Two independent experiments were performed.

4.6. Exploring the L-OEI-h Mechanism of Action

Liposome Preparation

Large unilamellar vesicles (LUVs), with 100 nm of diameter, were prepared by extrusion of multilamellar vesicles [54]. The liposomes were prepared according to methods previously described [55]. Briefly, lipid mixtures composed of adequate amounts of lipids (POPC and POPG) were prepared in chloroform to a final lipid concentration of 2 mM. The solvent was slowly vaporized under a nitrogen flux and the resulting lipid film was left in vacuum for 3 h to ensure the complete removal of chloroform. Afterwards, the lipid was resuspended in 2 mL of DPBS (Thermo Fisher Scientific) and freeze–thaw cycles (liquid nitrogen/water bath at 60 °C) were performed to re-equilibrate and homogenize the samples. LUVs were finally obtained by extrusion of the solutions at 50 °C with an Avanti Mini-Extruder (Merck, Darmstadt, Germany) using 100 nm pore size polycarbonate membranes. All lipid stock solutions were prepared in chloroform and the respective concentrations were determined by the colorimetric quantification of inorganic phosphate.

Liposome size was determined by dynamic light scattering (DLS) using a Nanosizer ZS (Malvern Instruments). The POPC/POPG vesicles were incubated with L-OEI-h for

5 min. Data was collected at 25 °C and a backscattering angle of 173°. Two independent experiments were performed.

Supplementary Materials: The following are available online at https://www.mdpi.com/2079-6382/10/1/56/s1, Figure S1: Evaluation of distinct virulence response of *K. pneumoniae* KPC(+) and OXA-48 (+) isolates in *G. mellonella*. Figure S2: Killing kinetics of *K. pneumonia* SYN4 OXA-48 (a) and SYN8 KPC (b) clinical isolates induced by L-OEI-h. Table S1: *K. pneumonia* clinical isolates origin and the minimum inhibitory concentration (MIC) values of trimethoprim (TM)/sulfamethoxazole (SM) antibiotics.

Author Contributions: Conceptualization, S.N.P., D.M.-H., V.D.B.B.; methodology, S.N.P., D.M.-H., V.D.B.B, R.F.P., M.M., J.B., M.J.S.; formal analysis, S.N.P., D.M.-H., V.D.B.B, M.J.S.; investigation, S.N.P., D.M.-H., R.F.P., M.M., J.B., M.J.S.; V.R.; writing—original draft preparation, S.N.P.; writing—review and editing, S.N.P., V.D.B.B, D.M.-H., M.J.S., G.S.; supervision, S.N.P., V.D.B.B. All authors have read and agreed to the published version of the manuscript.

Funding: This research was funded by Fundação para a Ciência e a Tecnologia (FCT, Portugal), Ministério da Ciência, Tecnologia e Ensino Superior (MCTES) through projects PTDC/MEC-ONC/29327/2017, UIDB/04565/2020 and SAICTPAC/0019/2015.

Data Availability Statement: The data presented in this study are available in the article and in the supplementary material.

Conflicts of Interest: The authors declare no conflict of interest.

References

1. Aslam, B.; Wang, W.; Arshad, M.I.; Khurshid, M.; Muzammil, S.; Rasool, M.H.; Nisar, M.A.; Alvi, R.F.; Aslam, M.A.; Qamar, M.U.; et al. Antibiotic resistance: A rundown of a global crisis. *Infect. Drug Resist.* **2018**, *11*, 1645–1658. [CrossRef]
2. Coates, A.R.; Halls, G.; Hu, Y. Novel classes of antibiotics or more of the same? *Br. J. Pharmacol.* **2011**, *163*, 184–194. [CrossRef]
3. Breijyeh, Z.; Jubeh, B.; Karaman, R. Resistance of Gram-Negative bacteria to current antibacterial agents and approaches to resolve it. *Molecules* **2020**, *25*, 1340. [CrossRef]
4. Theuretzbacher, U.; Outterson, K.; Engel, A.; Karlén, A. The global preclinical antibacterial pipeline. *Nat. Rev. Microbiol.* **2020**, *18*, 275–285. [CrossRef]
5. Ventola, C.L. The antibiotic resistance crisis: Part 1: Causes and threats. *PT* **2015**, *40*, 277–283.
6. Nordmann, P.; Cuzon, G.; Naas, T. The real threat of *Klebsiella pneumoniae* carbapenemase-producing bacteria. *Lancet Infect. Dis.* **2009**, *9*, 228–236. [CrossRef]
7. Molton, J.S.; Tambyah, P.A.; Ang, B.S.; Ling, M.L.; Fisher, D.A. The global spread of healthcare-associated multidrug-resistant bacteria: A perspective from Asia. *Clin. Infect. Dis.* **2013**, *56*, 1310–1318. [CrossRef]
8. Tzouvelekis, L.S.; Markogiannakis, A.; Psichogiou, M.; Tassios, P.T.; Daikos, G.L. Carbapenemases in *Klebsiella pneumoniae* and other *Enterobacteriaceae*: An evolving crisis of global dimensions. *Clin. Microbiol. Rev.* **2012**, *25*, 682–707. [CrossRef] [PubMed]
9. Peleg, A.Y.; Hooper, D.C. Hospital-acquired infections due to Gram-negative bacteria. *N. Engl. J. Med.* **2010**, *362*, 1804–1813. [CrossRef]
10. Halat, D.H.; Moubareck, C.A. The current burden of carbapenemases: Review of significant properties and dissemination among Gram-negative bacteria. *Antibiotics (Basel)* **2020**, *9*, 186. [CrossRef]
11. Mil-Homens, D.; Bernardes, N.; Fialho, A.M. The antibacterial properties of docosahexaenoic omega-3 fatty acid against the cystic fibrosis multiresistant pathogen *Burkholderia cenocepacia*. *FEMS Microbiol. Lett.* **2012**, *328*, 61–69. [CrossRef] [PubMed]
12. Cutuli, M.A.; Petronio, G.P.; Vergalito, F.; Magnifico, I.; Pietrangelo, L.; Venditti, N.; Di Marco, R. Galleria mellonella as a consolidated in vivo model hosts: New developments in antibacterial strategies and novel drug testing. *Virulence* **2019**, *10*, 527–541. [CrossRef] [PubMed]
13. Jander, G.; Rahme, L.G.; Ausubel, F.M. Positive correlation between virulence of *Pseudomonas aeruginosa* mutants in mice and insects. *J. Bacteriol.* **2000**, *182*, 3843–3845. [CrossRef] [PubMed]
14. Mil-Homens, D.; Barahona, S.; Moreira, R.N.; Silva, I.J.; Pinto, S.N.; Fialho, A.M.; Arraiano, C.M. Stress response protein BolA influences fitness and promotes *Salmonella enterica* serovar Typhimurium virulence. *Appl. Environ. Microbiol.* **2018**, *84*, e02850-17. [CrossRef]
15. Vilmos, P.; Kurucz, E. Insect immunity: Evolutionary roots of the mammalian innate immune system. *Immunol. Lett.* **1998**, *62*, 59–66. [CrossRef]
16. Hoffmann, J.A. Innate immunity of insects. *Curr. Opin. Immunol.* **1995**, *7*, 4–10. [CrossRef]
17. Papst, L.; Beović, B.; Pulcini, C.; Durante-Mangoni, E.; Rodríguez-Baño, J.; Kaye, K.S.; Daikos, G.L.; Raka, L.; Paul, M. Antibiotic treatment of infections caused by carbapenem-resistant Gram-negative bacilli: An international ESCMID cross-sectional survey among infectious diseases specialists practicing in large hospitals. *Clin. Microbiol. Infect.* **2018**, *24*, 1070–1076. [CrossRef]

18. Karakonstantis, S.; Kritsotakis, E.I.; Gikas, A. Treatment options for *K. pneumoniae*, *P. aeruginosa* and *A. baumannii* co-resistant to carbapenems, aminoglycosides, polymyxins and tigecycline: An approach based on the mechanisms of resistance to carbapenems. *Infection* **2020**, *48*, 835–851. [CrossRef]
19. Correia, V.G.; Bonifácio, V.D.B.; Raje, V.P.; Casimiro, T.; Moutinho, G.; da Silva, C.L.; Pinho, M.G.; Aguiar-Ricardo, A. Oxazoline-based antimicrobial oligomers: Synthesis by CROP using supercritical CO_2. *Macromol. Biosci.* **2011**, *11*, 1128–1137. [CrossRef]
20. McLaughlin, M.M.; Advincula, M.R.; Malczynski, M.; Barajas, G.; Qi, C.; Scheetz, M.H. Quantifying the clinical virulence of *Klebsiella pneumoniae* producing carbapenemase *Klebsiella pneumoniae* with a *Galleria mellonella* model and a pilot study to translate to patient outcomes. *BMC Infect. Dis.* **2014**, *14*, 31. [CrossRef]
21. Malanovic, N.; Lohner, K. Antimicrobial peptides targeting Gram-positive bacteria. *Pharmaceuticals (Basel)* **2016**, *9*, 59. [CrossRef] [PubMed]
22. Lohner, K. New strategies for novel antibiotics: Peptides targeting bacterial cell membranes. *Gen. Physiol. Biophys.* **2009**, *28*, 105–116. [CrossRef] [PubMed]
23. Loh, J.M.; Adenwalla, N.; Wiles, S.; Proft, T. *Galleria mellonella* larvae as an infection model for group A *streptococcus*. *Virulence* **2013**, *4*, 419–428. [CrossRef] [PubMed]
24. Carmona-Ribeiro, A.M.; de Melo Carrasco, L.D. Cationic antimicrobial polymers and their assemblies. *Int. J. Mol. Sci.* **2013**, *14*, 9906–9946. [CrossRef] [PubMed]
25. Mahlapuu, M.; Håkansson, J.; Ringstad, L.; Björn, C. Antimicrobial peptides: An emerging category of therapeutic agents. *Front Cell Infect. Microbiol.* **2016**, *6*, 194. [CrossRef] [PubMed]
26. Kaplan, J.B.; Velliyagounder, K.; Ragunath, C.; Rohde, H.; Mack, D.; Knobloch, J.K.; Ramasubbu, N. Genes involved in the synthesis and degradation of matrix polysaccharide in *Actinobacillus actinomycetemcomitans* and *Actinobacillus pleuropneumoniae* biofilms. *J. Bacteriol.* **2004**, *186*, 8213–8220. [CrossRef]
27. Matsuzaki, K. Why and how are peptide–lipid interactions utilized for self-defense? Magainins and tachyplesins as archetypes. *Biochimica Biophysica Acta (BBA) Biomembranes* **1999**, *1462*, 1–10. [CrossRef]
28. Kaplan, C.W.; Sim, J.H.; Shah, K.R.; Kolesnikova-Kaplan, A.; Shi, W.; Eckert, R. Selective membrane disruption: Mode of action of C16G2, a specifically targeted antimicrobial peptide. *Antimicrob. Agents Chemother.* **2011**, *55*, 3446–3452. [CrossRef]
29. Wimley, W.C. Describing the mechanism of antimicrobial peptide action with the interfacial activity model. *ACS Chem. Biol.* **2010**, *5*, 905–917. [CrossRef]
30. World Health Organization. Global Priority List of Antibiotic-Resistant Bacteria to Guide Research, Discovery, and Development of New Antibiotics. 2017. Available online: https://www.who.int/medicines/publications/global-priority-list-antibiotic-resistant-bacteria/en (accessed on 6 January 2021).
31. Palermo, E.F.; Lienkamp, K.; Gillies, E.R.; Ragogna, P.J. Antibacterial activity of polymers: Discussions on the nature of amphiphilic balance. *Angew. Chem. Int. Ed.* **2019**, *58*, 3690–3693. [CrossRef]
32. Kenawy, E.-R.; Worley, S.D.; Broughton, R. The chemistry and applications of antimicrobial polymers: A state-of-the-art review. *Biomacromolecules* **2007**, *8*, 1359–1384. [CrossRef]
33. Wang, G.; Li, X.; Wang, Z. APD3: The antimicrobial peptide database as a tool for research and education. *Nucleic Acids Res.* **2016**, *44*, D1087–D1093. [CrossRef]
34. Kuroda, K.; Caputo, G.A.; DeGrado, W.F. The role of hydrophobicity in the antimicrobial and hemolytic activities of polymethacrylate derivatives. *Chemistry* **2009**, *15*, 1123–1133. [CrossRef]
35. Palermo, E.F.; Kuroda, K. Chemical structure of cationic groups in amphiphilic polymethacrylates modulates the antimicrobial and hemolytic activities. *Biomacromolecules* **2009**, *10*, 1416–1428. [CrossRef]
36. Palermo, E.F.; Lee, D.K.; Ramamoorthy, A.; Kuroda, K. Role of cationic group structure in membrane binding and disruption by amphiphilic copolymers. *J. Phys. Chem. B* **2011**, *115*, 366–375. [CrossRef]
37. Al-Badri, Z.M.; Som, A.; Lyon, S.; Nelson, C.F.; Nusslein, K.; Tew, G.N. Investigating the effect of increasing charge density on the hemolytic activity of synthetic antimicrobial polymers. *Biomacromolecules* **2008**, *9*, 2805–2810. [CrossRef]
38. Lin, J.; Qiu, S.; Lewis, K.; Klibanov, A.M. Bactericidal properties of flat surfaces and nanoparticles derivatized with alkylated polyethylenimines. *Biotechnol. Prog.* **2002**, *18*, 1082–1086. [CrossRef]
39. Curtis, K.A.; Miller, D.; Millard, P.; Basu, S.; Horkay, F.; Chandran, P.L. Unusual salt and pH induced changes in polyethylenimine solutions. *PLoS ONE* **2016**, *11*, e0158147. [CrossRef]
40. Liu, L.; Xu, K.; Wang, H.; Tan, P.K.; Fan, W.; Venkatraman, S.S.; Li, L.; Yang, Y.Y. Self-assembled cationic peptide nanoparticles as an efficient antimicrobial agent. *Nat. Nanotechnol.* **2009**, *4*, 457–463. [CrossRef]
41. Yasir, M.; Dutta, D.; Willcox, M.D.P. Comparative mode of action of the antimicrobial peptide melimine and its derivative Mel4 against *Pseudomonas aeruginosa*. *Sci. Rep.* **2019**, *9*, 7063. [CrossRef]
42. Kwon, J.Y.; Kim, M.K.; Mereuta, L.; Seo, C.H.; Luchian, T.; Park, Y. Mechanism of action of antimicrobial peptide P5 truncations against *Pseudomonas aeruginosa* and *Staphylococcus aureus*. *AMB Express* **2019**, *9*, 122. [CrossRef]
43. Bengoechea, J.A.; Sa Pessoa, J. *Klebsiella pneumoniae* infection biology: Living to counteract host defences. *FEMS Microbiol. Rev.* **2019**, *43*, 123–144. [CrossRef]
44. Fleeman, R.M.; Macias, L.A.; Brodbelt, J.S.; Davies, B.W. Defining principles that influence antimicrobial peptide activity against capsulated *Klebsiella pneumoniae*. *Proc. Natl. Acad. Sci. USA* **2020**, *117*, 27620. [CrossRef]

45. Liu, X.; Tang, M.; Zhang, T.; Hu, Y.; Zhang, S.; Kong, L.; Xue, Y. Determination of a threshold dose to reduce or eliminate CdTe-induced toxicity in L929 cells by controlling the exposure dose. *PLoS ONE* **2013**, *8*, e59350. [CrossRef]
46. Venkatesh, M.; Barathi, V.A.; Goh, E.T.L.; Anggara, R.; Fazil, M.; Ng, A.J.Y.; Harini, S.; Aung, T.T.; Fox, S.J.; Liu, S.; et al. Antimicrobial activity and cell selectivity of synthetic and biosynthetic cationic polymers. *Antimicrob. Agents Chemother.* **2017**, *61*. [CrossRef]
47. Aguiar-Ricardo, A.; Bonifácio, V.D.B.; Casimiro, T.; Correia, V.G. Supercritical carbon dioxide design strategies: From drug carriers to soft killers. *Philos. Trans. A Math Phys. Eng. Sci.* **2015**, *373*. [CrossRef]
48. Burckhardt, I.; Zimmermann, S. Susceptibility testing of bacteria using Maldi-Tof Mass Spectrometry. *Front. Microbiol.* **2018**, *9*, 1744. [CrossRef]
49. Edwards-Jones, V.; Claydon, M.A.; Evason, D.J.; Walker, J.; Fox, A.J.; Gordon, D.B. Rapid discrimination between methicillin-sensitive and methicillin-resistant *Staphylococcus aureus* by intact cell mass spectrometry. *J. Med. Microbiol.* **2000**, *49*, 295–300. [CrossRef]
50. Wiegand, I.; Hilpert, K.; Hancock, R.E. Agar and broth dilution methods to determine the minimal inhibitory concentration (MIC) of antimicrobial substances. *Nat. Protoc.* **2008**, *3*, 163–175. [CrossRef]
51. Pankey, G.A.; Sabath, L.D. Clinical relevance of bacteriostatic versus bactericidal mechanisms of action in the treatment of Gram-positive bacterial infections. *Clin. Infect. Dis.* **2004**, *38*, 864–870. [CrossRef]
52. García-Armesto, M.R.; Prieto, M.; García-López, M.L.; Otero, A.; Moreno, B. Modern microbiological methods for foods: Colony count and direct count methods. A review. *Microbiologia* **1993**, *9*, 1–13.
53. Mangoni, M.L.; Papo, N.; Barra, D.; Simmaco, M.; Bozzi, A.; Di Giulio, A.; Rinaldi, A.C. Effects of the antimicrobial peptide temporin L on cell morphology, membrane permeability and viability of *Escherichia coli*. *Biochem. J.* **2004**, *380*, 859–865. [CrossRef]
54. Xu, M.; McCanna, D.J.; Sivak, J.G. Use of the viability reagent PrestoBlue in comparison with alamarBlue and MTT to assess the viability of human corneal epithelial cells. *J. Pharmacol. Toxicol. Methods* **2015**, *71*, 1–7. [CrossRef]
55. Pinheiro, M.; Lúcio, M.; Lima, J.L.; Reis, S. Liposomes as drug delivery systems for the treatment of TB. *Nanomedicine (Lond.)* **2011**, *6*, 1413–1428. [CrossRef]

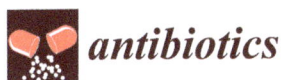

Article

Synthesis of Electrospun TiO$_2$ Nanofibers and Characterization of Their Antibacterial and Antibiofilm Potential against Gram-Positive and Gram-Negative Bacteria

Mohammad Azam Ansari [1], Hani Manssor Albetran [2], Muidh Hamed Alheshibri [3], Abdelmajid Timoumi [4], Norah Abdullah Algarou [5,6], Sultan Akhtar [5], Yassine Slimani [5], Munirah Abdullah Almessiere [5], Fatimah Saad Alahmari [7], Abdulhadi Baykal [7] and It-Meng Low [8,*]

1. Department of Epidemic Disease Research, Institute for Research & Medical Consultations (IRMC), Imam Abdulrahman Bin Faisal University, P.O. Box 1982, Dammam 31441, Saudi Arabia; maansari@iau.edu.sa
2. Department of Basic Sciences, College of Education, Imam Abdulrahman Bin Faisal University, P.O. Box 2375, Dammam 31451, Saudi Arabia; halbatran@iau.edu.sa
3. Basic Science Department, Deanship of Preparatory Year and Supporting Studies & Basic and Applied Scientific Research Center, Imam Abdulrahman Bin Faisal University, P.O. Box 1982, Dammam 31441, Saudi Arabia; mhalheshibri@iau.edu.sa
4. Physics Department, Faculty of Applied Science, Umm AL-Qura University, Makkah 24231, Saudi Arabia; timoumiabdelmajid@yahoo.fr
5. Department of Biophysics, Institute for Research & Medical Consultations (IRMC), Imam Abdulrahman Bin Faisal University, P.O. Box 1982, Dammam 31441, Saudi Arabia; nalgarou@iau.edu.sa (N.A.A.); suakhtar@iau.edu.sa (S.A.); yaslimani@iau.edu.sa (Y.S.); malmessiere@iau.edu.sa (M.A.A.)
6. Department of Physics, College of Science, Imam Abdulrahman Bin Faisal University, P.O. Box 1982, Dammam 31441, Saudi Arabia
7. Department of Nano-Medicine Research, Institute for Research & Medical Consultations (IRMC), Imam Abdulrahman Bin Faisal University, P.O. Box 1982, Dammam 31441, Saudi Arabia; fsalahmari@iau.edu.sa (F.S.A.); abaykal@iau.edu.sa (A.B.)
8. Department of Physics and Astronomy, Curtin University, GPO Box U1987, Perth, WA 6845, Australia
* Correspondence: j.low@curtin.edu.au; Tel.: +618-9266-7544; Fax: +61-8-9266-2377

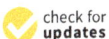

Received: 23 July 2020; Accepted: 1 September 2020; Published: 3 September 2020

Abstract: Recently, titanium dioxide (TiO$_2$) nanomaterials have gained increased attention because of their cost-effective, safe, stable, non-toxic, non-carcinogenic, photocatalytic, bactericidal, biomedical, industrial and waste-water treatment applications. The aim of the present work is the synthesis of electrospun TiO$_2$ nanofibers (NFs) in the presence of different amounts of air–argon mixtures using sol-gel and electrospinning approaches. The physicochemical properties of the synthesized NFs were examined by scanning and transmission electron microscopies (SEM and TEM) coupled with energy-dispersive X-ray spectroscopy (EDX), ultraviolet-visible spectroscopy and thermogravimetric analyzer (TGA). The antibacterial and antibiofilm activity of synthesized NFs against Gram-negative *Pseudomonas aeruginosa* and Gram-positive methicillin-resistant *Staphylococcus aureus* (MRSA) was investigated by determining their minimum bacteriostatic and bactericidal values. The topological and morphological alteration caused by TiO$_2$ NFs in bacterial cells was further analyzed by SEM. TiO$_2$ NFs that were calcined in a 25% air-75% argon mixture showed maximum antibacterial and antibiofilm activities. The minimum inhibitory concentration (MIC)/minimum bactericidal concentration (MBC) value of TiO$_2$ NFs against *P. aeruginosa* was 3 and 6 mg/mL and that for MRSA was 6 and 12 mg/mL, respectively. The MIC/MBC and SEM results show that TiO$_2$ NFs were more active against Gram-negative *P. aeruginosa* cells than Gram-positive *S. aureus*. The inhibition of biofilm formation by TiO$_2$ NFs was investigated quantitatively by tissue culture plate method using crystal violet assay and it was found that TiO$_2$ NFs inhibited biofilm formation by MRSA and *P. aeruginosa* in a dose-dependent manner. TiO$_2$ NFs calcined in a 25% air-75% argon mixture exhibited maximum biofilm formation inhibition of 75.2% for MRSA and 72.3% for *P. aeruginosa* at 2 mg/mL, respectively. The antibacterial and antibiofilm results suggest that TiO$_2$ NFs can be used to coat various inanimate objects, in food packaging and in waste-water treatment and purification to prevent bacterial growth and biofilm formation.

Keywords: TiO$_2$ nanofibers; electrospinning; biofilm prevention and control; multidrug-resistant bacteria; biomedical application

1. Introduction

Titanium dioxide (TiO$_2$) is among the investigated photocatalytic nanomaterials and is used extensively in diverse applications and for diverse purposes [1]. TiO$_2$ nanomaterials are widely used in waste-water treatment and purification, air-pollutant decomposition, implantable devices, air-conditioning filters, hydrophilic coatings, self-cleaning and self-disinfecting devices, pesticide degradation (e.g., herbicides, insecticides and fungicides) and in the production of hydrogen fuel [2,3]. TiO$_2$ is usually non-toxic, highly durable with a high refractive index, high absorption of light and a lower-cost production with antibacterial activity [4,5]. Because of its strong stability, TiO$_2$ materials can be applied easily on inanimate items, e.g., metal, glass and biomedical implants [5]. Recently, TiO$_2$ nanoparticles (NPs) have attracted increased interest in the scientific and industrial community because of their extensive applications in biological and pharmaceutical areas, purification of environmental sources, electronic system, solar energy cells, photocatalysts, photo-electrodes and gas sensors. TiO$_2$ NPs are proven to be employed in food technology, drugs, cosmetics, paint pigment, ointments and toothpaste [6,7]. Because of their cost-effective, safe, stable, non-toxic, non-carcinogenic, photo-induced super-hydrophobicity and antifogging properties, TiO$_2$ NPs have been used to kill bacteria, remove toxic and harmful organic elements from water and air and for self-sterilize glass surfaces [8–11].

However, it is difficult to separate TiO$_2$ NPs after a photochemical reaction, which limits their practical applications [12]. TiO$_2$ NPs aggregate easily in solution, which reduces their photocatalytic efficacy because of the decreased surface area. These limitations can be overcome by preparing TiO$_2$ nanofibers (NFs) using simple, rapid and cost-effective electrospinning (ES) methods [13–18]. TiO$_2$ NFs have gained increased attention because of their mesoporous structure [19], stability in solution, little or no aggregation, high surface to volume ratio that enhances photocatalytic reactions and their ease in separation and collection from solution after photochemical reactions [20,21]. However, the photocatalytic efficacy of TiO$_2$ NFs is comparatively low and is effective only under ultraviolet (UV) light because of their relatively large band-gap energy and low-ordered crystalline structure [22]. An exceptional feature of TiO$_2$ nanoparticles (NPs) is their photocatalytic activity that enhances the bacterial killing when exposed to UV light [7,23]. TiO$_2$ NPs tend to exist in three principal forms, namely brookite, rutile and anatase, and it has been reported that the anatase form has a high photocatalytic and antibacterial activity [23–26]. A major biomedical application of TiO$_2$ NPs is to prevent biofilm formation on medical devices that is related to infections and sepsis [3,27,28]. Several researchers have focused on the antibacterial and antibiofilm activities of TiO$_2$ NPs under UV light against standard bacterial strains, e.g., ATCC, MTCC and NCIM. However, limited work has been published on the antibacterial and antibiofilm activities of TiO$_2$ NFs without application of UV light against drug resistant isolates. The objective of present investigation is to explore the antibacterial and antibiofilm efficacies of TiO$_2$ NFs in dark against two major human pathogenic drug resistant bacteria i.e., Gram-positive *methicillin-resistant Staphylococcus aureus* (MRSA) and Gram-negative *Pseudomonas aeruginosa* by using different methods.

2. Experimental Methodology

2.1. Electrospinning and Heating Protocol

Both the sol-gel and electrospinning approaches were used to synthesize electrospun TiO_2 NFs. Briefly, Titanium isopropoxide (IV), acetic acid and ethanol were mixed and stirred with respect to volume ratio of 3:1:3. After that, 12% by weight of polyvinylpyrrolidone (PVP) was dissolved in the obtained TiO_2 solution. This mixed TiO_2/PVP sol-gel was then placed within a plastic syringe for electrospinning experiment. Additional details are provided in a preliminary study [15]. Thermal gravimetric analysis (TGA) and differential scanning calorimetry (DSC) for the non-isothermal heating of electrospun TiO_2 NFs were performed on a Mettler Teledo thermal gravimetric analyzer TGA/DSC. The samples were heated from ambient temperature to 900 °C at a rate of 10 °C/min with an argon protective gas of 20 mL/min in various mixtures of air and argon. The thermal experiments were carried out by utilizing alumina crucibles that were charged with 25 mg of sample and in mixtures of 50% air-50% argon, 25% air-75% argon and 100% argon. It is worth noting that the argon shielding gas is included in the relative percentage of air to argon gas. For safety reasons, samples that were contacted with 100% air were heated in an oven under the same conditions [29].

2.2. Characterization of Electrospun TiO_2 NFs

The morphological and structural properties of as-prepared NFs were characterized by SEM (FEI Inspect S50) and TEM (FEI Morgagni 268). The elemental composition was determined by energy-dispersive spectroscopy (EDX). A strong correlation can be established from the initial microstructure images. The TiO_2 grains were structured as microspheres and a complete description of the microstructure is provided. The microstructure relates to monitoring by three-dimensional imaging of the evolution of internal porosity as a function of annealing temperature. A Jasco V-670 UV–visible diffuse reflectance spectrophotometer (DRS) under a wavelength ranging between 200 and 750 nm was used to estimate the band gap energy (E_g) of various TiO_2 NFs.

The values of band gap energy (E_g) were calculated from the absorption spectra versus wavelength using the following expression:

$$E_g = \frac{hC}{\lambda_0} \quad (1)$$

In this expression, h is Planck's constant (6.626×10^{-34} J.s) and C is the speed of light (3×10^8 m/s). λ_0 (expressed in nm) is the cut off wavelength obtained from the absorption spectra [30]. Accordingly, λ_0 denotes the absorption edge wavelength, obtained from the offset wavelength derived and extrapolated from the low energy absorption band.

2.3. Evaluation of Antibacterial Activity of Electrospun TiO_2 NFs

2.3.1. Bacterial Culture

The laboratory strain of Gram-negative *Pseudomonas aeruginosa* PAO1 and Gram-positive methicillin resistant *Staphylococcus aureus* (MRSA) ATCC 33591 used in this study was obtained from Molecular Microbiology Laboratory, Institute for Research and Medical Consultations, Imam Abdulrahman Bin Faisal University, Dammam, Saudi Arabia. The bacterial strains preserved in glycerol cultures (−80 °C) were cultivated on Tryptic soy broth (TSB) at 37 °C in a shaker incubator before being used for microbial studies.

2.3.2. Investigation of Minimum Inhibitory and Minimum Bactericidal Concentration (MIC/MBC) Values of Electrospun TiO_2 NFs

The MIC values of TiO_2 NFs against *P. aeruginosa* and MRSA was estimated by serial two-fold dilutions of TiO_2 NFs from 32 to 1 mg/mL as described previously [31,32]. The determination of MBC values was also investigated as method described in previous studies [32,33].

2.4. Effect of TiO$_2$ NFs on Biofilm Formation

The antibiofilm potential of TiO$_2$ NFs against *P. aeruginosa* and MRSA biofilm was examined quantitatively in a sterilized 96-well polystyrene (flat bottom) microtiter tissue culture plate using crystal violet assay as described in our previous study [31,33].

2.5. Effect of TiO$_2$ NFs on the Morphology of P. aeruginosa and MRSA: SEM Analysis

Further, the effects of TiO$_2$ NFs on the morphological features of *P. aeruginosa* and *S. aureus* cells were analyzed by SEM. In Brief, ~10^6 CFU/mL of *P. aeruginosa* and *S. aureus* cells treated with 1 mg/mL of TiO$_2$ NFs for 18 h were incubated at 37 °C [33,34]. After incubation, the treated and untreated samples were centrifuged at 10,000 rpm for 15 min. The obtained pellets were washed with PBS (1×) three times and fixed with primary fixative (i.e., 2.5% glutaraldehyde) for 6 h at 4 °C and then further fixed with secondary fixative (i.e., 1% osmium tetroxide) for 1 h. After fixation, the samples were dehydrated by a series of ethanol [34,35]. The cells were then fixed on the aluminum stubs, dried in a desecrator and coated with gold. Finally, the treated and untreated samples were examined by SEM.

3. Results and Discussion

3.1. Effects of the Calcining Atmosphere on TiO$_2$ Colour

Figure 1 presents a gradual color change from white to dark grey after heat treatment in 100% air and in different mediums of air–argon compositions up to 100% argon medium. This change is likely because of oxygen vacancy defects. The change and the intensification of the color are mainly a result of defects associated with oxygen vacancies that rise from an increase in argon content [36].

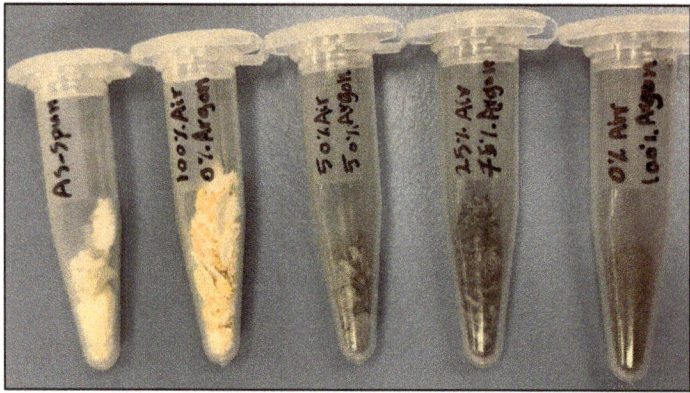

Figure 1. Color changes in electrospun titanium oxide (TiO$_2$) nanofibers (NFs) in argon-air mixtures.

3.2. Microstructure Analysis of the Prepared NFs

Figures 2 and 3 show the typical SEM and TEM micrographs of the as-spun TiO$_2$ and calcined NFs. The electrospinning process could produce good quality TiO$_2$ NFs, possibly without nodes and defects. The diameter of the as-spun fibers varied between 80 and 600 nm, whereas the estimated average thickness was ~400 nm (Figure 2a). Upon annealing in different mediums of air/argon (100%-0%, 50%-50%, 25%-75%, and 0%-100%), the fibers shrank, and their morphology changed slightly from smooth to rough. This figure also shows the presence of a heterogeneous matrix made up of agglomerated grains for the initial microstructure and leads to faster granular growth. The fibers size was between 50 and 300 nm (Figure 2b–e). Several thin-fibers of about 50 nm were perceived in specimens annealed under 25-75% air-argon. The quality and shape of fiber mats were preserved after calcination as clarified by the TEM images (Figure 3b–e) unlike the electrospun fibers that are often composed of oxide nanoparticles (Figure 3a) [37]. The as-spun fibers showed organic species, whereas the annealed fibers exhibited a solid morphology with high-quality individual particles in the range of 100 nm. The annealing of TiO_2 NFs at 900 °C in 50%-50% air-argon led to pure TiO_2 fibers formation, which was proven by EDX and TGA characterization techniques. In Figure 4, the EDX spectrum illustrates high-intensity O and Ti peaks and a small Pt peak from the platinum coating on the TiO_2 NFs heated in 50-50% air-argon, which is mainly similar to those observed in specimens annealed in 100% air, 25% air-75% argon, and 100% argon. Figure 5 shows the TGA result for samples heated under 50-50% air-argon medium. The PVP polymer and organic material are completely removed from the electrospun TiO_2 NFs at ~450 °C, and ~100 °C, respectively.

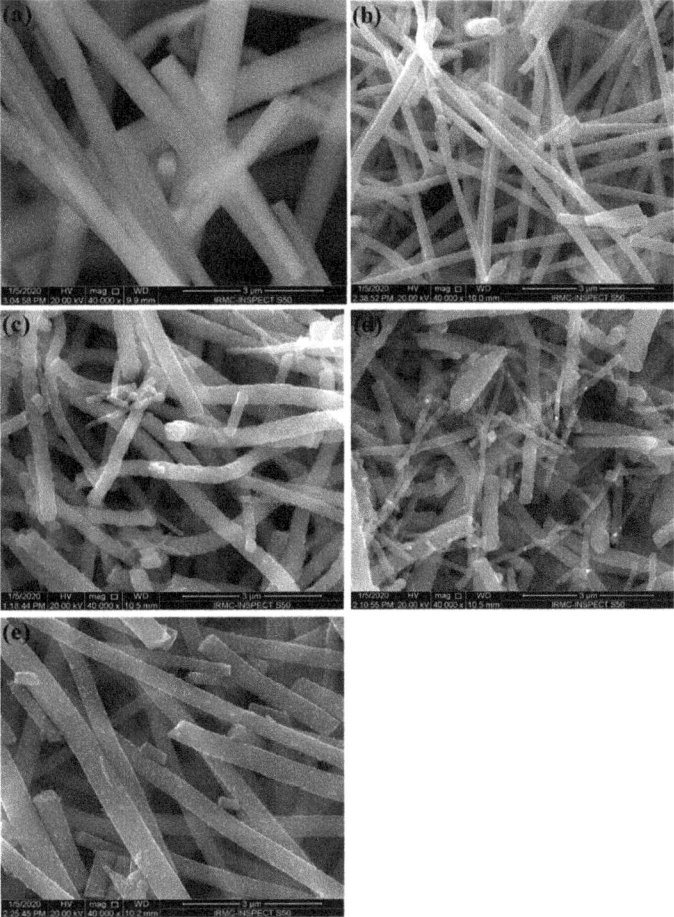

Figure 2. Scanning electron microscopy (SEM) of TiO_2 NFs calcined in different air and argon mixture. (**a**) As-spun TiO_2, (**b**) 100% Air, (**c**) 50% Air and 50% Argon, (**d**) 25% Air and 75% Argon and (**e**) 100% Argon.

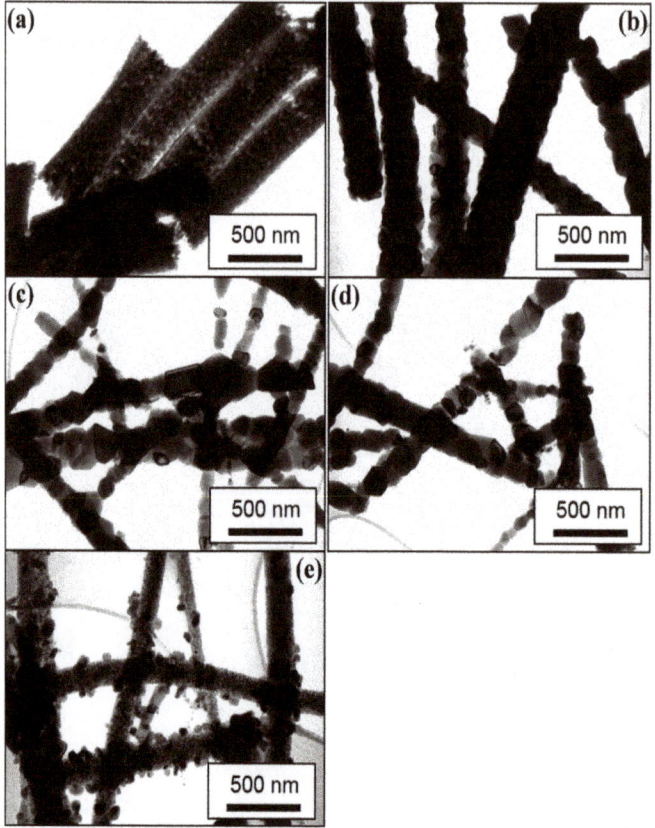

Figure 3. Transmission electron microscopy (TEM) of TiO_2 NFs calcined in different air and argon mixture. (**a**) As-spun TiO_2, (**b**) 100% Air, (**c**) 50% Air and 50% Argon, (**d**) 25% Air and 75% Argon and (**e**) 100% Argon.

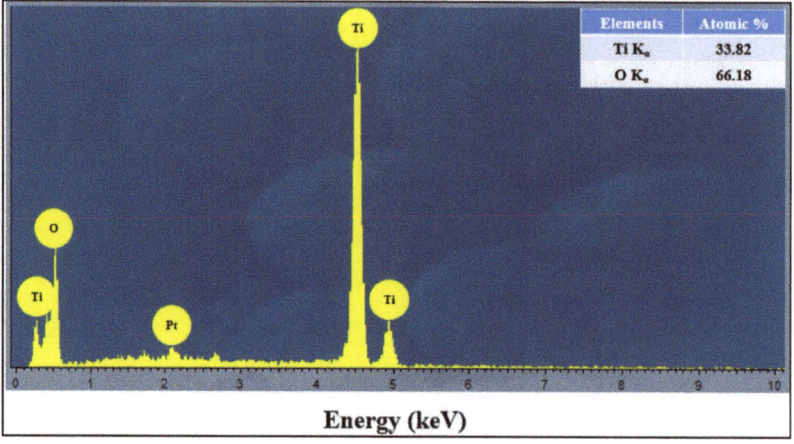

Figure 4. An energy-dispersive X-ray spectroscopy (EDX) spectrum of electrospun TiO_2 NFs prepared in 50% air-50% argon mixture.

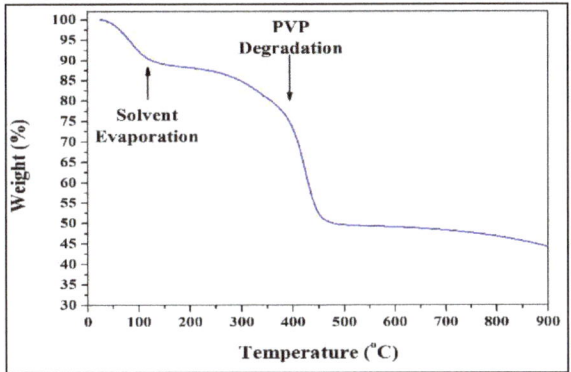

Figure 5. Thermogravimetric analysis (TGA) performed for electrospun TiO$_2$ NFs prepared under 50% air-50% argon mixture.

3.3. Wide-Band Gap Analysis of Calcined Electrospun TiO$_2$ NFs

Figure 6 shows the UV-vis DRS spectra of as-electrospun TiO$_2$ NFs calcinated in air-argon media at 900 °C and cooling to ambient temperature. Table 1 shows the values of band-gaps at room temperature for various TiO$_2$ NFs. The band-gap value reduced from 3.33 eV for as-spun and non-calcinated samples to about 3.09 eV for the ones calcinated in 100% air. Under various air-argon environments, the value of E_g decreased from about 3.09 to 2.18 eV with an increase in argon content. A previous study on similar specimens revealed that the growth of vacancies was minimal and the reduction of E_g value was ascribed to the increase in crystallinity [38]. The measured difference agrees with that weighted according to the concentration of pure anatase and rutile phases [38–40]. Alterations in levels and phase mixing and gradual development of oxygen vacancies are two factors that can reduce the band-gap energy with argon introduction. The measured energy gap was 2.18 eV for sample heated in 100% argon and for the phase composition for which the difference according to the concentration would be 3.05 eV. The difference of 0.87 eV is assigned to the development of oxygen vacancies and allows a greater density of charge carriers. The development of oxygen vacancies leads to the creation of Ti^{3+} centers or unpaired electrons that generate vacant states under the conduction band [41,42]. The development of oxygen vacancies for different argon concentrations has been previously discussed [38]. When the specimen is annealed in argon, oxygen disappears and the non-stoichiometric anatase (TiO$_{2-x}$) forms [43]. The formation of oxygen vacancy defects in titanium oxide is induced from the occurrence of new localized states of oxygen vacancies between the conduction and valence bands. The excitation of electrons from the valence band to the vacant oxygen states can be done in visible light. With rising argon amount, the effective E_g moves thoroughly to the red region, the specimen is being active under visible light and thus the E_g is reduced. So, the mutual effects of the formation of oxygen vacancies and crystallinity treatment have prolonged the excitation of light of electrospun TiO$_2$ NFs from ultraviolet to visible light range without the need of chemical doping.

Table 1. Band gap energies for as-electrospun TiO$_2$ nanofibers (non-calcinated), and TiO$_2$ NFs obtained after calcination at 900 °C in various air-argon media.

Calcination Conditions	E_g (eV)
As-electrospun	3.33
100% Air	3.09
50% Air and 50% Argon	2.94
25% Air and 75% Argon	2.91
100% Argon	2.18

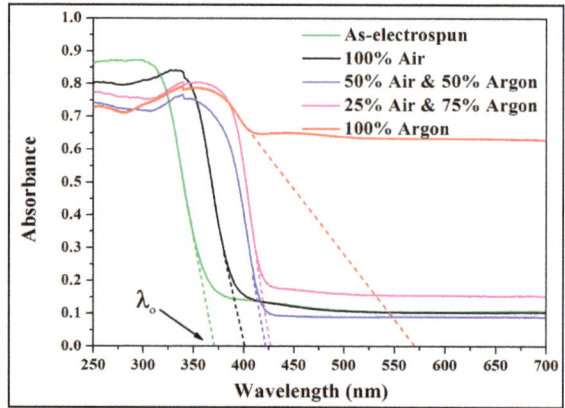

Figure 6. UV-vis diffuse reflectance spectrophotometer (DRS) spectra of electrospun TiO$_2$ NFs obtained before calcination and those obtained after calcination in various air-argon media.

3.4. Antibacterial and Antibiofilm Activity of TiO$_2$ NFs

3.4.1. MIC and MBC

The microbiocidal activities of TiO$_2$ photocatalysis were reported for the first time by Matsunaga and co-workers in 1985 [44]. They investigated the killing of bacteria and yeast cells in water by employing TiO$_2$-Pt photocatalysts in near-ultraviolet radiation. They reported that the inhibition of respiratory activity was the mechanism for cell death.

In this research work, the antibacterial property (MIC/MBC) of TiO$_2$ NFs calcined with different ratios of air–argon mixtures (i.e., 100% air, 50% air-50% argon, 25% air-75% argon, and 100% argon) has been investigated against *P. aeruginosa* and MRSA (Supplementary Figure S1). The MIC/MBC values of TiO$_2$ NFs heated with different ratios of air-argon mixtures against *P. aeruginosa* and MRSA are presented in Table 2. TiO$_2$ NFs heated in the presence of 25% air-75% argon showed a maximum antibacterial activity and MIC/MBC values against *P. aeruginosa* were 3 and 6 mg/mL and for MRSA it was 6 and 12 mg/mL, respectively (Table 2). Based on the MIC and MBC results, it was observed that Gram-negative *P. aeruginosa* was more susceptible to TiO$_2$ NFs than Gram-positive MRSA. These results agree with results from previous studies [45,46], and may occur owing to differences in their cell wall structures and to bacterial strain growth rate [45–47]. Pigeot-Rémy and co-workers [48] investigated the effects of TiO$_2$ particles against *E. coli* K-12 in the dark and reported that the attachment of NPs to bacterial surfaces causes membrane damage and perturbation, which may increase the permeability of the outer cell membrane and the resultant damage to the envelope of bacterial cells leads to bacterial cells death.

Table 2. Minimum inhibitory concentration (MIC) and minimum bactericidal concentration (MBC) (mg/mL) values of tested electrospun TiO$_2$ nanofibers against Methicillin resistant *S. aureus* and *P. aeruginosa*.

Electrospun TiO$_2$ Nanofibers Code	Calcination Conditions	Methicillin Resistant *S. aureus*		*P. aeruginosa*	
		MIC	MBC	MIC	MBC
(a)	100% Air	7	14	7	14
(b)	50% Air and 50% Argon	7	14	7	14
(c)	25% Air and 75% Argon	6	12	3	6
(d)	100% Argon	>16	>32	>16	>32

3.4.2. Effects of Electrospun TiO$_2$ NFs on the Morphology of Bacterial Cells

Morphological alterations in Gram-negative P. aeruginosa (Figure 7) and Gram-positive MRSA (Figure 8) after exposure to TiO$_2$ NFs were further examined by SEM. The untreated P. aeruginosa had a normal, rod-shaped structure and regular, smooth and intact cell surface (Figure 7). However, the morphology of *P. aeruginosa* cells was altered considerably, and cells were damaged to different extents after treatment with TiO$_2$ NFs. After 18 h of treatment, the cell envelope and cell wall were rough, irregular, abnormal in form and main damage was categorized by the creation of "pits" and depressions that probably lead to a loss of bacterial cell membrane integrity (Figure 7). Similarly, the untreated Gram-positive MRSA was normal with smooth and regular cell surfaces (Figure 8). However, MRSA cells treated with TiO$_2$ NFs exhibited noticeable alterations and damage and the clusters of NFs were linked and anchored on the surface of bacterial cells (Figure 8). Irregularities, shallows and depressions on the cell envelopes and cell walls of certain MRSA cells suggest that bacterial damage occurred (Figure 8). SEM analysis showed that TiO$_2$ NFs were more effective against P. aeruginosa bacterial cells in comparison with MRSA and were severely injured compared with Gram-positive MRSA. The obtained results may be due to morphological dissimilarities in the cell walls of bacteria. Gram-negative bacterial cells display thin layers of peptidoglycan that facilitate the mobility of metal-ion NPs within cells and facilitate the interaction among NPs and walls of bacterial cells. Gram-negative bacteria exhibit a negative charge due to their high content of lipopolysaccharides. This negative charge attracts and interacts with positive metal ions, which may lead to the NP penetration, intracellular damages and protein and DNA destruction [46]. It was suggested that the interaction of TiO$_2$ NPs with bacterial cells in the dark caused bacterial membrane integrity destruction, especially of lipopolysaccharides [48]. TiO$_2$ NPs form pores in bacterial cell walls and membranes, which increases the permeability and leads to cell death [10]. However, other published work has shown that the contact among metal oxides and bacterial cells provokes oxidation and formation of reactive oxygen groups including $O_2^{\bullet-}$, $^{\bullet}OH$, and H_2O_2. These free radicals attack bacteria cell walls and alter the membrane integrity and permeability, which leads to bacterial cell death [48–51]. It has been reported that the destruction of cell envelope by incorporation of TiO$_2$ NPs inside the cells damages bacterial DNA and RNA, which could provoke cell death [48]. The antimicrobial activity of TiO$_2$ in the absence of photoactivation has been also reported. Nakano and co-worker [51] stated that TiO$_2$ deactivates bacterial DNA and enzymes via coordination of electron-donor groups, like hydroxyls, indoles, carbohydrates, amides, and thiols in the absence of light. Pit formation in bacterial cell walls and envelopes that enhanced the permeability lead to bacterial cell death [51,52]. It has been reported that there is proportional relationship between the light and the antimicrobial activity of TiO$_2$. Senarathna et al [53] and Lee et al [54] reported that the presence of sunlight enhanced the antimicrobial activity of TiO$_2$ against S. aureus might be due to generation of free radicals [53,54].

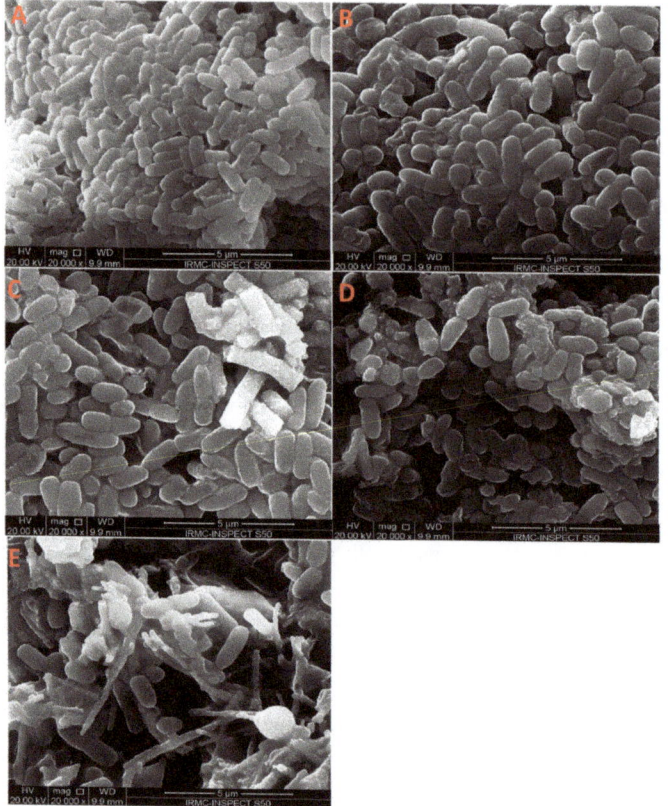

Figure 7. Effect of electrospun TiO$_2$ NFs on the morphological aspects of *P. aeruginosa* as examined by scanning electron microscopy: (**A**) control without any treatment and treated with TiO$_2$ calcined in (**B**) 100% Air, (**C**) 50% Air and 50% Argon, (**D**) 25% Air and 75% Argon; and (**E**) 100% Argon.

3.4.3. Inhibition of Biofilm Formation by TiO$_2$ NFs

The antibiofilm potential of TiO$_2$ NFs heated under different air-argon environments was evaluated at various amounts of 0.25, 0.5, 1.0 and 2.0 mg/mL against MRSA and *P. aeruginosa* biofilms using crystal violet microtiter assays in a 96-well flat-bottom polystyrene plate at OD595 nm. Plots in Figure 9A,B show that TiO$_2$ NFs inhibit the biofilms formation by MRSA and *P. aeruginosa* in a dose-dependent manner. It was reported that a rise in TiO$_2$ concentration provoked a reduction in the cultivability of bacteria [48]. As shown in Figure 9A,B, TiO$_2$ NFs heated in a 25% air-75% argon mixture exhibited the highest biofilm inhibition of about 75.2% for MRSA and 72.3% for *P. aeruginosa*, respectively at 2 mg/mL of TiO$_2$ NFs. These results agree with those reported in previous studies [55,56]. In a previous study, epoxy/Ag-TiO$_2$ nanocomposites were found to inhibit biofilm creation of *S. aureus* ATCC 6538 and *E. coli K-12* by 67% and 77%, respectively [56].

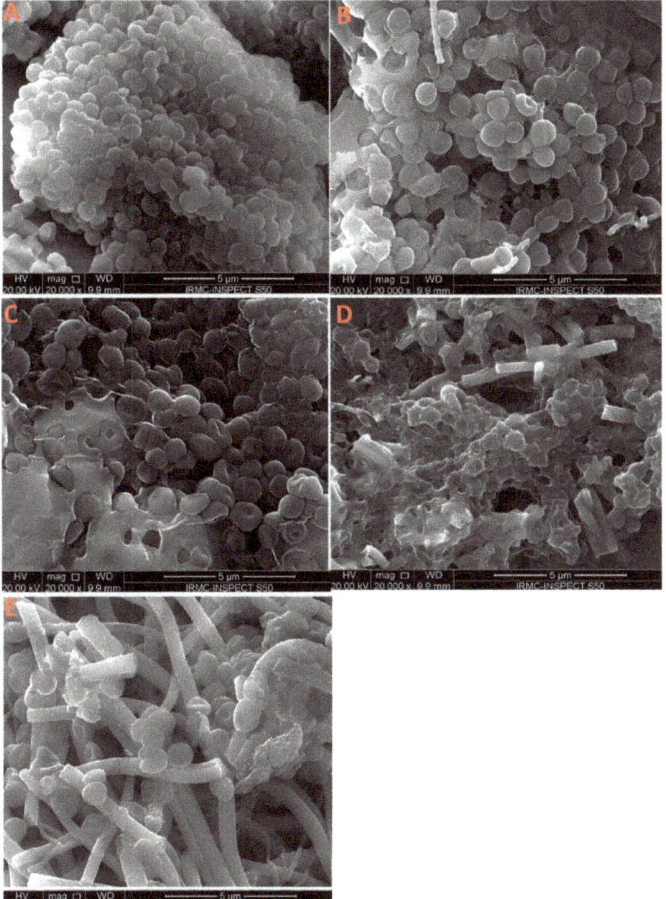

Figure 8. Effect of electrospun TiO$_2$ NFs on the morphological aspect of *S. aureus* as examined by scanning electron microscopy: (**A**) control without any treatment and treated with TiO$_2$ NFs calcined in (**B**) 100% Air; (**C**) 50% Air and 50% Argon; (**D**) 25% Air and 75% Argon, and (**E**) 100% Argon.

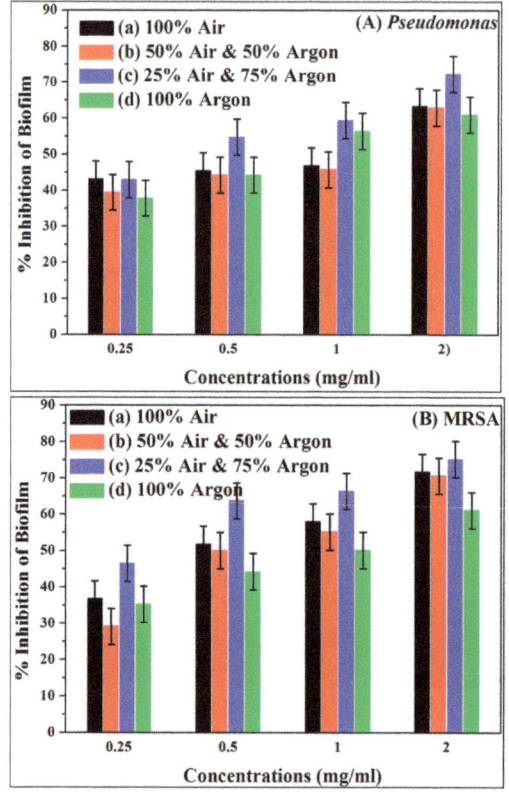

Figure 9. Effect of TiO$_2$ NFs calcined in various air–argon environments (a) 100% Air, (b) 50% Air and 50% Argon, (c) 25% Air and 75% Argon, and (d) 100% Argon on biofilm formation abilities of (**A**) *P. aeruginosa* and (**B**) methicillin-resistant *Staphylococcus aureus* (MRSA).

4. Conclusions

This study focuses on the heat treatment of TiO$_2$ NFs to develop photoactive titanium photocatalysis in the visible spectrum and to evaluate their antibacterial and antibiofilm potential against Gram-negative bacteria *P. aeruginosa* and Gram-positive MRSA. The E_g value was 3.09 eV for specimens heated in 100% air and 2.18 eV for the ones heated in 100% argon. The value of E_g decreased systematically with rising argon amount in the various air-argon mixtures. The increase in the amount of argon brings the state under the TiO$_2$ conduction band. TiO$_2$ NFs calcined in a 25% air-75% argon environment showed maximum antibacterial and antibiofilm activities. The MIC/MBC and SEM results show that TiO$_2$ NFs were more operative against Gram-negative *P. aeruginosa* than Gram-positive *S. aureus*. The inhibition of biofilm formation by TiO$_2$ NFs shows that TiO$_2$ NFs inhibit the biofilms formation by MRSA and *P. aeruginosa* in a dose-dependent manner. From the obtained data on antibacterial antibiofilm analysis, it has been concluded and suggested that TiO$_2$ NFs can be used in hydrophilic coatings, coating of various inanimate object surfaces, such as metals, glass, medical devices and equipment to prevent biofilm formation on medical devices or medical device-related infections and sepsis, and also can be applied in food packaging, wastewater treatment and purification, self-cleaning and self-disinfecting, killing of bacteria and the removal of toxic and damaging organic compounds from water and air.

Supplementary Materials: The following are available online at http://www.mdpi.com/2079-6382/9/9/572/s1, Figure S1: represents MHA plates showing MBC values of tested electrospun TiO_2 NFs in various air–argon environments.

Author Contributions: Conceptualization, H.M.A. and I.-M.L.; investigation, methodology, writing—original draft preparation H.M.A.; M.A.A. (Mohammad Azam Ansari) and S.A.; formal analysis, visualization, software, writing—review and editing, S.A.; M.H.A.; A.T.; N.A.A.; S.A.; Y.S.; M.A.A. (Munirah Abdullah Almessiere); F.S.A.; A.B.; I.-M.L.; data curation, S.A. and Y.S.; Supervision, I.-M.L. All authors have read and agreed to the published version of the manuscript.

Funding: The authors acknowledge financial support from Imam Abdulrahman Bin Faisal University (IAU-Saudi Arabia) through the project application No. 2020-086-CED. The authors thank all participants for their effort as well as for their insightful discussions.

Conflicts of Interest: The authors declare no conflict of interest.

References

1. Fujishima, A.; Rao, T.N.; Tryk, D.A. Titanium dioxide photocatalysis. *J. Photochem. Photobiol. C: Photochem. Rev.* **2000**, *1*, 1–21. [CrossRef]
2. Mills, A.; Le Hunte, S. An overview of semiconductor photocatalysis. *J. Photochem. Photobiol. A: Chem.* **1997**, *108*, 1–35. [CrossRef]
3. Gupta, S.M.; Tripathi, M. A review of TiO2 nanoparticles. *Chin. Sci. Bull.* **2011**, *56*, 1639–1657. [CrossRef]
4. Kamat, P. Photophysical, Photochemical and Photocatalytic Aspects of Metal Nanoparticles. *J. Phys. Chem. B* **2002**, *106*, 7729–7744. [CrossRef]
5. Mantravadi, H.B. Effectivity of Titanium Oxide Based Nano Particles on E. coli from Clinical Samples. *J. Clin. Diagn. Res.* **2017**, *11*, DC37–DC40. [CrossRef]
6. Awati, P.; Awate, S.; Shah, P.; Ramaswamy, V. Photocatalytic decomposition of methylene blue using nanocrystalline anatase titania prepared by ultrasonic technique. *Catal. Commun.* **2003**, *4*, 393–400. [CrossRef]
7. Othman, S.; Salam, N.R.A.; Zainal, N.; Basha, R.K.; Talib, R. Antimicrobial Activity of TiO2Nanoparticle-Coated Film for Potential Food Packaging Applications. *Int. J. Photoenergy* **2014**, *2014*, 1–6. [CrossRef]
8. Hashimoto, K.; Irie, H.; Fujishima, A. TiO2Photocatalysis: A Historical Overview and Future Prospects. *Jpn. J. Appl. Phys.* **2005**, *44*, 8269–8285. [CrossRef]
9. Fujishima, A.; Zhang, X.; Tryk, D.A. TiO2 photocatalysis and related surface phenomena. *Surf. Sci. Rep.* **2008**, *63*, 515–582. [CrossRef]
10. Haghi, M.; Hekmatafshar, M.; Janipour, M.B.; Gholizadeh, S.S.; Faraz, M.K.; Sayyadifar, F.; Ghaedi, M. Antibacterial effect of TiO2 nanoparticles on pathogenic strain of E. coli. *Int. J. Adv. Biotechnol. Res.* **2012**, *3*, 621–662.
11. Runa, S.; Khanal, D.; Kemp, M.L.; Payne, C.K. TiO2 Nanoparticles Alter the Expression of Peroxiredoxin Antioxidant Genes. *J. Phys. Chem. C* **2016**, *120*, 20736–20742. [CrossRef]
12. Schmidt, H.; Naumann, M.; Muller, T.; Akarsu, M. Application of spray techniques for new photocatalytic gradient coatings on plastics. *Thin Solid Film.* **2006**, *502*, 132–137. [CrossRef]
13. E Teo, W.; Ramakrishna, S. A review on electrospinning design and nanofibre assemblies. *Nanotechnology* **2006**, *17*, R89–R106. [CrossRef] [PubMed]
14. Albetran, H.; Dong, Y.; Low, I.M. Characterization and optimization of electrospun TiO2/PVP nanofibers using Taguchi design of experiment method. *J. Asian Ceram. Soc.* **2015**, *3*, 292–300. [CrossRef]
15. Albetran, H.; Haroosh, H.; Dong, Y.; Prida, V.M.; O'Connor, B.H.; Low, I.M. Phase transformations and crystallization kinetics in electrospun TiO2 nanofibers in air and argon atmospheres. *Appl. Phys. A* **2014**, *116*, 161–169. [CrossRef]
16. Albetran, H.; Low, I.M. Crystallization kinetics and phase transformations in aluminum ion-implanted electrospun TiO2 nanofibers. *Appl. Phys. A* **2016**, *122*. [CrossRef]
17. Albetran, H.; O'Connor, B.H.; Prida, V.M.; Low, I.M. Effect of vanadium ion implantation on the crystallization kinetics and phase transformation of electrospun TiO2 nanofibers. *Appl. Phys. A* **2015**, *120*, 623–634. [CrossRef]
18. Albetran, H.; Low, I. Parameters controlling the crystallization kinetics of nanostructured TiO2—An overview. *Mater. Today Proc.* **2019**, *16*, 25–35. [CrossRef]

19. Zhang, X.-W.; Xu, S.; Han, G. Fabrication and photocatalytic activity of TiO2 nanofiber membrane. *Mater. Lett.* **2009**, *63*, 1761–1763. [CrossRef]
20. Chandrasekar, R.; Zhang, L.; Howe, J.Y.; Hedin, N.E.; Zhang, Y.; Fong, H. Fabrication and characterization of electrospun titania nanofibers. *J. Mater. Sci.* **2009**, *44*, 1198–1205. [CrossRef]
21. Li, Q.; Satur, D.J.G.; Kim, H.; Kim, H.G. Preparation of sol–gel modified electrospun TiO2 nanofibers for improved photocatalytic decomposition of ethylene. *Mater. Lett.* **2012**, *76*, 169–172. [CrossRef]
22. Xu, S.; Li, A.; Poirier, G.; Yao, N. In Situ Mechanical and Electrical Characterization of Individual TiO2Nanofibers Using a Nanomanipulator System. *Scanning* **2012**, *34*, 341–346. [CrossRef] [PubMed]
23. Ahmad, R.; Sardar, M. TiO2 nanoparticles as an antibacterial agents against E. coli. *Int. J. Innov. Res. Sci. Eng. Technol.* **2013**, *2*, 3569–3574.
24. Albetran, H.; Low, I. Crystallization kinetics study of In-doped and (In-Cr) co-doped TiO2 nanopowders using in-situ high-temperature synchrotron radiation diffraction. *Arab. J. Chem.* **2020**, *13*, 3946–3956. [CrossRef]
25. Albetran, H.; Vega, V.; Prida, V.M.; Low, I.-M. Dynamic Diffraction Studies on the Crystallization, Phase Transformation, and Activation Energies in Anodized Titania Nanotubes. *Nanomaterials* **2018**, *8*, 122. [CrossRef]
26. Albetran, H.; Low, I.-M. Effect of indium ion implantation on crystallization kinetics and phase transformation of anodized titania nanotubes using in-situ high-temperature radiation diffraction. *J. Mater. Res.* **2016**, *31*, 1588–1595. [CrossRef]
27. Ravishankar, R.V.; Jamuna, B.A. Nanoparticles and their potential application as antimicrobials. In *Science against Microbial Pathogens: Communicating Current Research and Technological Advances*; Mendez-Vilas, A., Ed.; University of Mysore: Mysore, India, 2011; pp. 197–209.
28. Arora, H.; Doty, C.; Yuan, Y.; Boyle, J.; Petras, K.; Rabatic, B.; Paunesku, T.; Woloschak, G.E. Titanium Dioxide Nanocomposites. In *Nanomaterials for Life Sciences*; Kumar, C.S.S.R., Ed.; Wiley-VCH Verlag GmbH & Co KGaA: Weinheim, Germany, 2010; pp. 1–42.
29. Albetran, H.; O'Connor, B.; Low, I.-M. Effect of calcination on band gaps for electrospun titania nanofibers heated in air–argon mixtures. *Mater. Des.* **2016**, *92*, 480–485. [CrossRef]
30. Bhadwal, A.S.; Tripathi, R.; Gupta, R.K.; Kumar, N.; Singh, R.P.; Shrivastav, A. Biogenic synthesis and photocatalytic activity of CdS nanoparticles. *RSC Adv.* **2014**, *4*, 9484. [CrossRef]
31. Balasamy, R.J.; Ravinayagam, V.; Alomari, M.; Ansari, M.A.; Almofty, S.A.; Rehman, S.; Dafalla, H.; Marimuthu, P.R.; Akhtar, S.; Hamad, M. Cisplatin delivery, anticancer and antibacterial properties of Fe/SBA-16/ZIF-8 nanocomposite. *RSC Adv.* **2019**, *9*, 42395–42408. [CrossRef]
32. Sultan, A.; Khan, H.M.; Malik, A.; Ansari, A.; Azam, A.; Perween, N. Antibacterial activity of ZnO nanoparticles against ESBL and Amp-C producing gram negative isolates from superficial wound infections. *Int. J. Curr. Microbiol. App. Sci.* **2015**, *1*, 38–47.
33. Baig, U.; Ansari, M.A.; Gondal, M.; Akhtard, S.; Khan, F.A.; Falathaf, W.S. Single step production of high-purity copper oxide-titanium dioxide nanocomposites and their effective antibacterial and anti-biofilm activity against drug-resistant bacteria. *Mater. Sci. Eng. C* **2020**, *113*, 110992. [CrossRef] [PubMed]
34. Ali, F.A.A.; Alam, J.; Shukla, A.K.; Alhoshan, M.; Ansari, M.A.; Al-Masry, W.A.; Rehman, S.; Alam, M. Evaluation of antibacterial and antifouling properties of silver-loaded GO polysulfone nanocomposite membrane against Escherichia coli, Staphylococcus aureus, and BSA protein. *React. Funct. Polym.* **2019**, *140*, 136–147. [CrossRef]
35. Shukla, A.K.; Alam, J.; Ansari, M.A.; Alhoshan, M.; Alam, M.; Kaushik, A. Selective ion removal and antibacterial activity of silver-doped multi-walled carbon nanotube/polyphenylsulfone nanocomposite membranes. *Mater. Chem. Phys.* **2019**, *233*, 102–112. [CrossRef]
36. Gamboa, J.A.; Pasquevich, D.M. Effect of Chlorine Atmosphere on the Anatase-Rutile Transformation. *J. Am. Ceram. Soc.* **1992**, *75*, 2934–2938. [CrossRef]
37. Szilágyi, I.M.; Santala, E.; Heikkilä, M.; Pore, V.; Kemell, M.; Nikitin, T.; Teucher, G.; Firkala, T.; Khriachtchev, L.; Rasanen, M.; et al. Photocatalytic properties of WO3/TiO2 core/shell nanofibers prepared by electrospinning and atomic layer deposition. *Chem. Vap. Depos.* **2013**, *19*, 149–155. [CrossRef]
38. Albetran, H.; O'Connor, B.H.; Low, I.-M. Activation energies for phase transformations in electrospun titania nanofibers: Comparing the influence of argon and air atmospheres. *Appl. Phys. A* **2016**, *122*. [CrossRef]

39. Scanlon, D.O.; Dunnill, C.W.; Buckeridge, J.; Shevlin, S.A.; Logsdail, A.J.; Woodley, S.M.; Catlow, C.R.A.; Powell, M.J.; Palgrave, R.G.; Parkin, I.P.; et al. Band alignment of rutile and anatase TiO2. *Nat. Mater.* **2013**, *12*, 798–801. [CrossRef]
40. Natoli, A.; Cabeza, A.; Torre, Ángeles, G.; Aranda, M.A.G.; Santacruz, I.; Cabeza, A. Colloidal Processing of Macroporous TiO2 Materials for Photocatalytic Water Treatment. *J. Am. Ceram. Soc.* **2011**, *95*, 502–508. [CrossRef]
41. Nakamura, I.; Negishi, N.; Kutsuna, S.; Ihara, T.; Sugihara, S.; Takeuchi, K. Role of oxygen vacancy in the plasma-treated TiO2 photocatalyst with visible light activity for NO removal. *J. Mol. Catal. A: Chem.* **2000**, *161*, 205–212. [CrossRef]
42. Seo, H.; Baker, L.R.; Hervier, A.; Kim, J.; Whitten, J.L.; Somorjai, G.A. Generation of Highly n-Type Titanium Oxide Using Plasma Fluorine Insertion. *Nano Lett.* **2011**, *11*, 751–756. [CrossRef]
43. Andersson, S.; Collén, B.; Kuylenstierna, U.; Magnéli, A.; Pestmalis, H.; Åsbrink, S. Phase Analysis Studies on the Titanium-Oxygen System. *Acta Chem. Scand.* **1957**, *11*, 1641–1652. [CrossRef]
44. Matsunaga, T.; Tomoda, R.; Nakajima, T.; Wake, H. Photoelectrochemical sterilization of microbial cells by semiconductor powders. *FEMS Microbiol. Lett.* **1985**, *29*, 211–214. [CrossRef]
45. Nagalakshmi, M.; Karthikeyan, C.; Anusuya, N.; Brundha, C.; Basu, M.J.; Karuppuchamy, S. Synthesis of TiO2 nanofiber for photocatalytic and antibacterial applications. *J. Mater. Sci. Mater. Electron.* **2017**, *28*, 15915–15920. [CrossRef]
46. Azizi-Lalabadi, M.; Ehsani, A.; Divband, B.; Alizadeh-Sani, M. Antimicrobial activity of Titanium dioxide and Zinc oxide nanoparticles supported in 4A zeolite and evaluation the morphological characteristic. *Sci. Rep.* **2019**, *9*, 1–10. [CrossRef] [PubMed]
47. Vardanyan, Z.; Gevorkyan, V.; Ananyan, M.; Vardapetyan, H.; Trchounian, A. Effects of various heavy metal nanoparticles on Enterococcus hirae and Escherichia coli growth and proton-coupled membrane transport. *J. Nanobiotechnol.* **2015**, *13*, 1–9. [CrossRef]
48. Pigeot-Remy, S.; Simonet, F.; Errazuriz-Cerda, E.; Lazzaroni, J.; Atlan, D.; Guillard, C. Photocatalysis and disinfection of water: Identification of potential bacterial targets. *Appl. Catal. B: Environ.* **2011**, *104*, 390–398. [CrossRef]
49. Ranjan, S.; Ramalingam, C. Titanium dioxide nanoparticles induce bacterial membrane rupture by reactive oxygen species generation. *Environ. Chem. Lett.* **2016**, *14*, 487–494. [CrossRef]
50. Wang, D.; Zhao, L.; Ma, H.; Zhang, H.; Guo, L.-H. Quantitative Analysis of Reactive Oxygen Species Photogenerated on Metal Oxide Nanoparticles and Their Bacteria Toxicity: The Role of Superoxide Radicals. *Environ. Sci. Technol.* **2017**, *51*, 10137–10145. [CrossRef]
51. Chakra, C.S.; Mateti, S. Structural, Antimicrobial and Electrochemical Properties of Cu/TiO2 Nanocomposites. *J. Nanosci. Technol.* **2018**, *4*, 331–334. [CrossRef]
52. Nakano, R.; Hara, M.; Ishiguro, H.; Yao, Y.; Ochiai, T.; Nakata, K.; Murakami, T.; Kajioka, J.; Sunada, K.; Hashimoto, K.; et al. Broad Spectrum Microbicidal Activity of Photocatalysis by TiO2. *Catalysts* **2013**, *3*, 310–323. [CrossRef]
53. Senarathna, U.L.N.H.; Fernando, N.; Gunasekara, C.; Weerasekera, M.M.; Hewageegana, H.G.S.P.; Arachchi, N.D.; Siriwardena, H.D.; Jayaweera, P.M. Enhanced antibacterial activity of TiO2 nanoparticle surface modified with Garcinia zeylanica extract. *Chem. Cent. J.* **2017**, *11*, 7. [CrossRef] [PubMed]
54. Lee, W.S.; Park, Y.-S.; Cho, Y.-K. Significantly enhanced antibacterial activity of TiO 2 nanofibers with hierarchical nanostructures and controlled crystallinity. *Analyst* **2015**, *140*, 616–622. [CrossRef] [PubMed]
55. Alavi, M.; Karimi, N.; Valadbeigi, T.; Valadbaeigi, T. Antibacterial, Antibiofilm, Antiquorum Sensing, Antimotility, and Antioxidant Activities of Green Fabricated Ag, Cu, TiO2, ZnO, and Fe3O4 NPs via Protoparmeliopsis muralis Lichen Aqueous Extract against Multi-Drug-Resistant Bacteria. *ACS Biomater. Sci. Eng.* **2019**, *5*, 4228–4243. [CrossRef]
56. Santhosh, S.M.; Natarajan, K. Antibiofilm Activity of Epoxy/Ag-TiO2 Polymer Nanocomposite Coatings against Staphylococcus Aureus and Escherichia Coli. *Coatings* **2015**, *5*, 95–114. [CrossRef]

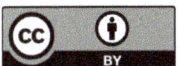 © 2020 by the authors. Licensee MDPI, Basel, Switzerland. This article is an open access article distributed under the terms and conditions of the Creative Commons Attribution (CC BY) license (http://creativecommons.org/licenses/by/4.0/).

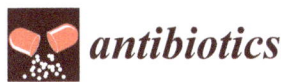 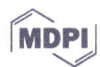

Communication

Biofilm Control Strategies: Engaging with the Public

Joanna Verran [1,*], Sarah Jackson [1], Antony Scimone [1], Peter Kelly [2] and James Redfern [3]

1. Department of Life Sciences, Faculty of Science and Engineering, Manchester Metropolitan University, Manchester M1 5GD, UK; S.L.Jackson10@stu.mmu.ac.uk (S.J.); T.Scimone@mmu.ac.uk (A.S.)
2. Surface Engineering Group, Faculty of Science and Engineering, Manchester Metropolitan University, Manchester M1 5GD, UK; peter.kelly@mmu.ac.uk
3. Department of Natural Sciences, Faculty of Science and Engineering, Manchester Metropolitan University, Manchester M1 5GD, UK; james.redfern.88@gmail.com
* Correspondence: J.Redfern@mmu.ac.uk

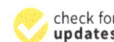

Received: 17 June 2020; Accepted: 29 July 2020; Published: 30 July 2020

Abstract: There are few peer-reviewed publications about public engagement with science that are written by microbiologists; those that exist tend to be a narrative of an event rather than a hypothesis-driven investigation. However, it is relatively easy for experienced scientists to use a scientific method in their approach to public engagement. This short communication describes three public engagement activities hosted by the authors, focused on biofilm control: hand hygiene, plaque control and an externally applied antimicrobial coating. In each case, audience engagement was assessed using quantitative and/or qualitative methods. A critical evaluation of the findings enabled the construction of a public engagement 'tick list' for future events that would enable a hypothesis-driven approach with more effective communication activities and more robust evaluation.

Keywords: Biofilm; Public Engagement; Outreach; Control Strategies; Oral Biofilm

1. Introduction

It is increasingly being recognised by 'experts' that science literacy is of key importance for the public [1]. At a time where antimicrobial resistance (AMR) continues to pose significant public health threats (or indeed, at a time of a global pandemic), an understanding of statistics, epidemiology and microbiology is even more desirable. As a subject, microbiology offers many topics with which we can engage non-experts, such as microbial diversity (including fungi, algae, protozoa and viruses as well as bacteria), beneficial microbes (for example, probiotics, fermented foods, the human microbiome), and messages that can influence behaviour in a positive manner (including vaccination, hand hygiene, antimicrobial stewardship) [2–4].

Biofilms (an assemblage of microbial cells that are irreversibly associated with a surface—not removed by gentle rinsing—and enclosed in a matrix of primarily polysaccharide material [5]) are of great importance to microbiologists, but also to many other professionals (such as engineers, biocide manufacturers, architects), and are found in a variety of environments (water distribution systems, industrial processing, hospitals). Biofilm research is multi-disciplinary, extensive and significant, with many applications. There are several research centres which focus on biofilm, such as the US-based Centre for Biofilm Engineering (http://www.biofilm.montana.edu/) and the UK-centred National Biofilm Innovation Centre (https://www.biofilms.ac.uk/), and conferences about biofilm are regular and not uncommon. Some individual researchers, research groups and research centres are keen to engage with external public audiences through outreach activities, although evidence of such activities (websites, articles, learning materials and other peer-reviewed outputs) is not easy to find. But why do we want the public to know about biofilms? And what does the 'public' need to know about biofilms?

How will we know if our activity has been effective? How can you identify good practice? How can you share success?

Science communication/public engagement can be seen as an emerging discipline, particularly for those scientists who have begun to question the effectiveness of their public engagement work. Evaluation of effectiveness using both quantitative and qualitative methods ('mixed methods') is strongly supported by education researchers [6,7], enabling the assessment of both reach (i.e., numbers) and impact (change in attitudes, perception). There are few peer-reviewed publications on the topic that are written by microbiologists: those that exist tend to be a narrative of an event rather than a hypothesis-driven investigation with appropriate evaluation. However, it is relatively easy for experienced scientists to use a scientific method in their approach to public engagement. This short communication describes three different biofilm-related public engagement activities hosted by the authors, who used lessons learned to develop a tick list for future events to enable more effective communication activities with more robust evaluation.

1.1. Activity One: 'Now Wash Your Hands'

'Now wash your hands' was developed as part of a University faculty family fun day during National Science and Engineering Week/Healthcare Science Week in the UK. The aim was to raise awareness of effective handwashing, whilst also engaging the participants in a discussion about the skin microbiome/biofilm. This event guarantees an audience of predominantly families who are likely to have an existing interest in science. Hand hygiene activities are well established as interactive learning activities with demonstrable public health impact (for example, as an intervention in reducing the spread of coronavirus [6]). In this activity, demonstrators (academic staff and student volunteers) engaged audiences to demonstrate surface contamination and effective handwashing (Figure 1). Thus, visitors at this activity (in a walkway area) had their hands 'contaminated' with a UV hand gel (www.hand-washing.com). This kit uses a fluorescent dye and ultraviolet light to illustrate the transmission of 'germs' from hands to other surfaces (and vice versa) and the importance of handwashing. In addition, the participants were invited to press their hands onto large agar plates for subsequent incubation to reveal the culturable microorganisms present on their skin. Of course, they were unable to see the results of this work until after incubation, thus images of plates pre-inoculated with microorganisms present on hands and mobile phones [7] were available to view, and post-incubation images of their own plates were uploaded to Flickr, a social media site that hosts images (http://tinyurl.com/howcleanareyourhands, Figure 2). Within a week from results going online, almost 100 downloads were recorded (the participants were provided with a card/web address), equivalent to the number of plates inoculated. From this, we deduced that visitors demonstrated interest and engagement with the activity. Throughout the activity, conversations were ongoing. It was unfortunate that these interactions were not noted in some form: informal observations revealed points of interest from the participants such as their inability to clean hands effectively (especially the adults!) and amazement at the mobile phone contamination. The handprint technique has been used as an engagement tool for other events, such as an art installation called 'Hands across the cultures' for registrants to a qualitative research conference and as part of the 'bioselfies' project (https://blogs.bl.uk/science/2020/02/introducing-bio-selfies-11-february-2020.html) initiated by the University of Salford. Flickr has been used for other events that require incubation of plates [8,9], and download numbers have on occasion exceeded the number of images posted, showing that the participants may have been sharing the findings with others. The fluorescent hand technique was used to illustrate person-to-person transmission by handshaking prior to a screening of the movie *Contagion* (directed by Soderbergh, 2011). One person 'contaminated' his/her hands, shook the hand of their neighbour, who shook her/his neighbour's hand and so on. Thus, the passing-on of fluorescence was used to illustrate the transmission of infection through poor hand hygiene, reinforcing the message as to how the movie pandemic was initiated (hand contact).

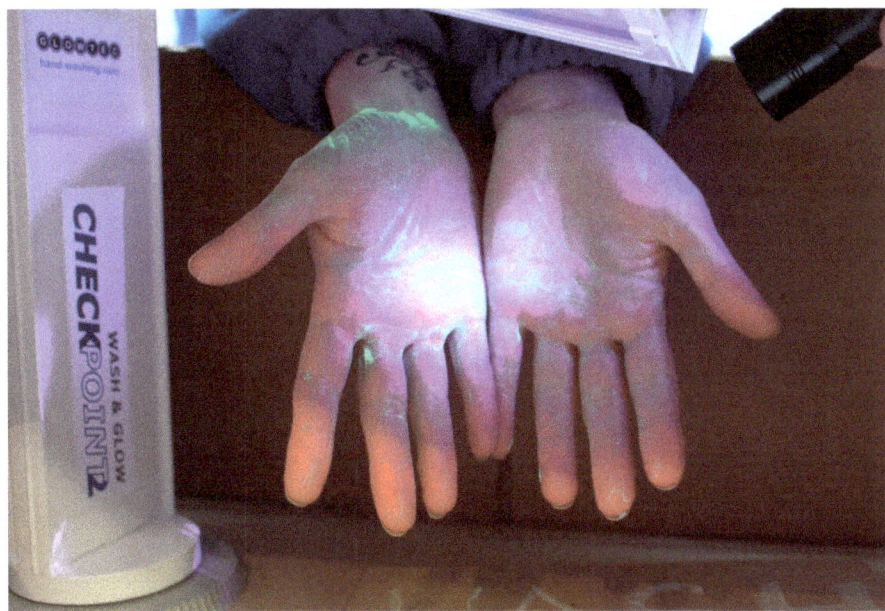

Figure 1. Activity one: 'Now wash your hands': the audience engaged in hands-on activities focusing on the topic of hand hygiene. Here, a participant's hands can be seen during the use of the UV glow gel.

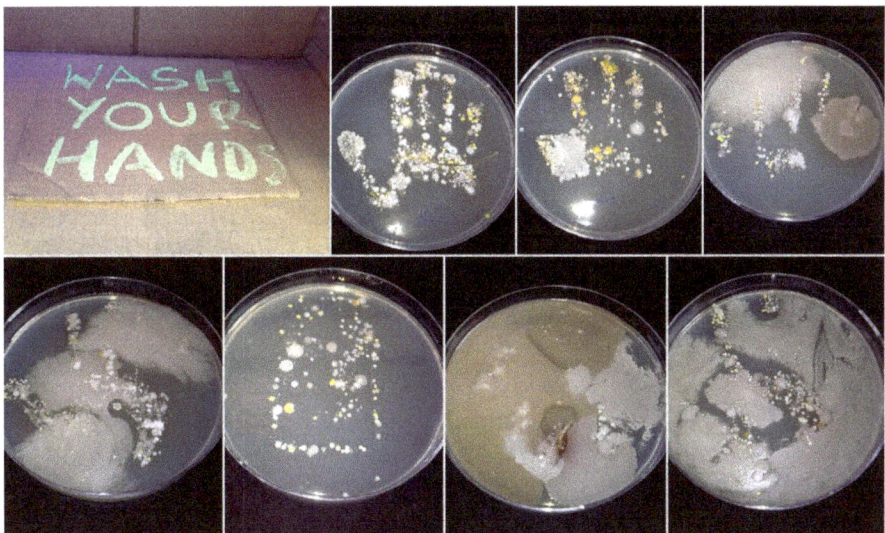

Figure 2. Example of the images uploaded to the Flickr page following the 'Now Wash Your Hands' event. Each image represents the handprint of one participant, revealing the range of microorganisms present on the hand.

Hand hygiene activities are common in microbiology engagement, the aim of the activity being primarily to inform, and hopefully to change, participants' behaviour so that effective handwashing techniques are employed. Explanation regarding the presence or importance of the skin microbiome/biofilm are likely rare (especially if the results are not available until a later date): the activity is inevitably more focused on the removal of temporary contaminants and on the importance of good handwashing. Some discussion could take place regarding the hygiene-versus-cleanliness hypothesis [10,11]. The Flickr method used for posting images and monitoring downloads at least gives an indication of interest, but much more could be made of this activity. It would also be interesting to know if the 'good handwashing' messages are retained and employed in the future. However, longitudinal studies are rare in this type of public engagement, probably because of the significant advanced planning required in terms of gaining approval for personal data access (e.g., emails) and also because only short-term awareness raising tends to be the primary aim of the activity.

1.2. Activity Two: Plaque Attack!

The plaque biofilm is one of the best-known medical biofilms [12,13], and oral hygiene advertising frequently provides cartoons of plaque being removed to demonstrate the effectiveness of a paste, mouthwash or brush. It is known that good toothbrushing helps to remove plaque [14] and should be carried out regularly. Different dentifrices claim varying activities, but virtually all formulations include fluoride (to 'strengthen the teeth') [15], and many contain antimicrobial agents (to reduce the number of microorganisms, with claims around gum health) [16].

'Plaque attack!' was a laboratory-based activity designed for children and their parents, taking place during Manchester Science Festival's family fun day at Manchester Metropolitan University. The aim of the event was to encourage good oral hygiene but also to captivate visitors with the components of the plaque biofilm as well as the laboratory and its equipment. Being time-consuming and space-limited, the participants had to register for the event, were limited to 3 groups of 20 participants, be escorted to the laboratory, provided with appropriate clothing and instruction and supervised at all times. Oral microbiology is a key research area in our laboratories, and the delivery team thought it would be valuable for visitors to encounter activity in a working (teaching) laboratory. The delivery team comprised PhD students, technical staff and an academic. Several activities were conducted as part of a 'round-robin' activity: sampling plaque (microscopy demonstration and take-home photo [ZIP Mobile Printer, Polaroid]); disclosing plaque (using commercially available disclosing tablets), with photographs taken before and after cleaning teeth (in a wash area adjacent to the laboratory); looking at cultures of oral bacteria on agar plates; investigating biofilm structure/building a biofilm (using 'Model Magic' [Crayola Bedford UK], a white air-drying modelling clay) (Figure 3a); and destroying a biofilm (using a water pistol to remove plaque (whose microorganisms were pre-constructed from Fimo, a multi-coloured clay which can be hardened in the oven [www.staedtler.com]) hampered by plaque matrix (a translucent hair gel) [17] (Figure 3b). The participants were provided with a basic information sheet on plaque and oral hygiene, onto which they could attach their Polaroid images. They were also given a bag containing complimentary toothbrush and toothpaste (courtesy of Unilever [www.unilever.co.uk]). At the end of the activity, they were asked for free text feedback on what they thought of the event, and the information was coded into categories to allow for comparison [18,19] (Figure 4). The participants were particularly engrossed in the microscopy demonstration, being able to see their own plaque at high magnification. They also clearly had fun 'destroying' the biofilm but were less interested in the more passive/less exciting activity (agar plates demonstration, building a biofilm). The free text provided by the participants (allowing more thorough insight compared to multiple-choice or leading questions such as 'give three things you have learned', or 'smiley face/sad face' evaluations [18,20]) gave valuable qualitative information that was used to inform subsequent activities.

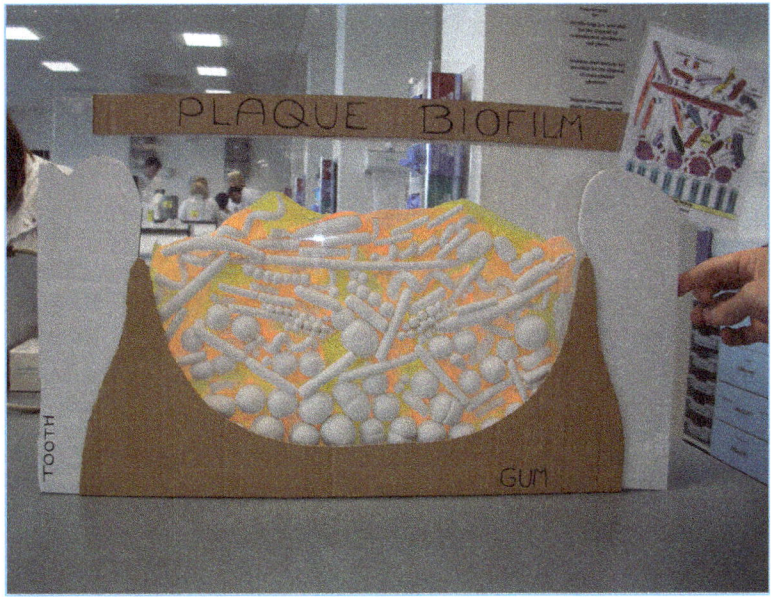

(a)

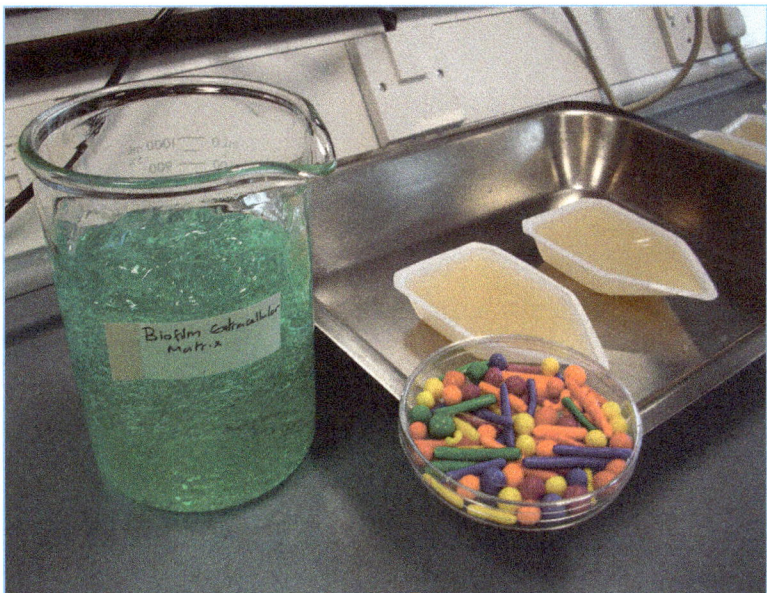

(b)

Figure 3. (**a**/**top**) Participants at the 'Plaque attack!' event were encouraged to create their own oral bacteria flora from modelling clay, which was assembled into the oral biofilm representation here shown. (**b**/**bottom**) Participants were encouraged to 'destroy a biofilm' by removing bacteria (coloured plastic pieces) encased in biofilm extracellular matrix (hair gel) with a spray bottle filled with water.

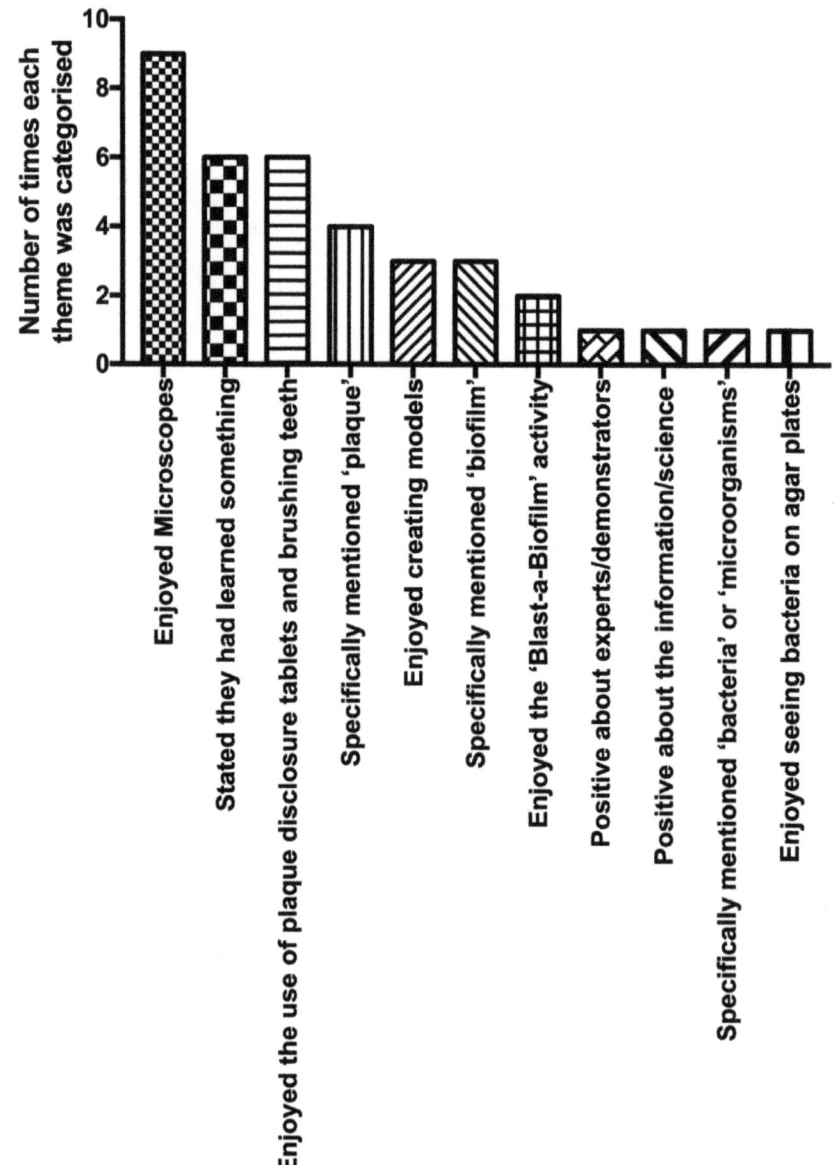

Figure 4. Themes identified from 'Plaque attack!' feedback. There was a total of 19 comments that were coded based on their focus—with each comment possibly being coded into more than one category.

1.3. Activity Three: A Photocatalytic Wall

Our research into titanium dioxide coatings included a range of laboratory-based studies that compared different titanium dioxide concentrations in paint formulations [21]. The work described in this paper was to see whether the effect of a photocatalyst in paint could be detected by the human eye. Thus, as part of a PhD project investigating the activity of photocatalytic surfaces, one of the external walls of the University was used to illustrate the effectiveness of titanium dioxide paints in terms of self-cleaning and reduction of the formation of biofilm on the wall material. Photocatalytic material such as titanium dioxide can exhibit self-cleaning, anti-fouling and antimicrobial properties in the presence of light, which makes these materials excellent candidates for incorporation into urban buildings and infrastructure [22–24]. The self-cleaning properties stem from their superhydrophilic nature—as, for instance, that of a liquid (e.g., rain) rolling off the surface of a continuous body. This sheeting carries away dirt and debris, cleaning the surface in the process—as seen in the Sydney Opera House [25]. Thus, biofilm formation on the surface is delayed or prevented.

In our study, the wall, comprising concrete panels (smaller panels 190 cm × 76 cm, larger panels 406 cm × 76 cm) on a 1970s University building, was west-facing (location on Chester Street, Manchester, UK M1 5GD). Six of the panels were painted with a siloxane external paint formulation that contained or lacked the photoactive pigment (kindly provided by Tronox, www.tronox.com). Our aim was to inform the passing public about our research (an interpretation panel was affixed to the wall), and on occasion, we encouraged passers-by to participate in a longitudinal subjective assessment of the impact of titanium dioxide-containing paint on the perceived cleanliness of the panel. This engagement activity was done directly by interview and indirectly using photographs at specific times over a 44-month period.

Initially there was no apparent difference in the brightness of the painted panels (Figure 5a). Members of the public attending a Manchester Science Festival event (October 2014) were asked to rank the painted panels in order of cleanliness/whiteness, with 1 being most clean, and 6 being least clean (n = 18). The experiment was also conducted via a social media platform (Facebook), with participants asked to assess whiteness using photographs (n = 48). The direct assessment was repeated after three years (n = 21). In all cases, the participants ranked two or three of the photocatalytic panels as the 'whitest'. In 2014, around 60% of the participants selected the three photocatalytic panels correctly. In 2017, this figure rose to 78%. After six years, the test-paint panels appeared whiter than the control panels (Figure 5b, May 2020).

The presence of the wall with its accompanying information panel at the side of the University Science and Engineering building provided a useful pointer to introduce visitors to some of the research ongoing in the faculty. The use of the public to assess the cleanliness of the wall proved unnecessary within a few months, when the impact of the test paint was apparent. The fact that almost all participants could discriminate between the panels after less than 12 months was also of interest. This approach might therefore be useful in the future for the assessment of test formulations.

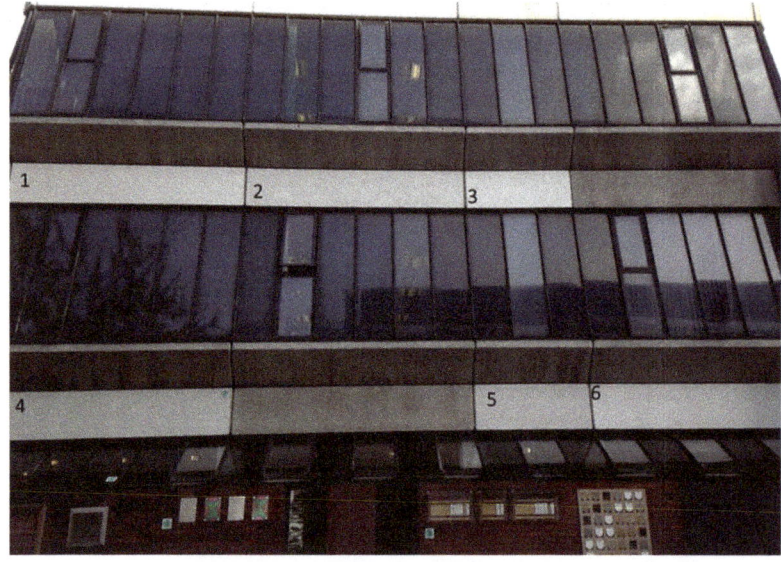

(a)

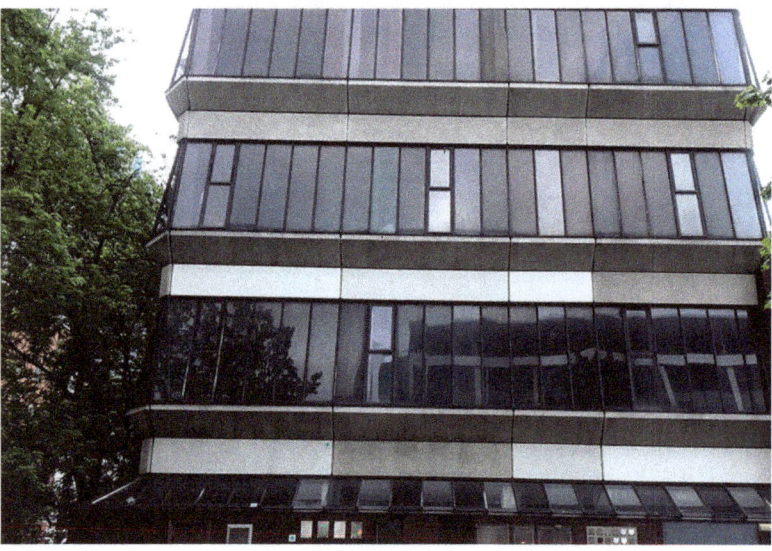

(b)

Figure 5. Images of the wall at Manchester Metropolitan University used in the study of photocatalytic paint (panels labelled 1–6). Panels 1, 3 and 6 were painted with photocatalytic paint, whilst panels 2, 4 and 5 were painted with paint that did not contain the photocatalytic agent. The image on the top (**a**) was taken in 2014, eight months following the application of the paint: whiteness/brightness difference between the two paint types is hard to distinguish. The lower image (**b**) was taken six years later (2020); panels painted with photocatalytic paint are visibly brighter compared to control paint panels.

2. Discussion

Much was learned from each event (as noted above), particularly through observation, in terms of what components participants like and engage with when discussing biofilm. In addition, quantitative evidence of engagement was derived from the 'Now wash your hands' event; qualitative evidence of enjoyment and engagement was obtained from 'Plaque attack', and the potential for acquisition of research data was indicated by the photocatalytic wall activity. These various outcomes informed how subsequent events for the public would take place, with more focus on design, delivery and evaluation.

More recently, there has been increasing effort to ensure that these criteria for effective public engagement are met. Microbiology has a particularly dynamic approach to public engagement, and many teams are now publishing the outcomes of their public engagement research in peer-reviewed journals, magazines or online. Yet, in a review of public engagement activity around AMR, a rich bedrock of activity was found only through personal contacts and communication rather than through a literature search [4]. It is even more important when talking to audiences about biofilms that intended messages are clear. Thus, we describe in Table 1 the planning of a hypothetical public engagement event designed to inform a large number of adults about biofilm and AMR. Our focus was on the combination of the two phenomena, which occurs, for example, when biofilms on medical devices present increased resistance to antibiotics [26]. In order to address this combined effect, it was first necessary to define the two phenomena separately. We particularly wished to avoid intrusive aspects of evaluation, relying instead on observation and other (subjective and objective) indicators from participants. We hope that this checklist may be useful for others who might wish to engage audiences with their biofilm/antibiotic research.

The National Biofilm Information Centre has recognised the importance of public engagement and is providing a hub for the dissemination of biofilm-focused outreach and engagement activities, which will enable, over time, ideas, expertise and outcomes to be shared and developed, in order to improve the effectiveness of engagement encounters for scientists and their audiences alike. We hope that our experiences in the area are of interest in this context.

Table 1. Checklist for public engagement events, with accompanying information detailing planning for a proposed event focusing on antimicrobial resistance (AMR) and biofilms.

	General Considerations	Example
Event	Audience, venue, time, date, numbers	Adults, evening, 3 hours, audience around 500 participants, drop-in marketplace format
Topic	Theme	AMR and biofilms
Aim/hypothesis		Aim: To engage the audience with the biofilm phenomenon and its relationship with AMR Hypothesis: That the audience will leave the event with an increased awareness of AMR and some knowledge of biofilms
The message	What specific message(s)	About AMR What biofilms are Why biofilms are important with regard to AMR
What will be happening	Focus activities on key messages, encourage active participation and engagement	Welcome table (guide to activities) Bitesize quotes about AMR on a pop-up stand iPad questionnaire used to lead discussion about AMR Screening of the film 'Catch' [4] Swabbing face/nasal area (anonymous) Rolling images of biofilm Discussion about biofilm Building biofilm using Bunch'ems (www.bunchems.com) Sign up to Antibiotic Guardians (www.antibioticguardian.com)

Table 1. *Cont.*

	General Considerations	Example
Personnel required	Ensure sufficient numbers of staff/students, all familiar with overall aims and activities and informed about key messages	**Welcome table: one person;** **AMR discussion: 2–3 people** What is AMR [27]? Why is it important? **Swabbing table: 2–3 people** **Biofilm discussion and activity: 3–4 people** What is a biofilm? How common are they/where are they? What do they look like? Why is AMR important in biofilms? - medical implants; - drug-resistant biofilms; - transmission of resistance through biofilm? Build biofilms with Bunch'ems **Floating support staff: 2 people** **Observers: 2 people [8]** **Estimate 12 personnel required**
Evaluation	Quantitative and qualitative assessment regarding achievement of aims	Survey of 'do you know what a biofilm is?' (yes/no) Survey of understanding/information about AMR Number of agar plates used Number of visitors to Flickr (presenting images of plates post-incubation) Qualitative observation of discussion/questions/activities Photographs/images of biofilms being built/Twitter hashtag usage #buildabiofilm Number of Antibiotic Guardian sign-ups/leaflets taken
Actions	Preparation in advance of the event	Health and safety documents/risk assessment List of staff/volunteers' names Ethical approval for survey, agar plates/swabs and observers Produce pop-up Develop yes/no test for prior knowledge of biofilms Provide substrata/backdrop for Bunch'ems (e.g., giant microscope slides, other surfaces) Practice building biofilms Produce biofilm slideshow Develop Q&A for iPad Identify key messages and provide them to the team (laminated) Sheet for observers Antibiotic Guardian information
Logistics		Arrival time and set up Staff rota Refreshments Transport of agar plates and other equipment Briefing pre-event, with key messages Debriefing post-event, fix date/time

3. Conclusions

Public engagement activities can be designed with clear aims that enable effective evaluation using both quantitative and qualitative methods. This is particularly important for complex phenomena such as biofilms and AMR.

Author Contributions: Conceptualization, J.V., P.K. and J.R.; Methodology, J.V., P.K., J.R.; Formal Analysis, J.V., J.R., A.S.; Investigation, J.V., J.R., A.S., S.J.; Resources, J.V. and P.K.; Writing – Original Draft Preparation, J.V. and J.R.; Writing – Review & Editing, J.V., A.S. and J.R.; Visualization, J.V., J.R. and A.S.; Supervision, J.V. and P.K.; Project Administration, J.V. All authors have read and agreed to the published version of the manuscript.

Funding: This research received no external funding

Conflicts of Interest: The authors declare no conflict of interest

References

1. Timmis, K.; Cavicchioli, R.; Garcia, J.L.; Nogales, B.; Chavarría, M.; Stein, L.; McGenity, T.J.; Webster, N.; Singh, B.K.; Handelsman, J.; et al. The urgent need for microbiology literacy in society. *Environ. Microbiol.* **2019**, *21*, 1513–1528. [CrossRef] [PubMed]
2. Carolan, K.; Verran, J.; Amos, M.; Crossley, M.; Redfern, J.; Whitton, N.; Louttit, D. Simfection: A digital resource for vaccination education. *J. Biol. Educ.* **2018**, *53*, 225–234. [CrossRef]
3. Redfern, J.; Burdass, D.; Verran, J. Practical microbiology in schools: A survey of uk teachers. *Trends Microbiol.* **2013**, *21*, 557–559. [CrossRef] [PubMed]
4. Redfern, J.; Bowater, L.; Coulthwaite, L.; Verran, J. Raising awareness of antimicrobial resistance among the general public in the uk: The role of public engagement activities. *JAC-Antimicrob. Resist.* **2020**, *2*, dlaa012. [CrossRef]
5. Donlan, R.M. Biofilms: Microbial life on surfaces. *Emerg. Infect. Dis.* **2002**, *8*, 881–890. [CrossRef]
6. Allegranzi, B.; Pittet, D. Role of hand hygiene in healthcare-associated infection prevention. *J. Hosp. Infect.* **2009**, *73*, 305–315. [CrossRef]
7. Verran, J. The microbial contamination of mobile communication devices. *J. Microbiol. Biol. Educ.* **2012**, *13*, 59–61. [CrossRef]
8. Verran, J.; Haigh, C.; Brooks, J.; Butler, J.A.; Redfern, J. Fitting the message to the location: Engaging adults with antimicrobial resistance in a world war 2 air raid shelter. *J. Appl. Microbiol.* **2018**, *125*, 1008–1016. [CrossRef]
9. Redfern, J.; Bowater, L.; Crossley, M.; Verran, J. Spreading the message of antimicrobial resistance: A detailed account of a successful public engagement event. *FEMS Microbiol. Lett.* **2018**, *365*, fny175. [CrossRef]
10. Bloomfield, S.F. Rsph and ifh call for a clean-up of public understanding and attitudes to hygiene. *Perspect. Public Health* **2019**, *139*, 285–288. [CrossRef]
11. Rook, G.A.W. 99th dahlem conference on infection, inflammation and chronic inflammatory disorders: Darwinian medicine and the 'hygiene' or 'old friends' hypothesis. *Clin. Exp. Immunol.* **2010**, *160*, 70–79. [CrossRef] [PubMed]
12. Lamfon, H.; Al-Karaawi, Z.; McCullough, M.; Porter, S.R.; Pratten, J. Composition of in vitro denture plaque biofilms and susceptibility to antifungals. *FEMS Microbiol. Lett.* **2005**, *242*, 345–351. [CrossRef] [PubMed]
13. Marsh, P.D.; Zaura, E. Dental biofilm: Ecological interactions in health and disease. *J. Clin. Periodontol.* **2017**, *44*, S12–S22. [CrossRef] [PubMed]
14. Penick, C. Power toothbrushes: A critical review. *Int. J. Dent. Hyg.* **2004**, *2*, 40–44. [CrossRef] [PubMed]
15. Bartlett, D.W.; Smith, B.G.; Wilson, R.F. Comparison of the effect of fluoride and non-fluoride toothpaste on tooth wear in vitro and the influence of enamel fluoride concentration and hardness of enamel. *Br. Dent. J.* **1994**, *176*, 346–348. [CrossRef] [PubMed]
16. Prasanth, M. Antimicrobial efficacy of different toothpastes and mouthrinses: An in vitro study. *Dent. Res. J.* **2011**, *8*, 85–94.
17. Marlow, V.L.; MacLean, T.; Brown, H.; Kiley, T.B.; Stanley-Wall, N.R. Blast a biofilm: A hands-on activity for school children and members of the public. *J. Microbiol. Biol. Educ.* **2013**, *14*, 252–254. [CrossRef]
18. Redfern, J.; Burdass, D.; Verran, J. Transforming a school learning exercise into a public engagement event: "The good, the bad and the algae". *J. Biol. Educ.* **2013**, *47*, 246–252. [CrossRef]
19. Verran, J.; Redfern, J.; Moravej, H.; Adebola, Y. Refreshing the public appetite for 'good bacteria': Menus made by microbes. *J. Biol. Educ.* **2018**, *53*, 34–46. [CrossRef]
20. Cohen, L.; Manion, L.; Morrison, K. *Research Methods in Education*, 7th ed.; Routledge: Oxon, UK, 2011.
21. Caballero, L.; Whitehead, K.A.; Allen, N.S.; Verran, J. Photoinactivation of *Escherichia coli* on acrylic paint formulations using fluorescent light. *Dyes Pigment.* **2010**, *86*, 56–62. [CrossRef]
22. Carp, O.; Huisman, C.L.; Reller, A. Photoinduced reactivity of titanium dioxide. *Prog. Solid State Chem.* **2004**, *32*, 33–177. [CrossRef]
23. Chen, J.; Poon, C.-S. Photocatalytic construction and building materials: From fundamentals to applications. *Build. Environ.* **2009**, *44*, 1899–1906. [CrossRef]
24. Smits, M.; Huygh, D.; Craeye, B.; Lenaerts, S. Effect of process parameters on the photocatalytic soot degradation on self-cleaning cementitious materials. *Catal. Today* **2014**, *230*, 250–255. [CrossRef]

25. Hanley, S. Secrets of the Sydney Opera House. Available online: https://greenbuildingelements.com/2017/01/30/secrets-sydney-opera-house/ (accessed on 3 October 2019).
26. Stewart, P.S.; William Costerton, J. Antibiotic resistance of bacteria in biofilms. *Lancet* **2001**, *358*, 135–138. [CrossRef]
27. O'Neill, J. *Tackling Drug-Resistant Infections Globally: Final Report and Recommendations*; Resistance, R.O.A., Ed.; Wellcome Trust: London, UK, 2016.

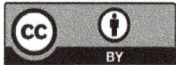

© 2020 by the authors. Licensee MDPI, Basel, Switzerland. This article is an open access article distributed under the terms and conditions of the Creative Commons Attribution (CC BY) license (http://creativecommons.org/licenses/by/4.0/).

MDPI
St. Alban-Anlage 66
4052 Basel
Switzerland
Tel. +41 61 683 77 34
Fax +41 61 302 89 18
www.mdpi.com

Antibiotics Editorial Office
E-mail: antibiotics@mdpi.com
www.mdpi.com/journal/antibiotics

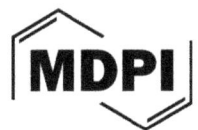

www.ingramcontent.com/pod-product-compliance
Lightning Source LLC
LaVergne TN
LVHW070458100526
838202LV00014B/1744